KU-825-692

Renal, bladder, prostate and testicular cancer

an update

Renal, bladder, prostate and testicular cancer
an update

The Proceedings of the VI Congress on Progress and
Controversies in Oncological Urology (PACIOU VI),
held in Rotterdam, The Netherlands, October 2000

Edited by

Karl H. Kurth, Gerald H. Mickisch and Fritz H. Schröder

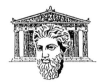

The Parthenon Publishing Group
International Publishers in Medicine, Science & Technology

NEW YORK   LONDON

Library of Congress Cataloging-in-Publication Data

Congress on Progress and Controversies in Oncological Urology (6th : 2000 : Rotterdam, Netherlands)
    Renal, bladder, prostate and testicular cancer : an update : the proceedings of the VIth Congress on Progress and Controversies in Oncological Urology (PACIOU VI) / edited by Karl H. Kurth, Gerald H. Mickisch and F.H. Schröder.
       p.   cm.
    Includes bibliographical references and index.
    ISBN 1-84214-067-1
    1. Genitourinary organs—Cancer—Congresses.   I. Kurth, Karl H. II. Mickisch, Gerald H. III. Schröder, F. H. IV. Title.
    [DNLM: 1. Kidney Neoplasms—Congresses. 2. Bladder Neoplasms—Congresses. 3. Prostatic Neoplasms—Congresses. 4. Testicular Neoplasms—Congresses.
WJ 358 C749r 2001]
RC280.G4 C596 2000
616.99′46—dc21

British Library Cataloguing in Publication Data
Renal, bladder, prostate and testicular cancer : an update : the proceedings of the VIth Congress on Progress and Controversies in Oncological Urology (PACIOU VI)
    1. Genitourinary organs — Cancer
    I. Kurth, Karl H. II. Mickisch, Gerald H.
    III. Schröder, F. H. IV. Congress on Progress and Controversies in Oncological Urology (6th)
    616.9′946

ISBN   1-84214-067-1

Published in the USA by
The Parthenon Publishing Group Inc.
One Blue Hill Plaza
PO Box 1564, Pearl River
New York 10965, USA

Published in the UK and Europe by
The Parthenon Publishing Group Ltd.
Casterton Hall
Carnforth
Lancs. LA6 2LA, UK

Copyright © 2001 Parthenon Publishing Group

No part of this publication may be reproduced in any form without permission from the publishers, except for the quotation of brief passages for the purpose of review

Typeset by AMA DataSet, Preston, UK

Printed and bound by
Butler & Tanner Ltd., Frome and London, UK

Contents

List of principal contributors

C. H. Bangma
Department of Urology
Academic Hospital Rotterdam
Dr. Molewaterplein 40
Rotterdam 3015 GD
The Netherlands

A. V. Bono
Department of Urology
Ospedale Di Circolo e Fondazione Macchi
Viale Borri 57
Varese 21100
Italy

A. V. D'Amico
Department of Radiotherapy/Oncology
Brigham and Women's Hospital
75 Francis Street, L-2 Level
Boston
MA 02115
USA

P. H. M. De Mulder
Department of Medical Oncology
Academic Hospital Nijmegen St Radboud
PO Box 9101
Nijmegen 6500 HB
The Netherlands

M. A. Eisenberger
Department of Oncology and Urology
John Hopkins University
School of Medicine/Bunting Blaustein
    Cancer Research Building
1650 Orleans Street, Suite 1M51
Baltimore
MD 21231-1000
USA

B. Guillonneau
Department of Urology
L'Institut Mutualiste Montsouris
42, Boulevard Jourdan
Paris 75014
France

F. C. Hamdy
BAUS Office of Education at the
    University of Sheffield
Department of Urology
Floor 1, Royal Hallamshire Hospital
Glossop Road
Sheffield S10 2JF
United Kingdom

A. Hobisch
Department of Urology
University of Innsbruck
Anichstrasse 35
Innsbruck A-6020
Austria

J. Hugosson
Department of Urology
Sahlgrenska University Hospital
Gôteborg S-413 45
Sweden

E. Huland
Tumor and Transplantation Immunology
University Hospital Eppendorf
Martinistrasse 52
Hamburg D-20246
Germany

P. Iversen
Department of Urology
Rigshospitalet
Blegdamsvej 9
Copenhagen DK-2100
Denmark

S. B. Kaye
Department of Medical Oncology
Royal Marsden Hospital
Downs Road
Sutton SM2 5PT
United Kingdom

M. Kriegmair
Department of Urology
Kreisklinik Ebersberg
Pfarrer Guggetcerstrasse 3
Ebersberg D-85560
Germany

K. H. Kurth
Department of Urology
Academic Medical Center
Meibergdreef 9
Amsterdam 1105 AZ
The Netherlands

D. L. Lamm
Department of Urology
WVU Health Science Center
PO Box 9251
Morgantown
WV 26506
USA

H. Lilja
Department of Laboratory Medicine
Division of Clinical Chemistry
University Hospital Malmö
Malmö S-205 02
Sweden

B. Ljungberg
Department of Urology and Andrology
Umea University Hospital
Umea S-901 85
Sweden

V. Narain
Department of Urology
Wayne State University
4160 John R. Suite 1017
Detroit
MI 48201
USA

G. H. J. Mickisch
Department of Urology
Academic Hospital and
Erasmus University Rotterdam
Dr. Molewaterplein 40
Rotterdam 3015 GD
The Netherlands

D. W. W. Newling
Department of Urology
AZVU
PO Box 7057
Amsterdam 1007 MB
The Netherlands

R. O. Northway
Department of Urology
Emory University School of Medicine
1365 Clifton Road, NE, Room 3225
Atlanta
GA 30322
USA

J. W. Oosterhuis
Erasmus University Rotterdam
Josephine Nefkens Instituut
Dr. Molewaterplein 50
Rotterdam 3015 GE
The Netherlands

S. J. Otto
Erasmus University Medical Center
Rotterdam
Department of Public Health
PO Box 1738
Rotterdam 3000 DR
The Netherlands

J. Rassweiler
Department of Urology
Klinikum Heilbronn GmbH
Gesundbrunnen 20
Heilbronn D-74074
Germany

F. H. Schröder
Department of Urology
Academic Hospital and
Erasmus University Rotterdam
Dr. Molewaterplein 40
Rotterdam 3015 GD
The Netherlands

M. S. Soloway
Department of Urology
University of Miami School of Medicine
PO Box 016960 (M814)
Miami
FL 33101
USA

C. S. Stewart
Department of Urology
Mayo Clinic Rochester
200 First St. S.W.
Rochester
MN 55905
USA

P. J. Van Cangh
Department of Urology
Cliniques Universitaires Saint Luc
10, Avenue Hippocrate
Brussels B-1200
Belgium

A. N. Vis
Department of Experimental Pathology
Erasmus University Rotterdam
Josephine Nefkens Institute
PO Box 1738
Rotterdam 3000 DR
The Netherlands

M. P. Wirth
Department of Urology
University Clinics 'Carl Gustav Carus'
Technical University of Dresden
Fetscherstrasse 74
Dresden D-01307
Germany

Foreword

You are confronted with the sixth monograph resulting from a congress in the series of *Progress and Controversies in Oncological Urology*. This event takes place every 2 years and the monograph which is in your possession now relates to the meeting that was held in October 2000 in Rotterdam.

The authors and Editors hope very much that, as in previous years, this monograph will serve as an important source of reference for you for the next 2 years. It represents an attempt to update the field of oncological urology with respect to the most important recent developments, controversies and important current knowledge.

The Editors are grateful to the authors who have all delivered excellent manuscripts within an extremely pressing timeline. Together with my co-editors, I hope very much that you will find reading the volume interesting and rewarding. Also, we hope very much that this monograph will stimulate you to participate in the next meeting on *Progress and Controversies in Oncological Urology*, which will be held in October 2002 in Rotterdam.

The editorial team and all the authors are grateful for the generous support of Schering AG which has made this publication possible.

Rotterdam, February 2001   *Fritz H. Schröder*

Section I

Testicular and renal cancer

Testicular germ cell tumors, an update: biology, prognostic factors and (molecular) diagnostics

1

J. W. Oosterhuis and L. H. J. Looijenga

Biology of testicular germ cell tumors

Anatomical localization and histology of human germ cell tumors

Human germ cell tumors (GCTs) comprise a heterogeneous group of neoplasms. They can occur in different anatomical locations, predominantly in the gonads (both ovary and testis) and in the midline of the body, including the retroperitoneal, mediastinal, head and neck, and hypothalamus/pineal gland regions (see reference 1 for review). This anatomical distribution has been related to the migration route followed by the primordial germ cells from the yolk sac to the gonadal ridge. The clinical behavior of these tumors depends on the sex of the patient, the age at clinical presentation and the histology of the tumor.

Within the testis, three groups of GCTs can be distinguished:

(1) The yolk sac tumors and teratomas of neonates and infants;

(2) The seminomas and non-seminomas;

(3) The spermatocytic seminomas.

It has been established that these different types of testicular germ cell tumors (TGCTs) are derived from cells belonging to the germ cell lineage, although the actual non-malignant counterparts are still a matter of debate. It is likely that the teratomas and yolk sac tumors of infants originate from an embryonic germ cell, while spermatocytic seminomas originate from a spermatogonial/spermatocyte type of cell. However, formal proof is lacking. In contrast, it has been established that the precursor of seminomas and non-seminomas is carcinoma *in situ* (CIS)[2], also referred to as intratubular germ cell neoplasia undifferentiated (IGCNU). In this review, we will mainly focus on the seminomas and non-seminomas, also known as TGCTs of adolescents and adults.

Epidemiology and histology of seminomas and non-seminomas

An increasing incidence (between 6 and 11/ 100 000) has been reported both for seminomas and non-seminomas during the past decades in white populations throughout the world (see reference 3 for review), with an annual increase of 3–6%. In some European countries, i.e. Denmark and Switzerland, the lifetime risk of developing a seminoma or non-seminoma is up to 1%. Blacks have a significantly lower risk, which is not increasing, although histology and age distribution are the same as in the white population[4].

While most patients with a seminoma present in their 4th decade of life, it is in the 3rd decade that patients present with a non-seminoma[5,6]. TGCTs containing both a seminomatous and a non-seminomatous component, known as combined tumors according to the British classification system[7], present at an age in between that of pure seminoma and non-seminoma[8]. Histologically, non-seminomas can be composed of different elements: embryonal carcinoma (the undifferentiated stem cell component), teratoma (the somatically differentiated component), yolk sac tumor and choriocarcinoma (the components of extra-embryonal differentiation)[9,10] (Figure 1). In

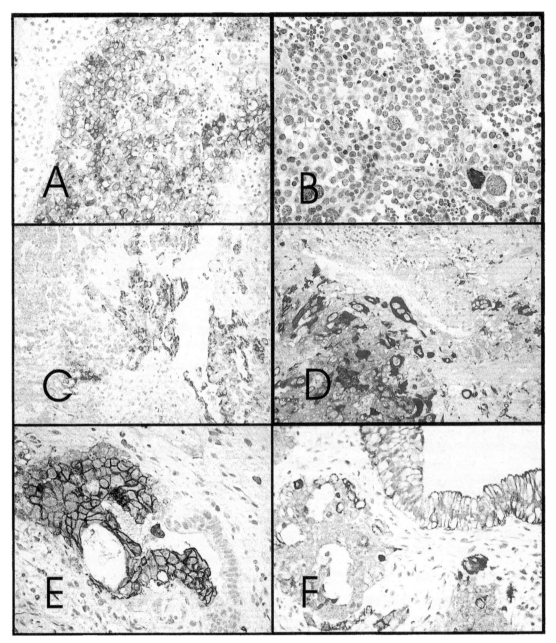

Figure 1 Representative examples of a seminoma, stained for alkaline phosphatase (A), a spermatocytic seminoma (B), a yolk sac tumor, stained for alpha-fetoprotein (C), a choriocarcinoma, stained for human chorionic gonadotropin (D), an embryonal carcinoma, stained for CD30 (E) and a teratoma, stained for cytokeratin (F)

fact, non-seminomas mimic embryonic and organ development to a certain level. To date, no parameters are available that predict the progression of CIS into a seminoma or non-seminoma. It has been suggested that CIS and seminoma cells lose their ability to develop into pluripotent stem cells over time[11,12]. Alternatively, the CIS cells or seminoma cells that have pluripotent potential are exhausted. This can explain the age difference between patients with a seminoma and those with a non-seminoma, and the intermediate age of patients with combined tumors, as the more aggressive non-seminomas manifest faster clinically.

Origin and epidemiology of CIS

The relatively young age of patients with a seminoma or a non-seminoma at clinical presentation suggests that exposure to certain factors early in development, possibly even during prenatal life, is involved in the pathogenesis of this cancer. This hypothesis is supported by the characteristics of the precursor cells of seminomas and non-seminomas, i.e. CIS[2]. CIS is composed of tumor cells located on the inner side of the basal membrane of the seminiferous tubules, under the tight junctions between the Sertoli cells, where the spermato-gonia are normally found[13]. The cells show similarities to embryonic germ cells, such as their positivity for alkaline phosphatase[14] (Figure 2), the stem cell factor receptor (c-KIT)[15] and their glycogen content[10]. Based on immunohistochemical findings, it has been suggested that the cell of origin of CIS is present in the gonad during normal development from around the 7–10th week of gestation[16]. That the initiating event leading to CIS happens during embryogenesis is also supported by the levelling off of the increasing incidence of seminomas and non-seminomas in cohorts of men born during or just before the second world war in Denmark, Norway and Sweden[17], as well as by the nature of some of the risk factors (see below). Moreover, about 5% of patients with a unilateral seminoma or non-seminoma have contralateral CIS (see reference 18 for review,

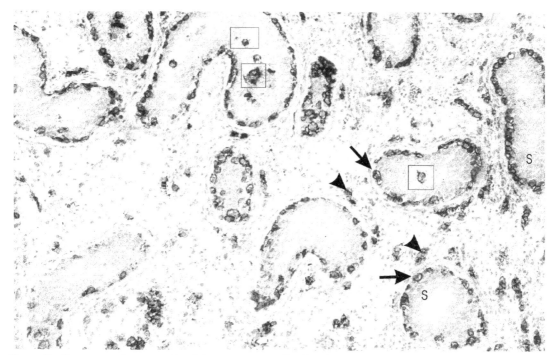

Figure 2 Representative example of the precursor cells of both seminoma and non-seminoma of the adult testis, known as carcinoma *in situ* (CIS). The cells are identified by detection of alkaline phosphatase reactivity on a frozen tissue section of testicular parenchyma adjacent to an invasive seminoma. Note the presence of the alkaline phosphatase-positive CIS cells at the inner basal membrane of the seminiferous tubules (indicted by an arrow), under the tight junctions present between the Sertoli cells (indicated by 'S'). Micro-invasive seminoma cells (indicated by an arrow-head) are also detectable, as well as CIS cells in the lumen of the seminiferous tubules (within the squares)

and below). This supports the model that the initiating events happen before the primordial germ cells reach the left and right gonadal blastema. Of special interest is the finding that the incidence of CIS in the general population is similar to the lifetime risk of developing a testicular seminoma or non-seminoma, indicating that CIS will always progress to invasiveness[19].

Risk factors for seminomas and non-seminomas

Several risk factors have been identified for TGCTs. The most important to date include cryptorchidism, infertility, familial history (see below), intersex (gonadal dysgenesis and androgen insensitivity) and low birth weight (see reference 3 for review). Patients with cryptorchidism have a 4–5-fold higher risk for seminoma or non-seminoma than individuals with scrotal testes. Bilateral cryptorchidism results in an even greater risk than unilateral cryptorchidism.

A possible link between sperm quality and development of a seminoma or non-seminoma is suggested by the finding that about 25% of patients with a unilateral seminoma or non-seminoma have severe abnormalities of spermatogenesis in their contralateral testis[20]. An association between sperm quality and the risk of developing a seminoma or non-seminoma has indeed been demonstrated[21]. In fact, Leydig cell function is impaired in patients with either a seminoma or a non-seminoma[22]. Moreover, a significantly lower number of children has been found in families of patients with either seminoma or non-seminoma prior to the diagnosis of malignancy, compared to a control group[23].

The relationship between the risk of developing a seminoma or non-seminoma and maternal age and birth order has been reported in multiple studies. This correlation might be related to the higher level of estrogens that occur during the first pregnancy compared to subsequent pregnancies[24]. A preterm effect has also been implied, which is related to a lower birth weight. Indeed, higher circulating estrogen levels have been found in mothers who have undergone preterm delivery[25]. The differences mentioned above between blacks and whites with regard to the incidence of seminoma and non-seminoma have been linked to a higher level of testosterone during early pregnancy in blacks compared to whites[26]. These data support the model that high estrogen levels may increase the risk of developing a seminoma or a non-seminoma, while high testosterone levels can reduce the risk.

Genetic predisposition

About 2% of patients with a seminoma or non-seminoma have an affected family member, indicating a genetic component in the development of this cancer. To date, two genome-wide linkage analyses have been performed. The first, a sib-pair analysis in 35 families, showed linkage to regions of chromosomes 1, 4, 5, 14 and 18[27]. A second genome-wide study by the International Familial Testis Cancer Linkage Consortium in 54 new families found, however, no evidence for linkage to chromosome 1, and a weaker indication for involvement of region 2 of chromosome 4 (4cen-q13)[28]. For the other region on chromosome 4 (p14-p13), and for chromosome 5, similar results were obtained. Both studies indicated linkage to chromosome 18. The latter study found linkage to the short arm of chromosome 2, and the telomeric region of 3q. A telomeric region of the long arm of chromosome 12 showed linkage when the results of both studies were combined, while no linkage was found in the separate studies. Another finding of interest is the fact that bilateral occurrence of the tumor is more frequent in familial than in sporadic cases (15 versus 5%)[29]. Indeed, most recently, linkage to Xq27 has been found for cryptorchidism and bilateral germ cell tumors, although the gene involved is still unknown[30].

Because families with a genetic predisposition are relatively few, linkage analysis is troublesome. Based on the characteristics of these families, the most likely mode of inheritance of this cancer is recessive, through constitutional inactivation of one allele of a tumor suppressor gene. The results to date indicate that probably a number of different genes may convey genetic predisposition.

Genomic changes of seminoma, non-seminoma and CIS

Seminomas, non-seminomas as well as CIS are consistently aneuploid[8,31,32]. This suggests that polyploidization is an early and important step in the development of these tumors. The cells of a seminoma and CIS are hypertriploid, while those of a non-seminoma, irrespective of histological composition, are hypotriploid. Using karyotyping (see reference 33 for review), more recently supported by *in situ* and comparative genomic hybridization (ISH and CGH)[34–38], a complex, but similar pattern of over- and under-representation of (parts of) chromosomes has been identified in seminomas and non-seminomas. Overall, chromosomes 4, 5, 11, 13, 18 and Y are under-represented, while chromosomes 7, 8, 12 and X are over-represented. Because seminomas and non-seminomas have a total DNA content around the triploid range, i.e. seminomas hypertriploid and non-seminomas hypotriploid, results obtained by CGH may not directly indicate the biologically important relative gains and losses. Therefore, we recently implemented a method to combine tailored normalization of the CGH data, based on ISH with region-specific probes[39]. This approach allowed us to obtain more information about the actual copy numbers of parts of chromosomes. In fact, we found novel chromosomal anomalies which remained undetected using the conventional CGH data analysis method, e.g. loss of chromosome 17 in seminoma compared to non-seminoma.

Using microdissection, DNA amplification and CGH, we investigated the chromosomal changes of various histological elements of both seminomas and non-seminomas[40]. Interestingly, some of the aberrations were restricted to particular histological elements, such as the loss of 6q in yolk sac tumors. This means that karyotyping and CGH of mixed non-seminomas without microdissection will, by definition, miss the histology-specific chromosomal anomalies.

Another interesting observation was that some of the histology-specific changes could already be observed in the adjacent CIS cells. This supports our model that CIS is 'one step behind' in the pathogenetic evolution of the invasive tumor[11,41].

The recurrent pattern of chromosomal gains and losses suggests that both activation of proto-oncogenes and inactivation of tumor suppressor genes are involved in the development of TGCTs. Some of the putative candidates have been studied, of which a summary is given below.

Proto-oncogenes   Several studies deal with the possible role of activation of proto-oncogenes in the development of seminomas and non-seminomas. *RAS* genes are rarely found to be mutated[42–44]. One study reported the presence of mutations in c-*KIT* in some cases[45]. Over-expression of c-*MYC* has been found in less than 10% of non-seminomas[46], and amplification of *MDM2* also in less than 10% of the tumors[47]. Cyclin D2 has been suggested as the candidate gene on 12p[48]. In conclusion, the role of activation of proto-oncogenes in the genesis of seminomas and non-seminomas has not yet been illucidated. In addition, activation of a proto-oncogene in the initiation of this cancer seems less unlikely (see also *Genetic predisposition*).

Tumor suppressor genes   Studies of loss of heterozygosity (LOH), a hallmark of the involvement of tumor suppressor genes, have given rather inconsistent results in cases of seminomas and non-seminomas, which might be related to their aneuploidy, as discussed by us elsewhere[49]. Several studies have been performed on chromosomes 1, 5, 11, 12 and 18[49–58]. Recurrent loss has been observed on 1p, in particular bands p13, p22, p31.3–p32 and 1q; in particular bands q32. Several regions on chromosome 5 show LOH, including p15.1–p15.2, q11, q14, q21 and q34–qter. Chromosome 12 contains two regions of interest, i.e. q13 and q22. In spite of the identification of homozygous deletions at 12q22, no candidate genes have yet been identified. Homozygous deletions have also been identified on the long arm of chromosome 18. Although *DCC* (deleted in colorectal cancer) may be a candidate[54,59,60], it has been indicated that loss of this gene is likely to be progression related. More recently, inactivating mutations of *SMAD4*, mapped to 18q, have been reported in a limited number of seminomas[61]. The other targets investigated with overall negative findings are: *NME1* and *2*[62], *APC, MCC, RB*[59,63], *WT1*[49,59] and *P53*[64-68]. However, hypermethylation of exon 1 of *p16* was found in about 50% of the tumors, which was related to no, or to a low level of, expression[69]. Moreover, a high incidence of homozygous deletions of *p16* has been reported in intracranial germinomas, the equivalent of testicular seminomas[70]. In addition, we studied the presence of genomic deletions by conventional detection of LOH by means of the polymerase chain reaction (PCR). This approach was applied to microdissected tumor cells of different histologies, including CIS. DNA was amplified using a universal amplification strategy[71]. Recurrent LOH was found at 3q27–q28, 5q31, 5q34–q35, 9p21–p22 and 12q22. Again, these anomalies were also found in the adjacent CIS cells. Interestingly, loss of 3q27–q28 was only, but consistently, detected in the pure embryonal carcinomas.

In summary, although interesting observations have been made, no convincing data based on studies on LOH, mutations and expression, to date, indicate a significant involvement of one of the studied known tumor suppressor genes in the initiation of testicular seminomas and non-seminomas.

Gain of 12p

The most consistent chromosomal anomaly in seminomas and non-seminomas, besides their aneuploidy, is gain of the short arm of chromosome 12. In fact, about 80% of the invasive tumors have extra copies of 12p due to the formation of an isochromosome (i(12p))[72] (Figure 3). The 20% of i(12p) negative tumors also show a gain of 12p, due to other chromosomal changes[73]. The consistent gain of 12p was supported by CGH results (see above). These data strongly indicate that the short arm of chromosome 12 contains a gene or genes of which extra copies are required for the development of the invasive tumor. Analysis of LOH on the long arm of chromosome 12 showed that polyploidization occurs prior to i(12p) formation[74]. In addition, it was demonstrated that i(12p) results from sister chromatin exchange[75]. Most recently, we have shown that the presence of extra copies of the short arm of chromosome 12 is related to invasive growth of the tumor[76], i.e. no gain of 12p is observed in CIS. Our current working model is that expression of apoptosis-suppressing genes mapped to 12p is relevant for the progression of CIS to an invasive tumor.

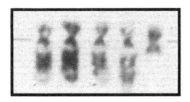 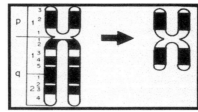 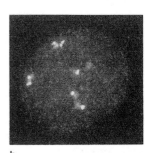

a   b

Figure 3   (a) Representative example of actual G-banding and schematic of a normal chromosome 12 (left within panel) and an isochromosome 12p (i(12p)) (right within panel). (b) The fluorescent *in situ* hybridization pattern with a probe specific for the centromeric region of chromosome 12 and the p-arm is also indicated. Note the presence of three normal chromosomes 12, and two isochromosomes

Conclusions on the biology of GCTs

The results available so far indicate that the invasive germ cell tumors, as well as their adjacent CIS, are aneuploid, containing a high number of chromosomal changes, both numerical and structural. Strikingly, CIS contains a significant number of changes also found in the invasive tumor. This supports our model that CIS is (only) 'one step behind' the invasive tumor, and this significantly hampers identification of the initiating genetic events in the pathogenesis of malignant germ cell tumors. It is worth noting that gain of 12p sequences is restricted to invasive TGCTs.

Animal models

The mouse teratocarcinoma is the most likely model for germ cell tumors of infants. Like those of their human counterparts, the mouse tumors present at prepubertal age, and lack CIS and seminomas. In addition, they are diploid, and can progress to a yolk sac tumor, with an aneuploid DNA content[77]. Canine seminomas are possibly the counterpart of human spermatocytic seminomas[78]. They have the same morphology and clinical presentation. In addition, no non-seminomatous elements or CIS have been reported. The tumors found in horses and rabbits might be of this same type. No convincing animal model exists as yet for seminomas and non-seminomas. The human papilloma virus (HPV)-type 16-transgenic[79] and glial cell line-derived neurotrophic factor (GDNF)-overexpressing mouse[80] might be of interest. These observations must be kept in mind when interpreting results of experiments in animal models on the possible role of endocrine disrupters (including estrogen) in gonadal development, and in the pathogenesis of testicular germ cell tumors.

Prognostic factors for testicular germ cell tumors

General

The teratomas of infants and spermatocytic seminomas are, generally, benign. Therefore, orchidectomy alone is mostly curative. However, spermatocytic seminomas may progress to sarcoma, a highly malignant tumor. When the yolk sac tumor component of infants is metastatic, it can be cured in the majority of patients using chemotherapy. Seminomas are highly sensitive to irradiation (see reference 81 for review). Thanks to the introduction of cisplatin-based chemotherapy, the survival of patients with metastatic seminoma, but even more impressively of patients with (metastatic) non-seminoma, increased significantly, with cure rates of up to 90%[82]. Criteria have been developed to distinguish non-seminoma patients with a good, intermediate and poor response[83]. Although these parameters are not informative on an individual basis, they separate the three groups as a whole. Patients with seminomas always fall in the good and inter-mediate prognostic group. Patients with refractory disease might benefit from high-dose chemotherapy[84].

Specific

When to biopsy the contralateral testis Since CIS is most probably formed during intrauterine growth (see above), and the treatable cancer in most cases manifests clinically after puberty, methods for early diagnosis and treatment might prevent progression of CIS to an invasive seminoma or non-seminoma, thereby prevent-ing possible progression to refractory disease. Moreover, it has been shown that CIS can be effectively eradicated using local irradiation, with limited side-effects (see above). In cases with CIS, 50% of patients will develop an invasive TGCT within 5 years. Given enough time, almost all CIS will become invasive. CIS is present in the contralateral testis in about 5% of the patients with a unilateral tumor (see above). Patients with cryptorchidism, atrophic testis or prior infertility have a higher risk of CIS in the contralateral testis. The exact numbers are unknown, but it is estimated that high-risk patients comprise 40–50% of the population with CIS. Altogether, about 50–60% of patients with a unilateral testis tumor will have no other risk factors for CIS[85]. Biopsy of the contralateral testis in men with a unilateral testis tumor is routinely done in most centers in Denmark, Germany and Austria, but is rarely carried out in the UK, the Netherlands and the USA. Another option, as is practiced in countries such as Norway, is to biopsy only those patients who have a high risk of contralateral CIS. The decision to do a contralateral biopsy is based on a combination of medical, psychosocial and cultural considerations. In patients who do not undergo a contralateral biopsy, the remaining testis should be followed up carefully. Self-evaluation by the patient is advised[86].

Several markers may be useful for early diagnosis[87–90], although as yet none have been applied in a clinical setting. In fact, detection of CIS cells or CIS-derived products in semen (Figure 2), would be the most interesting approach for a non-invasive screening method.

Predicting metastases in a clinical stage I TGCT For clinical stage I non-seminomatous TGCTs (NS-TGCTs) the risk of occult metastases is about 30%. Established factors predicting metastastic disease are lympho-vascular space invasion and percentage of embryonal carcinoma. Pathologists should be aware that intratubular embryonal carcinoma, retraction artifacts and implantation artifacts might mimic angioinvasive growth histo-logically. These difficulties probably account for

the differences in the reported prognostic value of this parameter. Ploidy and proliferation rate (determined by antibodies for MIB-1 and PCNA) may improve the prediction of metastases. For NS-TGCT there is no consensus on the best method for defining the risk of occult metastases and on how the information can be used for the clinical management of patients. In clinical stage I seminoma patients occult metastases are predicted by vascular invasion and tumor size. Again, it is not clear how these factors can be used in the clinic. Obviously they could serve to define a group of patients that could benefit from surveillance[86].

Predicting outcome in metastatic TGCT The goal of the efforts to predict outcome in metastatic TGCT is two-fold: to minimize toxicity in the good-risk patients, and to intensify treatment in the poor-risk patients[91]. The International GCT Consensus Criteria[83] are listed in Table 1. Seminoma patients never fall into the poor-risk category; on the other hand, all cases of mediastinal NS-GCT belong to the poor-risk category.

Predicting necrosis and fibrosis only in residual masses The most extensive study regarding this problem was carried out by Steyerberg and colleagues[92]. They concluded that pure necrosis

Table 1 Risk stratification from the International Germ Cell Cancer Collaborative Group

	Serum marker	Extent of disease
NS-GCTs		
Good risk	LDH, 1.5 × normal, hCG < 5000 mIU/ml and AFP < 1000 ng/ml	no evidence of non-pulmonary metastases
Intermediate risk	LDH 1.5–10 × normal, hCG 5000–50 000 mIU/ml, or AFP 1000–10 000 ng/ml	no evidence of non-pulmonary metastases
Poor risk	LDH > 10 × normal, hCG > 50 000 mIU/ml, AFP > 10 000 ng/ml	evidence of non-pulmonary metastases
Seminomas		
Good risk		no evidence of non-pulmonary metastases
Intermediate risk		evidence of non-pulmonary metastases

NS-GCTs, non-seminomatous germ cell tumors; LDH, lactacte dehydrogenase; hCG, human chorionic gonadotropin; AFP, alpha-fetoprotein can be predicted on the basis of absence of teratoma in the testis[93]; normal levels of alpha-fetoprotein (AFP) and human chorionic gonadotropin (hCG), but elevated levels of lactate dehydrogenase (LDH) before chemotherapy; a small pre-chemotherapy or post-chemotherapy tumor mass (≤ 2 cm in diameter); and a large shrinkage of the mass during chemotherapy ($\geq 90\%$). On the other hand, cancer cannot reliably be predicted or adequately discriminated from mature teratoma. Prediction models for the histology of residual masses are proposed to refine the selection of patients who should undergo lymph node dissection[94].

Prognostic value of histological findings in residual masses When only necrosis, fibrosis and teratoma are found histologically, the risk of progressive disease is low. It is important that the teratoma component is radically removed because of the risk of development of growing teratoma or a non-germ-cell malignancy. A poor prognostic sign is the finding of viable non-teratomatous GCT, in particular when this component is incompletely resected. The same is true for a non-germ cell malignancy (e.g. carcinoma, sarcoma or primitive neuroectodermal tumor (PNET). The diagnosis of a non-germ cell malignancy requires that there be evidence of stromal invasion or confluent growth. The organoid growth pattern of mature teratoma is disturbed. The outcome depends on the type of secondary non-germ-cell malignancy. PNET, for example, has a poor prognosis while a nephroblastoma-like tumor does not[86].

New diagnostic and prognostic markers The most specific marker for TGCT is over-representation of the short arm of the chromosome, either as isochromosome 12p or as other aberrations involving 12p material. These chromosomal aberrations can be used to demonstrate the germ cell origin of secondary non-germ-cell malignancies, and of poorly differentiated midline tumors which cannot be reliably classified on the basis of morphology and immunohistochemistry (see reference 95 for review). Similarly, the teratomatous or non-neoplastic nature of an epidermoid cyst of the testis can be unequivocally demonstrated on the basis of these chromosomal characteristics. The 1.5-kb transcript of platelet-derived growth factor α-receptor gene is a specific marker for GCT except teratoma, including CIS[88]. Its use for the non-invasive detection of CIS cells in seminal fluid, using reverse transcriptase-PCR, is under investigation[96].

The search for new, molecular prognostic markers is a big challenge. It should be borne in mind that new, tumor-based molecular markers must have independent prognostic significance when compared with conventional patient-based markers (e.g. LDH and hCG levels) and conventional pathological criteria. None of the markers under study stands up to this test.

References

1. Oosterhuis JW, Looijenga LHJ, van Echten J, *et al.* Chromosomal constitution and developmental potential of human germ cell tumors and teratomas. *Cancer Genet Cytogenet* 1997; 95:96–102
2. Skakkebæk NE. Possible carcinoma-*in-situ* of the testis. *Lancet* 1972;1:516–17
3. Swerdlow AJ. In Jones WG, Appleyard I, Harnden P, Joffe JK, eds. *Germ Cell Tumours IV.* London: John Libbey, 1998:3–8
4. Moul JW, Schanne FJ, Thompson IM, *et al.* Testicular cancer in blacks. A multicenter experience. *Cancer* 1994;73:388–93
5. Adami HO, Bergström R, Möhner M, *et al.* A testicular cancer in nine northern european countries. *Int J Cancer* 1994;59:33–8

6. Bergström R, Adami H-O, Mohner M, *et al.* Increase in testicular cancer incidence in six European countries: a birth cohort phenomenon. *J Natl Cancer Inst* 1996;88:727–33

7. Pugh RCB, ed. *Pathology of the Testis.* Oxford: Blackwell, 1976:245–58

8. Oosterhuis JW, Castedo SMMJ, De Jong B, *et al.* Ploidy of primary germ cell tumors of the testis. Pathogenetic and clinical relevance. *Lab Invest* 1989;60:14–20

9. Ulbright TM. Germ cell neoplasms of the testis. *Am J Surg Pathol* 1993;17:1075–91

10. Mostofi FK, Sesterhenn IA. *Histological Typing of Testis Tumours.* Berlin: Springer, 1998

11. Oosterhuis JW, Looijenga LHJ. The biology of human germ cell tumours: retrospective speculations and new prospectives. *Eur Urol* 1993; 23:245–50

12. Skakkebæk NE, Raipert-de Meyts E, Jørgensen N, *et al.* Germ cell cancer and disorders of spermatogenesis: an environmental connection? *APMIS* 1998;106:3–12

13. Gondos B. Ultrastructure of developing and malignant germ cells. *Eur Urol* 1993;23:68–75

14. Roelofs H, Manes T, Millan JL, *et al.* Heterogeneity in alkaline phosphatase isozyme expression in human testicular germ cell tumors. An enzyme-/immunohistochemical and molecular analysis. *J Pathol* 1999;189:236–44

15. Rajpert-De Meyts E, Skakkebæk NE. Expression of the c-kit protein product in carcinoma-*in-situ* and invasive testicular germ cell tumours. *Int J Androl* 1994;17:85–92

16. Jørgensen N, Rajpert-De Meyts E, Graem N, *et al.* Expression of immunohistochemical markers for testicular carcinoma *in situ* by normal fetal germ cells. *Lab Invest* 1995;72:223–31

17. Møller H. Decreased testicular cancer risk in men born in wartime. *J Natl Cancer Inst* 1989; 81:1668–9

18. Dieckmann KP, Skakkebaek NE. Carcinoma *in situ* of the testis: review of biological and clinical features. *Int J Cancer* 1999;83:815–22

19. Giwercman A, Müller J, Skakkebæk NE. Prevalence of carcinoma-*in situ* and other histopathological abnormalities in testes from 399 men who died suddenly and unexpectedly. *J Urol* 1991;145:77–80

20. Berthelsen JG, Skakkebaek NE. Gonadal function in men with testis cancer. *Fertil Steril* 1983;39:68–75

21. Jacobsen R, Bostofte E, Engholm G, *et al.* Risk of testicular cancer in men with abnormal semen characteristics: cohort study. *Br Med J* 2000; 321:789–92

22. Petersen PM, Giwercman A, Skakkebæk NE, *et al.* Gonadal function in men with testicular cancer. *Semin Oncol* 1998;25:224–33

23. Møller H, Skakkebæk NE. Risk of testicular cancer in subfertile men: case–control study. *Br Med J* 1999;318:559–62

24. Bernstein L, Depue RH, Ross RK, *et al.* Higher maternal levels of free estradiol in first compared to second pregnancy: early gestational differences. *J Natl Cancer Inst* 1986;76:1035–9

25. McGregor JA, Jackson GM, Lachelin GC, *et al.* Salivary estriol as risk assessment for preterm labor: a prospective trial. *Am J Obstet Gynecol* 1995;173:1337–42

26. Henderson BE, Bernstein L, Ross RK, *et al.* The early *in-utero* oestrogen and testosterone environment of blacks and whites: potential effects on male offspring. *Br J Cancer* 1988;57: 216–18

27. Leahy MG, Tonks S, Moses JH, *et al.* Candidate regions for a testicular cancer susceptibility gene. *Hum Mol Genet* 1995;4:1551–5

28. Bishop DT. Candidate regions for testicular cancer susceptibility genes. *APMIS* 1998;106: 64–72

29. Heimdal K, Ohlsson H, Tretli S, *et al.* Familial testicular cancer in Norway and southern Sweden. *Br J Cancer* 1996;73:964–9

30. Rapley EA, Crockford GP, Teare D, *et al.* Localization to Xq27 of a susceptibility gene for testicular germ-cell tumours. *Nature Genet* 2000; 24:197–200

31. De Graaff WE, Oosterhuis JW, De Jong B, *et al.* Ploidy of testicular carcinoma *in situ. Lab Invest* 1992;66:166–8

32. El-Naggar AK, Ro JY, McLemore D, *et al.* DNA ploidy in testicular germ cell neoplasms. Histogenetic and clinical implications. *Am J Surg Pathol* 1992;16:611–18

33. Sandberg AA, Meloni AM, Suijkerbuijk RF. Reviews of chromosome studies in urological tumors. 3. Cytogenetics and genes in testicular tumors. *J Urol* 1996;155:1531–56

34. Korn MW, Olde Weghuis DEM, Suijkerbuijk RF, *et al.* Detection of chromosomal DNA gains and losses in testicular germ cell tumors by comparative genomic hybridization. *Genes Chromosom Cancer* 1996;17:78–87

35. Mostert MC, Van de Pol M, Olde Weghuis D, *et al.* Comparative genomic hybridization of germ cell tumors of the adult testis; confirmation of karyotypic findings and identification of a 12p-amplicon. *Cancer Genet Cytogenet* 1996;89: 146–52

36. Ottesen AM, Kirchhoff M, Rajpert De-Meyts E, *et al.* Detection of chromosomal aberrations in seminomatous germ cell tumours using comparative genomic hybridization. *Genes Chromosom Cancer* 1997;20:412–18

37. Summersgill B, Goker H, Wber-Hall S, *et al.* Molecular cytogenetic analysis of adult

testicular germ cell tumours and identification of regions of consensus copy number change. *Br J Cancer* 1998;77:305–13

38. Rosenberg C, Bakker Schut T, Mostert MC, *et al.* Chromosomal gains and losses in testicular germ cell tumors of adolescents and adults investigated by a modified CGH approach. *Lab Invest* 1999;79:1447–51

39. Rosenberg C, Bakker Schut T, Mostert MC, *et al.* Comparative genomic hybridization in hypotriploid/hyperdiploid tumors. *Cytometry* 1997;29:113–21

40. Looijenga LHJ, Rosenberg C, Van Gurp RJHLM, *et al.* Comparative genomic hybridization of microdissected samples from different stages in the development of a seminoma and nonseminoma. *J Pathol* 2000;191:187–92

41. Looijenga LHJ, Gillis AJM, Van Putten WLJ, *et al.* In situ numeric analysis of centromeric regions of chromosomes 1, 12, and 15 of seminomas, nonseminomatous germ cell tumors, and carcinoma *in situ* of human testis. *Lab Invest* 1993;68:211–19

42. Ridanpää M, Lothe RA, Önfelt A, *et al.* K-ras oncogene codon 12 point mutations in testicular cancer. *Environ Health Perspect* 1993; 101:185–7

43. Olie RA, Looijenga LHJ, Boerrigter L, *et al.* N- and KRAS mutations in human testicular germ cell tumors: incidence and possible biological implications. *Genes Chromosom Cancer* 1995;12: 110–16

44. Moul JW, Theune SM, Chang EH. Detection of ras mutations in archival testicular germ cell tumors by polymerase chain reaction and oligonucleotide hybridization. *Genes Chromosom Cancer* 1992;5:109–18

45. Tian Q, Frierson HF Jr, Krystal GW, *et al.* Activating c-kit gene mutations in human germ cell tumors. *Am J Pathol* 1999;154:1643–7

46. Schmidt B, Ackermann R, Hartmann M, *et al.* Alterations of the metastasis suppressor gene nm23 and the proto-oncogene c-myc in human testicular germ cell tumors. *J Urol* 1997;158: 2000–5

47. Riou G, Barrois M, Prost S, *et al.* The p53 and mdm-2 genes in human testicular germ-cell tumors. *Mol Carcinog* 1995;12:124–31

48. Houldsworth J, Reuter V, Bosl GJ, *et al.* Aberrant expression of cyclin D2 is an early event in human male germ cell tumorigenesis. *Cell Growth Differ* 1997;8:293–9

49. Looijenga LHJ, Abraham M, Gillis AJM, *et al.* Testicular germ cell tumors of adults show deletions of chromosomal bands 11p13 and 11p15.5, but no abnormalities within the zinc-finger regions and exons 2 and 6 of the Wilms' tumor 1 gene. *Genes Chromosom Cancer* 1994; 9:153–60

50. Lothe RA, Hastie N, Heimdal K, *et al.* Frequent loss of 11p13 and 11p15 loci in male germ cell tumours. *Genes Chromosom Cancer* 1993;7:96–101

51. Mathew S, Murty VVVS, Bosl GJ, *et al.* Loss of heterozygosity identifies multiple sites of allelic deletions on chromosome 1 in human male germ cell tumors. *Cancer Res* 1994;54:6265–9

52. Murty VVVS, Li RG, Mathew S, *et al.* Replication error-type genetic instability at 1q42–43 in human male germ cell tumors. *Cancer Res* 1994;54:3983–5

53. Murty VVVS, Houldsworth J, Baldwin S, *et al.* Allelic deletions in the long arm of chromosome 12 identify sites of candidate tumor suppressor genes in male germ cell tumors. *Proc Natl Acad Sci USA* 1992;89:11006–10

54. Murty VVVS, Li RG, Houldsworth J, *et al.* Frequent allelic deletions and loss of expression characterize the DCC gene in male germ cell tumors. *Oncogene* 1994;9:3227–31

55. Murty VVVS, Renault B, Falk CT, *et al.* Physical mapping of a commonly deleted region, the site of a candidate tumor suppressor gene, at 12q22 in human male germ cell tumors. *Genomics* 1996;35:562–70

56. Murty VVVS, Reuter VE, Bosl GJ, *et al.* Deletion mapping identifies loss of heterozygosity at 5p15.1–15.2, 5q11 and 5q34–35 in human male germ cell tumors. *Oncogene* 1996;12:2719–23

57. Bala S, Oliver H, Renault B, *et al.* Genetic analysis of the APAF1 gene in male germ cell tumors. *Genes Chromosom Cancer* 2000;28:258–68

58. Peng HQ, Liu L, Goss PE, *et al.* Chromosomal deletions occur in restricted regions of 5q in testicular germ cell cancer. *Oncogene* 1999;18: 3277–83

59. Peng H-Q, Bailey D, Bronson D, *et al.* Loss of heterozygosity of tumor suppressor genes in testis cancer. *Cancer Res* 1995;55:2871–5

60. Strohmeyer D, Langenhof S, Ackermann R, *et al.* Analysis of the DCC tumor suppressor gene in testicular germ cell tumors: mutations and loss of expression. *J Urol* 1997;157: 1973–6

61. Bouras M, Tabone E, Bertholon J, *et al.* A novel SMAD4 gene mutation in seminoma germ cell tumors. *Cancer Res* 2000;60:922–8

62. Backer JM, Murty VVVS, Potla L, *et al.* Loss of heterozygosity and decreased expression of NME genes correlate with teratomatous differentiation in human male germ cell tumors. *Biochem Biophys Res Commun* 1994;202: 1096–103

63. Strohmeyer T, Reissmann P, Cordon-Cardo C, *et al.* Correlation between retinoblastoma gene expression and differentiation in human testicular tumors. *Proc Natl Acad Sci USA* 1991;88:6662–6

64. Peng HQ, Hogg D, Malkin D, *et al.* Mutations of the p53 gene do not occur in testis cancer. *Cancer Res* 1993;53:3574–8
65. Heimdal K, Lothe RA, Lystad S, *et al.* No germline TP53 mutations detected in familial and bilateral testicular cancer. *Genes Chromosom Cancer* 1993; 6:92–7
66. Fleischhacker M, Strohmeyer T, Imai Y, *et al.* Mutations of the p53 gene are not detectable in human testicular tumors. *Mod Pathol* 1994;7: 435–9
67. Schenkman NS, Sesterhenn IA, Washington L, *et al.* Increased p53 protein does not correlate to p53 gene mutations in microdissected human testicular germ cell tumors. *J Urol* 1995;154: 617–21
68. Guillou L, Estreicher A, Chaubert P, *et al.* Germ cell tumors of the testis overexpress wild-type p53. *Am J Pathol* 1996;149:1221–8
69. Chaubert P, Guillou L, Kurt AM, *et al.* Frequent p161NK4 (MTS1) gene inactivation in testicular germ cell tumors. *Am J Pathol* 1997;151:859–65
70. Iwato M, Tachibana O, Tohma Y, *et al.* Alterations of the INK4a/ARF locus in human intracranial germ cell tumors. *Cancer Res* 2000;60:2113–15
71. Faulkner SW, Leigh DA, Oosterhuis JW, *et al.* Allellic loss in carcinoma *in situ* and testicular germ cell tumours of adolescents and adults: evidence in support of the linear progression model. *Br J Cancer* 2000;83:729–36
72. Van Echten-Arends J, Oosterhuis JW, Looijenga LHJ, *et al.* No recurrent structural abnormalities in germ cell tumors of the adult testis apart from i(12p). *Genes Chromosom Cancer* 1995;14:133–44
73. Suijkerbuijk RF, Sinke RJ, Meloni AM, *et al.* Overrepresentation of chromosome 12p sequences and karyotypic evolution in i(12p)-negative testicular germ-cell tumors revealed by fluorescence *in situ* hybridization. *Cancer Genet Cytogenet* 1993;70:85–93
74. Geurts van Kessel A, Van Drunen E, De Jong B, *et al.* Chromosome 12q heterozygosity is retained in i(12p)-positive testicular germ cell tumor cells. *Cancer Genet Cytogenet* 1989:40: 129–34
75. Sinke RJ, Suijkerbuijk RF, De Jong B, *et al.* Uniparental origin of i(12p) in human germ cell tumors. *Genes Chromosom Cancer* 1993;6: 161–5
76. Rosenberg C, Van Gurp RJHLM, Geelen E, *et al.* Overrepresentation of the short arm of chromosome 12 is related to invasive growth of human testicular seminomas and nonseminomas. *Oncogene* 2000;19:5858–62
77. Van Berlo RJ, Oosterhuis JW, Schrijnemakers E, *et al.* Yolk-sac carcinoma develops spontaneously as a late occurrence in slow-growing teratoid tumors produced from transplanted 7-day mouse embryos. *Int J Cancer* 1990;45:153–5
78. Looijenga LHJ, Olie RA, Van der Gaag I, *et al.* Seminomas of the canine testis; counterpart of spermatocytic seminoma of men? *Lab Invest* 1994;71:490–6
79. Kondoh G, Murata Y, Aozasa K, *et al.* Very high incidence of germ cell tumorigenesis (seminomagenesis) in human papillomavirus. Type 16 transgenic mice. *J Virol* 1991;65:3335–9
80. Meng X, Lindahl M, Hyvonen ME, *et al.* Regulation of cell fate decision of undifferentiated spermatogonia by GDNF. *Science* 2000:287: 1489–93
81. Gospodarowicz MK, Sturgeon JFG, Jewett MAS, *et al.* Early stage and advanced seminoma: role of radiation therapy, surgery, and chemotherapy. *Semin Oncol* 1998;25:160–73
82. Bokemeyer C, Schmoll HJ. Treatment of testicular cancer and the development of secondary malignancies. *J Clin Oncol* 1995;13:283–92
83. International Germ Cell Cancer Collaborative Group. International Germ Cell Consensus Classification: a prognostic factor-based staging system for metastatic germ cell cancers. *J Clin Oncol* 1997;15:594–603
84. Bokemeyer C, Kollmannsberger C, Harstrick A, *et al.* Treatment of patients with cisplatin-refractory testicular germ-cell cancer. German Testicular Cancer Study Group (GTCSG). *Int J Cancer* 1999;83:848–51
85. Rørth M, Rajpert-de Meyts E, Skakkebæk NE, *et al.* Carcinoma *in situ* of the testis. *Scand J Urol* 2000;205:166–86
86. Ulbright TM. Testis risk and prognostic factors. The pathologist's perspective. *Urol Clin North Am* 1999;26:611–26
87. Giwercman A. Clausen OPF, Bruun E, *et al.* The value of quantitative DNA flow cytometry of testicular fine-needle aspirates in assessment of spermatogenesis: a study of 137 previously maldescended human testes. *Int J Androl* 1994;17:35–42
88. Mosselman S, Looijenga LHJ, Gillis AJM, *et al.* Aberrant platelet-derived growth factor α-receptor transcript as a diagnostic marker for early human germ cell tumors of the adult testis. *Proc Natl Acad Sci USA* 1996;93:2884–8
89. Meng FJ, Zhou Y, Giwercman A, *et al.* Fluorescence *in situ* hybridization analysis of chromosome 12 anomalies in semen cells from patients with carcinoma *in situ* of the testis. *J Pathol* 1998;186:235–9
90. Salanova M, Gandini L, Lenzi A, *et al.* Is hyperdiploidy of immature ejaculated germ cells predictive of testis malignancy? A comparative study in healthy normozoospermic, infertile, and testis tumor suffering subjects. *Lab Invest* 1999;79:1127–35

91. McCaffrey JA, Bajorin DF, Motzer RJ. Risk assessment for metastatic testis cancer: *Urol Clin North Am* 1998;25:389–95

92. Steyerberg EW, Keizer HJ, Fossa SD, *et al.* Prediction of residual retroperitoneal mass histology after chemotherapy for metastatic nonseminomatous germ cell tumor: multivariate analysis of individual patient data from six study groups. *J Clin Oncol* 1995; 13:1177–87

93. Oosterhuis JW, Suurmeyer AJH, Sleyfer DTh, *et al.* Effects of multiple-drug chemotherapy (Cis-Diammine-Dichloroplatinum, Bleomycin, and Vinblastine) on the maturation of retroperitoneal lymph node metastases of nonseminomatous germ cell tumors of the testis. *Cancer* 1983;51;408–16

94. Steyerberg EW, Keizer HJ, Habbema JD. Prediction models for the histology of residual masses after chemotherapy for metastatic testicular cancer. ReHiT Study Group. *Int J Cancer* 1999;83;856–9

95. Looijenga LHJ, Oosterhuis JW. Pathogenesis of testicular germ cell tumors. *Rev Reprod* 1999; 4:90–100

96. Oosterhuis JW, Gillis AJ, van Roozendaal CE, *et al.* The platelet-derived growth factor alpha-receptor 1.5 kb transcript: target for molecular detection of testicular germ cell tumours of adolescents and adults. *APMIS* 1998;106: 207–13, discussion 213–15

Surgery for testicular cancer – indications, technique and results

2

A. Hobisch, G. Janetschek, R. Peschel, L. Höltl, A. Hittmair, H. Rogatsch and G. Bartsch

Introduction

Testicular cancer is the most common malignancy in young men aged 15–35 years. Moreover, carcinoma of the testis has become one of the neoplasms with the highest curability. Patients presenting with clinical stage I disease have a cure rate of nearly 100% and patients with advanced disease achieve complete remission rates of over 90%. These high-cure rates are a result of platinum-based chemotherapy and surgery. Surgery remains a major factor in the overall management planning and its role is three-fold. First, radical orchidectomy establishes the diagnosis and controls the primary tumor. Second, retroperitoneal lymph node dissection has consistently been the single most important factor in determining the stage of the disease. Third, surgery has become an integral adjuvant to inductive platinum-based chemotherapy in patients with an advanced testicular tumor. In this respect, retroperitoneal lymph node dissection has an important role in the management of both low- and high-stage testicular cancer.

Radical orchidectomy

The first step in the treatment of testicular cancer is to perform a radical orchidectomy. An incision of the skin above and parallel to the inguinal ligament is performed. After incision of the external oblique fascia, the spermatic cord can be bluntly dissected. Care should be taken not to cut the ilioinguinal nerve. The cord is dissected to the internal ring and then clamped with a non-crushing clamp. Next, the testicle is pushed upward and the gubernacular attachments are ligated. Now the cord can be ligated at the internal ring using non-absorbable sutures. The ends of the sutures should be kept sufficiently long for later identification during lymph node dissection. The non-touch maneuver, by clamping the spermatic cord prior to testicular manipulation, is a time-honored and, probably, prudent technique. However, the necessity of this maneuver has no scientific validity. Tumor cells are probably escaping continually and manipulation may not add any more adverse consequences. In doubtful cases in which testicular exploration is necessary and a long wait for pathological diagnosis is required, this fact should be kept in mind[1].

Organ-preserving tumor enucleation

Radical orchidectomy is the standard therapy for testicular tumors. If these tumors occur in a single testis, or bilaterally, the consequences are azoospermia and hormonal deficiency. In contrast to previous therapies, many tumors such as those occurring in kidney and breast cancer are now treated by organ-preserving tumor enucleation. Therefore, some centers perform an organ-preserving tumor enucleation. By considering quality-of-life issues, it is the intention of these centers to prevent young patients from lifelong androgen supplementation and loss of fertility. Intraoperatively, an exploration of the testis is performed under cold ischemia with the testicle packed in crushed ice. After localization of the tumor using ultrasound, the tunica albuginea is incised above the tumor.

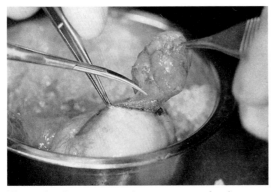

Figure 1 Organ-preserving tumor enucleation

While monitoring with ultrasound, the tumor can now be enucleated and resected with a small edge of adjacent parenchyma by bipolar forceps (Figure 1). Usually, the enucleation is technically quite easy, since a pseudocapsule surrounds these small tumors and, by using bipolar forceps, bleeding can successfully be avoided. Subsequently, biopsies of each side-wall and from the tumor bed are taken. After conscientious hemostasis, the parenchymal defect is filled with hemostyptic material and the tunica albuginea is closed using 5×0 monocryl sutures. The first data reported by Weissbach, Heidenreich and our group[2–4] look very promising. Based on these reports, the guidelines for organ-preserving tumor enucleation are: organ-confined tumor < 25 mm, enucleation under cold ischemia, frozen sections, multiple biopsies of the tumor bed and adjacent parenchyma, normal pre-operative endocrine function, negative biopsies and, in cases of testicular intraepithelial neoplasia (TIN), radiation therapy of the testis.

Retroperitoneal lymph node dissection

Indications

Although we have made tremendous advances in the treatment of testicular cancer, many controversies exist concerning the different therapeutic strategies at the different stages of these tumors. Despite the development of modern technologies to detect metastases[5–7], the clinical stage I of non-seminomatous germ cell tumors is inaccurate in about 30% of

patients. Therefore, in various centers, the therapy for clinical stage I patients differs; retroperitoneal lymph node dissection[8–18], surveillance[19–24] or primary chemotherapy[25–28] are all used. Many centers make their decision for treatment of clinical stage I tumors according to risk factors[29–34]. In case of stage II tumors, various therapeutic strategies are also used including primary retroperitoneal lymph node dissection with adjuvant chemotherapy, retroperitoneal lymph node dissection and chemotherapy only in cases of a relapse, primary chemotherapy followed by retroperitoneal lymph node dissection, or primary chemotherapy and retroperitoneal lymph node dissection only in cases of a residual tumor[12,34–44]. Retroperitoneal lymph node dissection offers patients two benefits: on the one hand, in the form of a staging lymphadenectomy, it offers the possibility of an accurate staging of clinical stage I tumors and, on the other hand, it offers the probability of surgical cure in patients with low-volume retroperitoneal metastases. Furthermore, retroperitoneal lymph node dissection is used following inductive chemotherapy in patients presenting with bulky tumors. Retroperitoneal lymph node dissection can be performed using a transabdominal or a thoracoabdominal approach.

Neuroanatomy of the sympathetic trunk

The long-term morbidity of retroperitoneal lymph node dissection is primarily due to a lesion of the postganglionic nerve fibers from the ganglia Th12 to L3, resulting in loss of ejaculation. In 1951, Whitelaw and Smithwick demonstrated in their study on secondary effects of sympathectomy that resection of the L1, L2 and L3 ganglia on one side and L1 and L2 on the contralateral side results in aspermia of up to 54%[45]. Resection of the L1, L2 and L3 ganglia on one side only did not result in aspermia (Figure 2). In an effort to preserve these fibers, several medical centers have, subsequently, developed a number of modifications, including the nerve-sparing or the template technique. The incidence of loss of

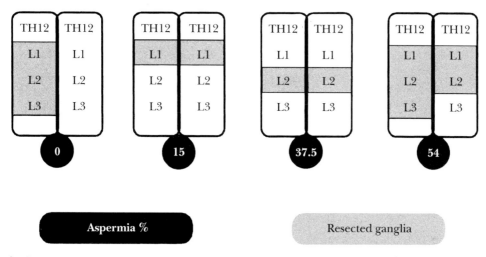

Figure 2 Percentage of aspermia after resection of sympathetic ganglia according to Whitelaw and Smithwick[45]

ejaculation is directly related to the extent and operative technique of the retroperitoneal lymph node dissection. The mapping studies of retroperitoneal lymph nodes by Weissbach and Boedefeld[46] and Donohue and colleagues[47] were an essential precondition for modifying the boundaries of dissection in order to achieve a good compromise between radical surgery and preservation of antegrade ejaculation.

Colleselli and co-workers[48] performed an anatomical study on neuroanatomy of the sympathetic ganglia and nerve fibers to serve as a basis for possible modifications of retroperitoneal lymph node dissection. For this anatomical study, 12 retroperitoneal cadaver specimens were dissected with the help of a magnifying lens. They found that the sympathetic trunk consists of a series of spindle-shaped ganglia, which are interconnected by short interganglionic rami. This trunk extends from the base of the skull down to the tip of the coccyx on either side of the spinal column (Figure 3). The right sympathetic trunk is situated dorsally to the inferior vena cava, while the left trunk is located dorsally and laterally to the abdominal aorta. The transverse rami connect the two sympathetic trunks. The lumbar splanchnic nerves are the continuation of postganglionic fibers of the lumbar ganglia. They travel to the para-aortic nerve plexuses and eventually reach the superior hypogastric plexus (Figure 4). On the right side, the nerve fibers run dorsally to the inferior vena cava at the level of the second to fourth lumbar vertebrae and unite with the left para-aortic fibers caudal to the inferior mesenteric artery. Furthermore, the lower margin of the L3 ganglion was found to be situated approximately 1 cm above the origin of the inferior mesenteric artery (Figure 3).

Boundaries of dissection

For years, bilateral radical retroperitoneal lymph node dissection was the standard therapy for non-seminomatous testicular cancer. This technique was modified to spare the nerves either by preparation of the nerves themselves or by using a template technique. Using these techniques avoids, in the majority of patients, loss of ejaculation without loss of oncological efficiency. Many different techniques are used in different centers such as nerve sparing on both sides, template technique on the side of the tumor and nerve sparing on the contralateral side, or a simple template technique on the side of the tumor. The boundaries of dissection used in our department are described below.

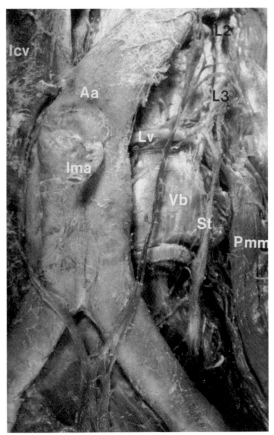

Figure 3 Anatomical dissection and detailed view of L3 ganglion and postganglionic nerve fibers. Icv, inferior caval vein; Aa, abdominal aorta; Ima, inferior mesenteric artery; Lv, lumbar vein; St, sympathetic truncus; Vb, vertebra; L2, L2 ganglion; Pm, psoas muscle

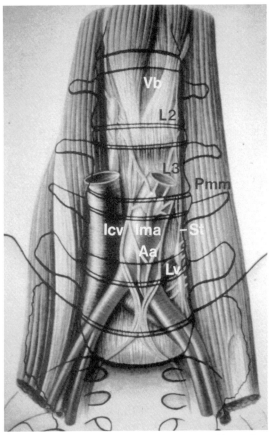

Figure 4 Sympathetic trunk and nerve fibers. Icv, inferior caval vein; Aa, abdominal aorta; Ima, inferior mesenteric artery; Lv, lumbar vein; St, sympathetic truncus; Vb, vertebra; L2, L2 ganglion; Pm, psoas muscle

In cases of clinical stage I non-seminomatous testicular tumor, modified nerve-preserving lymph node dissection using the template technique is performed in order to preserve ejaculatory function. In a prospective multi-center study, Weissbach and Boedefeld[46] assessed the localization of solitary metastases by mapping their primary landing sites. Based on the results of this study, the boundaries of dissection for right and left testicular tumors were defined (Figures 5 and 6).

In stage IIb patients, modified retro-peritoneal lymph node dissection using a template technique is performed within the boundaries proposed by Hobisch and colleagues[12]. The boundaries of dissection were determined on the basis of the volume of retroperitoneal metastases according to the mapping of Donohue and co-workers[47], the neuroanatomy of the sympathetic ganglia and nerve fibers as assessed in the anatomical study described by Colleselli and colleagues[48] and the results of the investigations by Whitelaw and Smithwick[45].

In cases of right testicular tumors, the lymph nodes from the right iliac vessels, in the paracaval and interaortocaval zones, are thoroughly resected as far as the right renal hilus. In addition, the lymph nodes in the pre- and para-aortic zones above the origin of the inferior mesenteric artery up to the left renal hilus are also resected (Figure 7).

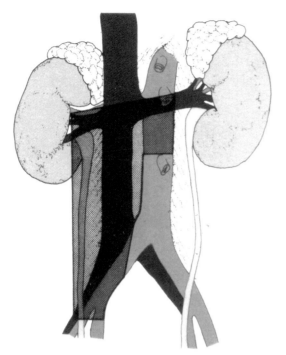

Figure 5 Boundaries of dissection according to Weissbach and Boedefeld[46] for a right-sided stage I tumor

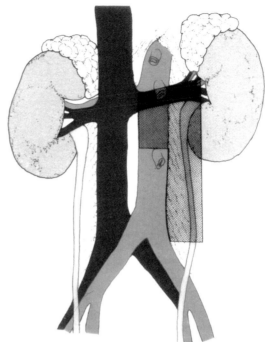

Figure 6 Boundaries of dissection according to Weissbach and Boedefeld[46] for a left-sided stage I tumor

For left testicular tumors, the lymph nodes from the left iliac vessels and the para-aortic zone are resected as far as the left renal hilus. In addition, the lymph nodes in the pre-aortic, interaortocaval and paracaval zones are resected above the origin of the inferior mesenteric artery up to the right renal hilus (Figure 8). By using this operative technique, the corresponding contralateral L3 and/or L2 ganglia as well as their postganglionic fibers can be preserved.

Primary landing site of retroperitoneal metastases

Donohue and colleagues[47] and Weissbach and Boedefeld[46] described boundaries for retroperitoneal lymph node dissection, based on the localization of primary metastases. Since, at that time, radical retroperitoneal lymph node dissection was the standard technique, they did not mention whether the primary metastases are invariably ventral to the lumbar vessels or whether the retrocaval and retroaortal lymphatic tissue may also be the site of primary lymph node metastases. There is controversy as to whether or not transection of the lumbar vessels and removal of the tissue behind is mandatory for retroperitoneal lymph node dissection in clinical stage I disease. Therefore, we analyzed our patients in whom retroperitoneal lymph node dissection was performed for small-volume retroperitoneal metastases. The analysis of our material shows that the site of the primary metastases of a non-seminomatous testicular tumor is always ventral to the lumbar vessels. Thus, we believe that transection of the lumbar vessels and removal of the tissue behind is not mandatory for diagnostic retroperitoneal lymph node dissection in clinical stage I cases[4–9]. In our series of laparoscopic staging lymphadenectomy in patients with clinical stage I disease, none of the first 29 patients had positive nodes dorsal to the lumbar vessels. In the additional series of 49 patients, the lumbar vessels were not transected

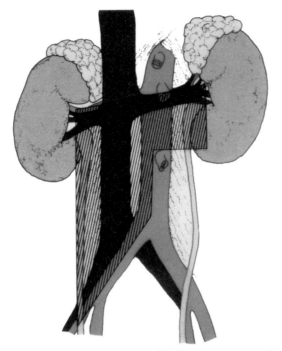

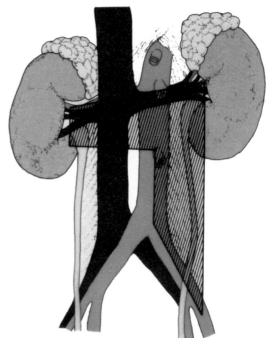

Figure 7 Template of modified retroperitoneal lymph node dissection according to Colleselli and colleagues[48] for a right-sided low-volume testicular tumor

Figure 8 Template of modified retroperitoneal lymph node dissection according to Colleselli and colleagues[48] for a left-sided low-volume testicular tumor

and the tissue behind was not removed. No retroperitoneal relapse has occurred to date (follow-up is 44.7 months).

Technique of retroperitoneal lymph node dissection

Right side The patient is placed supine and extended. Incision of the skin goes from the xiphoid to slightly below the pubis. The falciforme ligament is divided to allow upward displacement of the liver. The peritoneum is incised at the white line of Toldt beginning at the cecum and following on to the foramen of Winslow. Then the Kocher maneuver must be performed. Now the vena cava, which is surrounded by lymphatic tissue can be identified clearly. The incision is next continued around the cecum to the left by sharp and blunt dissection of the root of the mesentery up to the ligament of Treitz. At this point, the inferior mesenteric vein can be

ligated. The undersurface of the bowel, cecum, duodenum and pancreas can be mobilized cephalad. Here, the superior mesenteric artery can be identified.

If nerve-sparing retroperitoneal lymph node dissection is planned, the sympathetic trunk should first be identified and the postganglionic nerves separated. Vessel loops are placed around these nerve fibers. If there is a doubt about the clear identification of the nerves, electrostimulation of these fibers while observing the bladder neck is very helpful[50,51].

Now, dissection of the the lymph node is begun by using the 'split-and-roll' technique described by Donohue[52] in which the nodal package is split on the ventral surfaces of the inferior vena cava, aorta and renal vessels. This maneuver starts on the anterior aspect of the vena cava at the level of the renal hilus. The spermatic vein on the left side is divided. During surgery all the lymphatic vessels should be clipped. Then the split-and-roll technique is used to dissect the aorta downwards ending at the bifurcation of the left external and internal iliac artery. The inferior mesenteric artery should never be dissected or divided. Next, the tissue under the aorta below the renal artery is dissected. If necessary the lumbar arteries should be ligated and divided for better hemostasis. The interaortocaval tissue is dissected and, if necessary, the lumbar veins are ligated and divided. It may be necessary to suture-ligate the lumbar vessels at the posterior body wall foramina, especially in cases of bulky tumors. The surrounding tissue from the right renal vein and the vena cava is dissected. The right spermatic vein is ligated at its origin on the vena cava and dissected down to the internal inguinal ring. The tissue between the ureter and the vena cava is dissected down to the right common iliac artery and the first part of the right external iliac artery. Now the wound should be inspected for bleeding and residual tissue or tumor. The peritoneum should be brought back to the root of the mesentery as the bowel is replaced. Then the wound is closed in layers without bringing in drainage[52].

Left side For retroperitoneal lymph node dissection of a left-sided testicular tumor, the colon descendens is reflected medially and the splenocolic attachments and the mesocolon are divided. This technique allows an exposure as far as the left renal and iliac vessels. In the case of a left-sided tumor, the left spermatic vein is dissected down to the internal inguinal ring[52].

Laparoscopic approach

Because of the high cure rates, reduction of morbidity was the next goal in the treatment of testicular cancer. Therefore, some centers have changed open surgical retroperitoneal lymph node dissection to a laparoscopic approach in clinical stage I disease and in low-volume stage II tumors after chemotherapy[13–15,17,53–56]. The technique for laparoscopic retroperitoneal lymph node dissection, as performed at our department, is described.

Right side The patient is placed with the right side elevated 45°. Four or five 10-mm trocars are required. The camera-bearing laparoscope is introduced via the umbilical port. Two trocars for the surgeon are placed slightly lateral to the rectus muscle, 5 cm above and below the umbilicus. One or two trocars for the assistant are placed more laterally in the anterior axillar line (Figure 9). In rare cases, an additional trocar is useful. The peritoneum is incised along the line of Toldt from the cecum to the right colic flexure. This incision is carried cephalad parallel to the transverse colon and along the vena cava all the way up to the hepatoduodenal ligament. The colon and duodenum are deflected medially, allowing direct access to the retroperitoneal space. The next step is dissection of the spermatic vein from the inner inguinal ring to its opening in the vena cava. Then, the lymphatic tissue surrounding the vena cava is split open and, by rolling the vena cava, the anterior and lateral surfaces can be dissected free. Once the right and the left renal veins have been dissected, the right renal artery is exposed and the right ureter is separated from the nodal package down to its junction with the iliac artery. At this point, the package is clipped and transected. Next, the tissue overlying the right common iliac artery and the aorta is split in a cephalad direction. Care must be taken to preserve the inferior mesenteric artery. Cephalad to the artery, the lymphatic tissue is dissected along the left border of the aorta. The right renal artery can now be identified. The renal

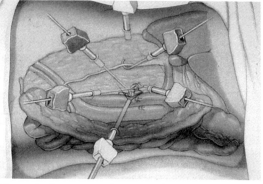

Figure 9 Laparoscopic approach of retroperitoneal lymph node dissection

artery is the cephalad border of dissection. The lymphatic tissue is dissected down to the lumbar vessels. These vessels are not dissected but freed totally from surrounding tissue, so that the interaortocaval lymphatic tissue can be removed totally with an endobag. The next step is dissection of the paracaval lymphatic tissue between the ureter and the vena cava. Finally, the colon and duodenum are brought back to their normal anatomical positions and fixed with an extracorporal knotted suture. Drainage of the retroperitoneum is not required[53].

Left side   On the left side, usually four 10-mm trocars are used, since it is necessary to retract the bowel only in rare cases. The template for left-sided tumors is smaller, and includes all lymphatic tissue cephalad to the inferior mesenteric artery. The interaortocaval nodes are not dissected. The boundaries of dissection are, cephalad, the renal vessels, laterally, the ureter and, caudally, the junction of the ureter with the left iliac artery[53].

Laparoscopic retroperitoneal lymph node dissection in stage IIb disease after chemotherapy   In our clinic, a unilateral laparoscopic retroperitoneal lymph node dissection is performed within the template described for the primary landing site. Bilateral retroperitoneal lymph node dissection is not attempted. The templates for right- and left-sided tumors are the same as for clinical stage I disease. In all of our patients, the residual tumor was located within these templates. The operative technique is essentially the same as for stage I tumors[53].

Results

Between August 1992 and August 2000, 137 patients underwent laparoscopic nerve-preserving retroperitoneal lymph node dissection in our department. A total of 78 out of these 137 patients presented with clinical stage I disease and 59 patients with stage II disease (most of them with stage IIb). Lymph nodes were positive in 24.4% of clinical stage I cases (pathological stage II). Histology of the 59 postchemotherapy laparoscopic retroperitoneal lymph node dissections revealed an active tumor in 1(1.7%) case and mature teratoma in 22 (37.3%) cases. Mean follow-up is 44.7 months. The ejaculation rate of all 137 patients was 100% obtained by performing a modified unilateral template dissection. Recurrences occurred in only two (1.5%) out of the 137 patients (one in the lung and one in the retroperitoneum because of a false negative histology); both are free of disease at present and no patient died. The results of our quality-of-life study showed that open surgery impaired the quality of life much more than laparoscopic retroperitoneal lymph node dissection[57,58]. Laparoscopic retroperitoneal lymph node dissection has proved to have both surgical and oncological efficacy.

References

1. Presti JC. Radical orchiectomy. In Hinman FJ, ed. *Atlas of Urologic Surgery*. Philadelphia: W.B. Saunders Company, 1998:380–4
2. Heidenreich A, Stark L, Derschum W, *et al.* Organ saving therapy of bilateral testicular tumor. *Urologe A* 1993;32:43–8
3. Heidenreich A, Holtl W, Albrecht W, *et al.* Testis-preserving surgery in bilateral testicular germ cell tumours. *Br J Urol* 1997;79:253–7
4. Maneschg C, Rogatsch H, Neururer R, *et al.* Follow-up of organ preserving tumor enucleation in testicular tumors. *J Urol* 2000; 163:144
5. Albers P, Bender H, Yilmaz H, *et al.* Positron emission tomography in the clinical staging of patients with Stage I and II testicular germ cell tumors. *Urology* 1999;53:808–11

6. Corral DA, Varma DG, Jackson EF, *et al.* Magnetic resonance imaging and magnetic resonance angiography before postchemotherapy retroperitoneal lymph node dissection. *Urology* 2000;55:262–6

7. Fernandez EB, Moul JW, Foley JP, *et al.* Retroperitoneal imaging with third and fourth generation computed axial tomography in clinical stage I nonseminomatous germ cell tumors. *Urology* 1994;44:548–52

8. Donohue JP, Foster RS, Rowland RG, *et al.* Nerve-sparing retroperitoneal lymphadenectomy with preservation of ejaculation. *J Urol* 1990;144:287–91, discussion 291–2

9. Donohue JP, Thornhill JA, Foster RS, *et al.* Retroperitoneal lymphadenectomy for clinical stage A testis cancer (1965 to 1989): modifications of technique and impact on ejaculation. *J Urol* 1993;149:237–43

10. Foster RS, Roth BJ. Clinical stage I nonseminoma: surgery versus surveillance. *Semin Oncol* 1998;25:145–53

11. Foster RS, Donohue JP. Retroperitoneal lymph node dissection for the management of clinical stage I nonseminoma. *J Urol* 2000;163:1788–92

12. Hobisch A, Colleselli K, Ennemoser O, *et al.* Modified retroperitoneal lymphadenectomy for testicular tumor: anatomical approach, operative technique and results. *Eur Urol* 1993;23(Suppl 2):39–43

13. Janetschek G, Hobisch A, Holtl L, *et al.* Retroperitoneal lymphadenectomy for clinical stage I nonseminomatous testicular tumor: laparoscopy versus open surgery and impact of learning curve. *J Urol* 1996;156:89–93, discussion 94

14. Janetschek G, Hobisch A, Peschel R, *et al.* Laparoscopic retroperitoneal lymph node dissection for clinical stage I nonseminomatous testicular carcinoma: long-term outcome. *J Urol* 2000;163:1793–6

15. Nelson JB, Chen RN, Bishoff JT, *et al.* Laparoscopic retroperitoneal lymph node dissection for clinical stage I nonseminomatous germ cell testicular tumors. *Urology* 1999; 54:1064–7

16. Richie JP. Clinical stage 1 testicular cancer: the role of modified retroperitoneal lymphadenectomy. *J Urol* 1990;144:1160–3

17. Winfield HN. Laparoscopic retroperitoneal lymphadenectomy for cancer of the testis. *Urol Clin North Am* 1998;25:469–78

18. Hermans BP, Sweeney CJ, Foster RS, *et al.* Risk of systemic metastases in clinical stage I nonseminoma germ cell testis tumor managed by retroperitoneal lymph node dissection. *J Urol* 2000;163:1721–4

19. Dunphy CH, Ayala AG, Swanson DA, *et al.* Clinical stage I nonseminomatous and mixed germ cell tumors of the testis. A clinicopathologic study of 93 patients on a surveillance protocol after orchiectomy alone. *Cancer* 1988;62:1202–6

20. Freedman LS, Parkinson MC, Jones WG, *et al.* Histopathology in the prediction of relapse of patients with stage I testicular teratoma treated by orchidectomy alone. *Lancet* 1987;2:294–8

21. Peckham MJ, Barrett A, Husband JE, *et al.* Orchidectomy alone in testicular stage I non-seminomatous germ-cell tumours. *Lancet* 1982;2:678–80

22. Raghavan D, Colls B, Levi J, *et al.* Surveillance for stage I non-seminomatous germ cell tumours of the testis: the optimal protocol has not yet been defined. *Br J Urol* 1988;61:522–6

23. Sturgeon JF, Jewett MA, Alison RE, *et al.* Surveillance after orchidectomy for patients with clinical stage I nonseminomatous testis tumors. *J Clin Oncol* 1992;10:564–8

24. Thompson PI, Nixon J, Harvey VJ. Disease relapse in patients with stage I nonseminomatous germ cell tumor of the testis on active surveillance. *J Clin Oncol* 1988;6:1597–603

25. Cullen MH, Stenning SP, Parkinson MC, *et al.* Short-course adjuvant chemotherapy in high-risk stage I nonseminomatous germ cell tumors of the testis: a Medical Research Council report. *J Clin Oncol* 1996;14:1106–13

26. Horwich A. Primary chemotherapy: how does it compare with surgery? *Semin Urol Oncol* 1996; 14:34–5

27. Pont J, Albrecht W, Postner G, *et al.* Adjuvant chemotherapy for high-risk clinical stage I nonseminomatous testicular germ cell cancer: long-term results of a prospective trial. *J Clin Oncol* 1996;14:441–8

28. Studer UE, Fey MF, Calderoni A, *et al.* Adjuvant chemotherapy after orchiectomy in high-risk patients with clinical stage I non-seminomatous testicular cancer. *Eur Urol* 1993;23:444–9

29. Moul JW, McCarthy WF, Fernandez EB, *et al.* Percentage of embryonal carcinoma and of vascular invasion predicts pathological stage in clinical stage I nonseminomatous testicular cancer. *Cancer Res* 1994;54:362–4

30. Heidenreich A, Sesterhenn IA, Moul JW. Prognostic risk factors in low stage testicular germ cell tumors: unanswered questions regarding clinically useful prognosticators for extra-testicular disease [editorial; comment]. *Cancer* 1997;79:1641–5, discussion 1646

31. Albers P, DeRiese WT, Ulbright TM, *et al.* Prognostic factors in patients with pathological stage I non-seminomatous testicular germ cell tumors and tumor recurrence during follow-up. *Urol Res* 1995;23:211–13

32. Albers P, Bierhoff E, Neu D, *et al.* MIB-1 immunohistochemistry in clinical stage I nonseminomatous testicular germ cell tumors predicts patients at low risk for metastasis. *Cancer* 1997;79:1710–16

33. de Riese WT, Albers P, Walker EB, *et al.* Predictive parameters of biologic behavior of early stage nonseminomatous testicular germ cell tumors. *Cancer* 1994;74:1335–41

34. Ondrus D, Matoska J, Belan V, *et al.* Prognostic factors in clinical stage I nonseminomatous germ cell testicular tumors: rationale for different risk-adapted treatment. *Eur Urol* 1998;33:562–6

35. Behnia M, Foster R, Einhorn LH, *et al.* Adjuvant bleomycin, etoposide and cisplatin in pathological stage II non-seminomatous testicular cancer. The Indiana University experience. *Eur J Cancer* 2000;36:472–5

36. Coogan CL, Foster RS, Rowland RG, *et al.* Postchemotherapy retroperitoneal lymph node dissection is effective therapy in selected patients with elevated tumor markers after primary chemotherapy alone. *Urology* 1997;50:957–62

37. Donohue JP, Thornhill JA, Foster RS, *et al.* The role of retroperitoneal lymphadenectomy in clinical stage B testis cancer: the Indiana University experience (1965 to 1989). *J Urol* 1995;153:85–9

38. Foster RS, Donohue JP. Can retroperitoneal lymphadenectomy be omitted in some patients after chemotherapy? *Urol Clin North Am* 1998; 25:479–84

39. Herr HW. Does necrosis on frozen-section analysis of a mass after chemotherapy justify a limited retroperitoneal resection in patients with advanced testis cancer? *Br J Urol* 1997;80: 653–7

40. Motzer RJ, Bosl GJ. Role of adjuvant chemotherapy in patients with stage II nonseminomatous germ-cell tumors. *Urol Clin North Am* 1993;20:111–16

41. Motzer RJ. Adjuvant chemotherapy for stage II nonseminomatous testicular cancer: what is its role? *Semin Urol Oncol* 1996;14:30–3

42. Richie JP, Kantoff PW. Is adjuvant chemotherapy necessary for patients with stage B1 testicular cancer? *J Clin Oncol* 1991;9:1393–6

43. Steyerberg EW, Donohue JP, Gerl A, *et al.* Residual masses after chemotherapy for metastatic testicular cancer: the clinical implications of the association between retroperitoneal and pulmonary histology. Re-analysis of Histology in Testicular Cancer (ReHiT) Study Group. *J Urol* 1997;158:474–8

44. Weissbach L, Bussar-Maatz R, Flechtner H, *et al.* RPLND or primary chemotherapy in clinical stage IIA/B nonseminomatous germ cell tumors? Results of a prospective multicenter trial including quality of life assessment. *Eur Urol* 2000;37:582–94

45. Whitelaw GP, Smithwick RH. Some secondary effects of sympathectomy – with particular reference to distribution of sexual function. *N Engl J Med* 1951;245:121–30

46. Weissbach L, Boedefeld EA. Localization of solitary and multiple metastases in stage II nonseminomatous testis tumor as basis for a modified staging lymph node dissection in stage 1. *J Urol* 1987;138:77–82

47. Donohue JP, Zachary JM, Maynard BR. Distribution of nodal metastases in nonseminomatous testis cancer. *J Urol* 1982;128:315–20

48. Colleselli K, Poisel S, Schachtner W, *et al.* Nerve-preserving bilateral retroperitoneal lymphadenectomy: anatomical study and operative approach. *J Urol* 1990;144:293–7; discussion 297–8

49. Höltl L, Hobisch A, Knapp R, *et al.* Where are the primary landing sites for retroperitoneal metastases from testicular tumor? *J Urol* 1997;157:303

50. Huland H, Dieckmann KP, Sauerwein D. Nerve sparing retroperitoneal lymphadenectomy with intraoperative electrostimulation in patients with nonseminomatous testicular tumors. *Urologe A* 1992;31:1–7

51. Recker F, Goepel M, Otto T, *et al.* An intraoperative seminal and prostate emission test as a control for nerve-sparing procedures in primary and secondary retroperitoneal lymphadenectomy. *Br J Urol* 1996;77:133–7

52. Donohue JP. Retroperitoneal lymph node dissection. In Hinman FJ, ed. *Atlas of Urologic Surgery*. Philadelphia: W.B. Saunders Company, 1998:385–403

53. Janetschek G, Hobisch A, Peschel R, *et al.* Laparoscopic retroperitoneal lymph node dissection. *Urology* 2000;55:136–40

54. Rassweiler JJ, Seemann O, Henkel TO, *et al.* Laparoscopic retroperitoneal lymph node dissection for nonseminomatous germ cell tumors: indications and limitations. *J Urol* 1996; 156:1108–13

55. Rassweiler JJ, Frede T, Lenz E, *et al.* Long-term experience with laparoscopic retroperitoneal lymph node dissection in the management of low-stage testis cancer. *Eur Urol* 2000;37:251–60

56. Rukstalis DB, Chodak GW. Laparoscopic retroperitoneal lymph node dissection in a patient with stage 1 testicular carcinoma. *J Urol* 1992;148:1907–9, discussion 1909–10

57. Biebl W, Tönnemann J, Janetschek G, *et al.* Quality of life after laparoscopic versus open retroperitoneal lymphadenectomy for testicular tumor – the patients' view. *J Urol* 1999;161:181

58. Hobisch A, Tönnemann J, Janetschek G, *et al.* Morbidity and quality of life after open versus laparoscopic retroperitoneal lymphadenectomy for testicular tumour – the patient's view. In Jones WG. Appleyard I, Harnden P, *et al.*, eds. *Germ Cell Tumours. IV.* London: John Libbey & Co. Ltd., 1998:277–9

Chemotherapy for testicular cancer: present standards and future advances

3

S. B. Kaye

Introduction

In 1981, Einhorn described testicular cancer as the 'model for a curable neoplasm'[1]. In 2000 this continues to be true. What has changed over the past 20 years? The answer is that, thanks to a series of clinical trials (mostly randomized), a number of clear statements can be made about the management of the disease which now form the basis of recommended treatment throughout the world. Areas of controversy do, however, still exist, but the major effort now should be to ensure that all patients with testicular cancer are managed in specialist units, where the results of therapy have been shown to be optimal[2].

Present standards

Following inguinal orchidectomy, expert pathology review and disease staging with computerized tomography (CT) scanning, and serial tumor marker (including lactate dehydrogenase) estimation, management recommendations are based on disease stage and primary tumor pathology (seminoma or teratoma). The 1997 International Germ Cell Cancer Collaborative Group (IGCCCG) classification provides an agreed framework for selecting the treatment approach for patients with metastatic disease (good, intermediate, poor prognosis – with over 90%, 70–80% and 40–50% prospect of cure, respectively; see Table 1)[3].

For stage I seminoma patients, standard therapy comprises prophylactic irradiation of the para-aortic lymph nodes (total dose of 30 Gy in 3 weeks)[4]. Ongoing trials are examining lower doses of radiotherapy and the alternative of adjuvant chemotherapy with the single agent carboplatin. Preliminary data have suggested that either one or two doses of carboplatin are likely to be effective in preventing disease relapse[5], and the result of a recently completed randomized trial including over 1200 patients (Medical Research Council (MRC)/European Organization for Research and Treatment of Cancer (EORTC)) is awaited eagerly.

For clinical stage I teratoma patients, disparity exists between those countries in which retroperitoneal lymph node dissection is routinely practised (mainly the USA) and those where it is not (much of Europe). Two courses of adjuvant chemotherapy (with bleomycin, etoposide and cisplatin (BEP)) are given to patients at high risk of relapse, either lymph node positive patients at retroperitoneal lymph node dissection (pathological stage II)[6], or, in the absence of retroperitoneal lymph node dissection, those with vascular invasion in the primary tumor[7]. Either policy results in a cure rate approaching 100%. Patients with a lesser risk of relapse (no vascular invasion) are generally followed by a policy of surveillance in European centers, but the relapse rate is still of the order of 10–15%, and monthly review, with tumor marker estimation, is mandatory for the first year post-orchidectomy.

For metastatic testicular teratoma and a good prognosis (based on IGCCCG criteria which involve tumor marker levels and presence/absence of visceral metastases), three courses of BEP rather than four are now standard treatment[8]. This recommendation is based on the results of a large randomized MRC/EORTC trial, completed in April 1998, which included

Table 1 Classification of the prognostic variables for metastatic disease by the International Germ Cell Cancer Collaborative Group (IGCCCG)

Prognosis	Markers
Good	
Non-seminoma	
testis/retroperitoneal primary	AFP < 1000 ng/ml
and good markers	*and* hCG < 1000 ng/ml (5000 IU/l)
and no non-pulmonary visceral metastases*	*and* LDH < 1.5 × N
Seminoma	
any primary site	
and any markers	
and no non-pulmonary visceral metastases*	
Intermediate	
Non-seminoma	
testis/retroperitoneal primary	AFP = 1000–10 000 ng/ml
and intermediate markers	*or* hCG = 1000–10 000 ng/ml (5000–50 000 IU/l)
and no non-pulmonary visceral metastases*	*or* LDH = 1.5–10 × N
Seminoma	
any primary site	
and any markers	
and no non-pulmonary visceral metastases*	
Poor	
Non-seminoma	
mediastinal primary site or	AFP > 10 000 ng/ml
testis/retroperitoneal with	*or* hCG > 10 000 ng/ml (50 000 IU/l)
either non-pulmonary visceral metastases*	*or* LDH > 10 × N
or poor markers	

* Non-pulmonary visceral metastases refers to liver, bone, brain and skin.
AFP, α-fetoprotein; hCG, human chorionic gonadotropin; LDH, lactate dehydrogenase; N, upper limit of normal

812 patients, randomized to either three or four courses of BEP. With a median follow-up of 25 months, the 2-year progression-free survival was 90.4% and 89.4%, respectively. A second randomization, to either a 2- or 5-day cisplatin regimen (100 mg/m^2 in both cases) showed no difference (2-year progression-free survival of 89.4% and 88.9%, respectively). The 2-day cisplatin regimen led to a slightly higher rate of ototoxicity, but is often preferred on grounds of convenience.

In that trial, there was no evidence of major bleomycin pulmonary toxicity. However, this can be a problem. Our own studies in Glasgow have indicated that lethal pulmonary toxicity occurs at a rate of 2.7%. Interestingly, in our review of 180 patients receiving bleomycin as part of BEP chemotherapy in a 5-year period in our unit, the only deaths due to pulmonary toxicity (five in all) occurred in patients aged over 40 years, in whom the mortality rate (five out of 47) was an alarming 10.6%[9]. Accordingly, we would recommend withholding bleomycin in this age group unless there were good grounds to use it, e.g. poor prognosis disease. If bleomycin is contraindicated, because of age or poor renal function, four courses of etoposide and cisplatin (EP) are an alternative.

For metastatic testicular teratoma with intermediate and poor prognosis, four courses of BEP are recommended. Our previous studies in this group of patients have so far failed to show a benefit from more intensive schedules. A large randomized trial compared BEP with a novel schedule (bleomycin, vincristine, cisplatin (BOP)/etoposide, ifosfamide, cisplatin (VIP)) in over 400 cases, and no difference was observed[10]. Importantly, however, clear differences did emerge when an analysis was performed according to where patients were treated[11]. More than half of the patients in the trial were actually treated in institutes which entered a total of less than five patients. Their survival, corrected for IGCCCG risk factors, was significantly worse than the others ($p = 0.009$), raising questions of the appropriateness of current referral patterns (Figure 1).

For metastatic testicular seminoma, radiotherapy to abdominal lymph nodes is acceptable for patients with stage IIA and some stage IIB patients; otherwise chemotherapy with EP or BEP is recommended, along the lines of treatment for teratoma.

Future issues

More accurate testicular cancer staging, with positron emission tomography (PET) scans to avoid unnecessary adjuvant chemotherapy will become an important issue. Preliminary data from Denmark have indicated a high level of sensitivity for 2[18F]fluoro-2-deoxy-D-glucose

(FDG)-PET scans in detecting metastatic testicular tumor in patients with normal CT scans[12]. If this is confirmed in larger studies, the technique holds considerable promise in more accurate disease staging and appropriate treatment selection.

A second application of PET scanning under current evaluation is the investigation of patients with disease relapse based on marker elevation with normal CT scans. These patients pose difficult management problems, and surgery can play a major role. Localization of tumor recurrence through PET scanning may, therefore, be especially valuable.

The potential for surveillance for patients with stage I seminoma deemed to be of low risk of recurrence will be carefully explored. The risk of recurrence in stage I seminoma, based on histological grounds, is not so firmly established as for stage I non-seminoma. However, careful analyses, performed by Canadian investigators, have indicated that tumor size and involvement of the rete testis are the major prognostic

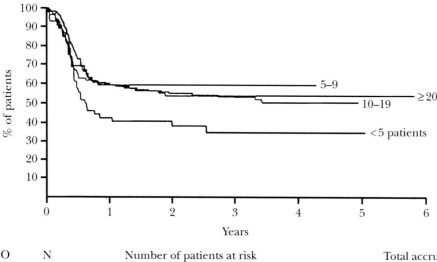

O	N	Number of patients at risk					Total accrual
34	55	22	16	7	5	1	<5
21	52	30	23	15	3	0	5–9
81	174	100	83	59	19	0	10–19
44	99	56	43	37	27	7	≥20

Figure 1 Kaplan–Meier estimate of failure-free survival according to total accrual of patients by the treating institution, in a trial by the Medical Research Council/European Organization for Research and Treatment of Cancer comparing bleomycin, etoposide and cisplatin (BEP) with bleomycin, vincristine and cisplatin (BOP)/etoposide, ifosfamide and cisplatin (VIP). O, observed events; N, number of patients at risk

factors[13], and prospective trials of surveillance and adjuvant therapy for 'high-risk' patients, are being planned.

Further reduction in the toxicity of chemotherapy with BEP, e.g. routine prophylactic antibiotics to prevent neutropenic sepsis is being explored in ongoing randomized trials, and changes in bleomycin schedules to reduce pulmonary toxicity are also being considered. Interestingly, bleomycin was first given by prolonged infusion schedules in the initial testicular cancer regimens[14]. Although no randomized trials have ever been done, the impression is that this may be a more effective way of delivering the drug than by bolus/intermittent schedules. Moreover, there is some evidence to suggest that pulmonary toxicity may be reduced with infusional schedules[15], and a randomized trial is currently under discussion.

Further improvements in the cure rate of patients with intermediate and poor prognosis are being sought, through randomized trials examining the addition of other drugs, e.g. taxol[16], and the use of high-dose chemotherapy. As regards taxol, a feasibility study confirmed that its addition to BEP is safe and acceptable to most patients[17]. An EORTC/MRC trial in intermediate-prognosis patients is currently comparing treatment using four courses of 'taxol-BEP' with four courses of BEP. As regards high-dose chemotherapy, numerous feasibility studies have been carried out, using single or multiple treatments in relapsed or refractory patients. Many investigators do feel that, for selected patients with relapsed disease, this intensive approach may have a role. However, its true utility can only be assessed properly in randomized trials; these are now ongoing both in the USA and Europe in first-line treatment for poor-risk patients, and in patients with disease relapse.

Further improvements are also anticipated in the 'salvage' therapy of those 10–20% of patients who require repeat treatment for recurrent tumor. Data from our own unit in Glasgow confirm that the treatment of relapse is continuing to improve (currently about 50% of relapsed patients may still receive curative treatment[18]), but they also point to the importance of surgery. Those patients with late relapse are particularly problematic, because the disease then is rarely chemocurable, and surgery does play a key role.

Recently, considerable progress has been made in identifying the gene(s) responsible for testicular cancer, by careful study of families with a strong family history of the disease. This may eventually lead to alternative and less toxic forms of treatment. In addition, a better understanding of the mechanisms underlying testicular cancer's exquisite chemosensitivity would be an important step in moving other more common cancers into this curable category, and such work is making good progress[19].

References

1. Einhorn LH. Testicular cancer as a model for a curable neoplasm. *Cancer Res* 1981;41:3275–8
2. Harding MJ, Paul J, Gillis C, *et al.* Management of malignant teratoma; does referral to a specialist unit matter. *Lancet* 1993;341:999–1022
3. IGCCCG International Germ Cell Consensus Classification. *J Clin Oncol* 1997;15:594–603
4. Fossa SD, Horwich A, Russell JM, *et al.* Optimal planning target volume for Stage I testicular seminoma. A MRC randomized trial. *J Clin Oncol* 1999;17:146–54
5. Oliver R, Edmonds P, Ong J. Pilot studies of 2 and 1 course carboplatins as adjuvant for Stage I seminoma. *Int J Radiat Oncol Biol Phys* 1994; 29:3–8
6. Williams SD, Stablein DM, Einhorn LH, *et al.* Immediate adjuvant chemotherapy vs observation with treatment at relapse in pathological

stage II testicular cancer. *N Engl J Med* 1987; 317:1433–8

7. Cullen MH, Stenning SC, Parkinson MC, *et al.* Short course adjuvant chemotherapy in high risk stage I NSGCTT. *J Clin Oncol* 1996;14:1106–13

8. de Wit R, Roberts JT, Wilkinson P, *et al.* Is 3 BEP equivalent to 3 BEP-1 EP in good prognosis germ cell cancer? An EORTC/MRC Phase III study. *Proc Am Soc Clin Oncol* 1999;18:309a

9. Simpson AB, Paul J, Graham J, *et al.* Fatal bleomycin toxicity in West of Scotland 1991–95. A review of patients with germ cell tumours. *Br J Cancer* 1998;78:1061–6

10. Kaye SB, Mead GM, Fossa S, *et al.* BEP vs. BOP/VIP for poor prognosis NSGCT: result of an MRC/EORTC randomized trial. *J Clin Oncol* 1998;16:692–701

11. Collette L, Sylvester R, Stennings SP, *et al.* Impact of the treating institution on survival of patients with 'poor-prognosis' metastatic nonseminoma. European Organization for Research and Treatment of Cancer Genito-Urinary Tract Cancer Collaborative Group and the Medical Research Council Testicular Cancer Working Party. *J Natl Cancer Inst* 1999;91:839–46

12. Cremerius U, Effert P, Adam G, *et al.* FDG-PET for detection and therapy control of metastatic germ cell tumour. *J Nucl Med* 1998;39:815–22

13. Warde P, von der Masse H, Horwich A, *et al.* Prognostic factors for relapse in Stage I seminoma managed by surveillance. *Proc Am Soc Clin Oncol* 1998;17:309a

14. Samuels M, Johnston DE, Holoye P. Continuous intravenous bleomycin therapy with vinblastine in Stage III testicular neoplasia. *Cancer Chem Rep* 1975;59:563–70

15. Sammash J, Oliver R, Rezaaek R, *et al.* Bolus v. infusional bleomycin for germ cell cancer. *Proc Am Soc Clin Oncol* 1999;18:327a

16. Motzer R. Paclitaxel in salvage therapy for germ cell tumours. *Semin Oncol* 1997;24(Suppl 15): 83–5

17. de Wit R, Louwerens M, de Mulder P, *et al.* A dose finding study of paclitaxel added to fixed doses of BEP in patients with adverse prognosis germ cell cancer. *Proc Am Soc Clin Oncol* 1998; 17:322a

18. de Bono JS, Paul J, Simpson A, *et al.* Improving the outcome of salvage treatment for non-seminomatous germ cell tumours (NSGCT). *Br J Cancer* 2000;73:425–30

19. Koberle B, Masters JR, Hartley JA, *et al.* Defective repair of cisplatin-induced DNA damage caused by reduced XPA protein in testicular germ cell tumours. *Curr Biol* 1999;9:273–6

Section II

Renal carcinoma

Prognostic factors and treatment decisions in renal cell carcinoma

B. Ljungberg

4

Introduction

Renal cell carcinoma is the most common renal tumor accounting for approximately 85% of all renal malignancies. Metastatic renal cell carcinoma is one of the more therapy-resistant malignancies. Around 60% of the patients who are clinically diagnosed will die due to the disease because of progressive disease and metastatic spread[1]. Factors that predict the course of the disease are needed in order to better characterize the malignancy. Intensive pathological and genetic studies have resulted in the recognition of distinctive types of tumor with presumed different cellular origin, different phenotypes and different clinical characteristics[2]. Over the past decades, alternative therapes with promising response rates such as immune-based therapies have been evaluated[3]. Other promising therapies that use gene and vaccine treatment strategies are in development[4]. One important tool for improving the treatment of renal cell carcinoma is to use such prognostic tumor factors for the identification of patients eligible to enter into the studies, for identifying treatment options and for assessing patients' response to therapy.

Genetics

Renal cell carcinoma is characterized by heterogeneous morphology and heterogeneous biological behavior. Tumors with similar morphology and spread often have a different clinical course. Conventional histopathological grading gives little insight into tumorogenesis and little assistance in predicting the clinical behavior of the disease[5]. During the past decades, the recognition of collecting duct carcinoma and chromophobe renal cell carcinoma as specific entities was the first step in defining renal cell carcinoma subtypes[6]. Recent advances in the understanding of the genetics underlying the pathogenesis have resulted in the recognition of distinct types of tumor. The identification of specific genetic alterations has led to the classification of subtypes such as the papillary and conventional renal cell carcinomas. Such a classification, based on genetic features, was first suggested by Kovacs and colleagues[7]. The knowledge of specific genetic alterations underlying different renal cell carcinoma types resulted in the first consensus for a new classification system, reached in 1996 at the Heidelberg conference[2]. Four different tumor types were defined: conventional (non-papillary), papillary, chromophobe and collecting duct carcinoma. There is also a group of tumors that will remain unclassified. Based on these data, it can be hypothesized that a difference exists between the subtypes regarding clinical behavior and response to therapy. Conventional (non-papillary) renal cell carcinoma is characterized by the occurrence of a deletion of chromosome 3p[8]. The mutation of the *VHL* gene occurs exclusively in this type[9]. Duplication of chromosome band 5q22 and deletion of chromosome arms 6q, 8p, 9p and 14q are other characteristic alterations[10]. Papillary renal cell carcinoma generally has trisomies in different combinations including trisomy of chromosome 7 and 17[7,11]. Trisomy of chromosomes 3q, 8, 12, 16 and 20 and the loss of the Y chromosome are other common alterations in this tumor type[8,11]. The papillary (chromophil) renal cell carcinoma are often bilateral and/or multifocal. Chromophobe renal cell carcinoma is characterized by having a low chromosome number with a combination of loss of heterozygosity at chromosomes 1, 2, 6, 10, 13, 17, 21 and X[12,13], and a hypodiploid DNA content is frequently found[14]. Collecting duct carcinoma is a rare, highly malignant renal neoplasm comprising 1–2% of the cases of renal cell carcinoma. No specific genetic alterations have been established for this tumor type. Verdofer and co-workers[15] found a loss of DNA sequences involving chromosomes 1, 2, 9, 11 and 18 detected by comparative genomic hybridization and a gain of DNA sequences affecting chromosomes 16 and 20. In another study, a frequent deletion on chromosome 1q was demonstrated[16].

Renal cell carcinoma types

Our group has demonstrated a significant difference in clinical behavior between the different renal cell carcinoma types, results that have also recently been confirmed by Moch and co-workers[17,18]. Conventional renal cell carcinomas, about 75% of the kidney tumors, have, as a group, a poorer prognosis than papillary renal cell carcinomas, results that confirm previous studies indicating that papillary renal cell carcinomas have a better prognosis than solid renal cell carcinomas[19,20]. Patients with chromophobe renal cell carcinoma survive longer and have less advanced disease than patients with conventional or papillary renal cell carcinoma[17,21]. In conventional renal cell carcinomas, tumor progression has been associated with additional genetic alterations such as duplication of chromosome 5q22 and deletions at chromosomes 6q23, 8p, 9p and 14q regions[10,22]. In papillary renal cell carcinoma, trisomy of chromosome 3/3q and loss of chromosome Xp have been found to be associated with more malignant behavior of the tumors[11,23,24]. Thus, specific genetic alterations underlie the pathogenesis and aggressiveness of specific tumor phenotypes. At present technical developments allow a genetic approach, using molecular tools such as microsatellite primers, to diagnose the tumor-specific regions. The use of the different renal cell carcinoma types can be one important step for the understanding of the variability of renal cell carcinoma. Furthermore, the different tumor types might respond unequally to immunotherapy and other treatment modalities and renal cell carcinoma types could be used for stratification in randomized studies.

Other genetic alterations

Other molecular genetic alterations that may provide prognostic information have rarely been reported in renal cell carcinoma. In contrast to alterations of the *VHL* gene that appear to occur early in the tumor development, alterations in the *p53* suppressor gene appear to be late events associated with malignancy and/or metastasis[25,26]. In renal cell carcinoma, the role of *p53* remains undetermined and diverging results have been presented concerning the prognostic significance of mutated *p53*[27,28]. In a recent study, we found a correlation between *p53* overexpression and advanced and poorly differentiated tumors, supporting previous results[29]. Papillary renal cell carcinoma had 44% *p53* overexpression compared to around 15% for conventional and chromophobe renal cell carcinomas. A correlation between *p53* overexpression and an adverse prognosis was found only in papillary and chromophobe renal cell carcinoma but not in conventional renal cell carcinoma. These results are contrary to the findings of Moch and colleagues[28], who showed that *p53* overexpression in conventional renal cell carcinoma was associated with a poor prognosis.

Similarly, alterations in *p15/16* tumor suppressor genes, which inhibit cell cycle progression, are found in renal cell carcinoma-derived cell lines but not in primary tumors, suggesting that these alterations occur in cells as a function of adaptation to autonomous growth *in vitro*[30].

Pathological factors

Tumor stage

Clinical stage, which demonstrates the anatomical extent of the malignancy, is still the most important and powerful prognostic factor[31,33]. The International Union against Cancer (UICC) tumor, node, metastasis (TNM) classification system is the most frequently used staging system today. This staging system takes into account tumor size, growth beyond the renal capsule, local spread into veins, lymph node and adrenal metastases and distant metastatic spread. These factors all indicate an unfavorable clinical course for the patients. Patients with tumors confined to the kidney have 85–95% 5-year survival rates whereas those with distant metastases have an extremely poor prognosis with 5-year survival rates of < 5%[33–36]. The prognostic impact of tumor vein invasion has been unclear and contradictory reports have appeared[31,33,37,38]. In a prospective study from our department, the frequency of tumor thrombus invasion was 36%, significantly higher than the 15–20% previously reported[39]. The survival rate for patients with vena caval thrombus formation was the same as that for patients with renal vein invasion only. Thus, an aggressive surgical approach to completely resect a tumor thrombus that is invading the atrium appears to be as justified as performing a nephrectomy in cases of invasion of the renal vein only. For patients with metastatic spread, vein invasion also showed significant prognostic information indicating that vein invasion itself is an adverse factor in progression. Our study also showed, in contrast to previous studies, that the survival time for patients with vein invasion was almost identical to the survival time for patients with adrenal gland and lymph node metastasis[31,33,38]. Montie and co-workers[40] studied 68 patients with a tumor thrombus extending into the inferior vena cava and concluded that survival was not dependent on lymph node status. The finding that the level of tumor thrombus formation was not associated with any survival difference confirms previous results found when the thrombus was resected completely[33,37]. In contrast, other authors have found that the level confers further prognostic significance[40,41]. Microscopic infiltration into adjacent venules and microvessel invasion was also shown to be an important predictor

of progression, confirming our results[42,43]. Thus, vein invasion itself, irrespective of level of invasion and thrombus formation, seems to be one factor of importance for the biological property of a tumor.

Perinephric fat and lymph node metastases Patients with perinephric fat invasion when compared to those with organ-confined disease have a significantly worse prognosis with about a 50% 5-year survival rate[31,44]. Lymph node involvement indicates an even worse survival impact. The survival rate for patients with lymph node metastases ranges from 5–30% at 5 years[45,46]. In an autopsy study, Johnsen and Hellsten[47] found that almost all cases with lymphatic spread had additional distant metastases. Therefore, the value of systemic lymphadenectomy has been discussed. Schafhauser and colleagues[48] concluded that 4% of patients benefit from extensive lymphadenectomy with prolonged survival. In a randomized phase III study by the European Organization for Research and Treatment of Cancer (EORTC), it was found that complete lymph node dissection did not add morbidity when performed during a radical nephrectomy. In that study, the incidence of unsuspected lymph node metastases was low (3.3%) following a proper preoperative staging[49].

Patients with adrenal gland metastases in most cases also have distant or lymph node metastases[50]. Sandock and co-workers[51] have concluded that ipsilateral adrenalectomy should be performed only if a lesion is seen preoperatively on a radiological work-up or if gross disease is seen at the time of nephrectomy. However, its removal may not benefit the patient.

Distant metastases Patients with metastatic disease have a dismal prognosis with 5-year survival rates between 2 and 10%[31,32,52]. Patients with synchronous presentation of the metastatic disease have a longer survival time compared to those with asynchronous diagnosis of the metastatic disease. Survival is generally better in patients with solitary metastases than in those with multiple metastatic sites[53]. A 5-year survival rate of 23% has been reported for patients with solitary metastases at diagnosis after surgical extirpation of both the primary tumor and the metastasis[54]. Selected patients with solitary, especially lung and bone metastases, may have longer survival times with up to 45–50% 5-year survival rates[55]. Prolonged survival has also been reported for selected cases with solitary brain and skeletal metastases[54,56]. Repeated extirpations of recurrent metastases in selected cases can also imply long survival times[57].

Histopathology

A number of grading systems have been defined using cell type, necrosis pattern, growth pattern and nuclear shape. Most of the currently used grading systems are based on nuclear morphology and have also been shown to give independent prognostic information mostly secondary to stage in significance[31,44,58–60]. Although nuclear grade has been shown to be an independent prognostic factor there is a lack of uniformity and objectivity due to inter-observer variation, which has reduced its application. In addition, cell type and histopathological pattern have been shown to give reliable prognostic information[45,61,62]. Nuclear morphometry might be more objective and reproducible than conventional grading systems. However, few results have been published regarding the prognostic significance of morphometry in renal cell carcinoma. Carducci and co-workers[63] found that the range of ellipticity was a significant predictor of tumor recurrence, while Gutierrez and colleagues found that nuclear area and size were factors correlated to survival[64].

Tumor size

The role of tumor size in the clinical outcome seems to be stage-dependent. Also, small tumors < 3 cm have local tumor invasion and are diagnosed with metastatic disease[65,66]. Thus, preoperative and pathological staging are important in order to use the significant prognostic information provided by the tumor size[67,68]. Tumor size is especially important in patients with organ-confined tumors who are possible candidates for nephron-sparing surgery.

DNA ploidy and S phase

DNA ploidy is another variable with prognostic significance. Due to the frequent heterogeneity in renal cell carcinoma, ploidy determination based on a single sample might give inaccurate information of the DNA content[32,69]. Using multiple sample analysis, a significant difference in survival time was demonstrated between patients with diploid and those with aneuploid TNM-stage I and II tumors[34]. A similar result was obtained by del Vecchio and associates[70] in contrast to the negative results obtained in other studies that only analyzed one tumor sample[71,72]. In TNM-stage III tumors, DNA ploidy has not shown any prognostic information. In the group of patients with metastatic disease, homogeneously diploid tumors were associated with a significantly better prognosis than aneuploid tumors[34]. There is a positive association between DNA ploidy and tumor cell kinetics with lower S-phase fractions and longer potential tumor doubling times in diploid compared with aneuploid clones[73–75]. In a study of *in vivo* labelling with iododeoxyuridine, the shortest potential tumor doubling time detected within a tumor was of high prognostic significance[75]. Different proliferation methods such as S-phase analysis, Ki-67 and proliferating cell nuclear antigen expression give similar information although they monitor different compartments on the cell cycle[76,77]. Also cyclin A, which indicates a relative S-phase activity, is associated with the clinical outcome in patients with renal cell carcinoma[76,78].

Cell cycle regulation

Deregulation of the cell cycle is one key aberration that has been observed linked to growth control resulting in increased proliferation and an inability to arrest cells with DNA damage[79,80]. The cell cycle machinery consists of proteins including cyclins, cyclin-dependent kinases (CDKs), CDK-inhibitors and specific substrates that can be phosphorylated. The most important checkpoint in the cell cycle is the G_1/S transition where the decision is taken to proceed into the S phase. Cyclins D and E are involved in the G_1/S transition. Hedberg and colleagues have observed that a large proportion of renal cell carcinomas had a high cyclin D1 protein content potentially indicating an overexpression and activation of this proto-oncogene[81]. Surprisingly, a high cyclin D1 protein content was related to a favorable prognosis in conventional renal cell carcinoma, whereas tumors with low or downregulated cyclin D1 seemed to be more aggressive. Further studies on cyclin D3 and E might give new insights into the regulation of cell proliferation in renal cell carcinoma.

Angiogenesis

Tumor angiogenesis is one important factor for tumor development and progression. Tumors that grow more than 1 mm need new vessels for progressive growth. Stimulators of angiogenesis such as vascular endothelial growth factor (VEGF) have been suggested to play an important role in tumorigenesis. In a recent study, Jacobsen and co-workers[82] found a correlation between serum VEGF levels and tumor progression, especially for patients with vein invasion. Baccala and colleagues have suggested that serum $VEGF_{165}$ could be used as a biomarker for the follow-up of patients with renal cell carcinoma[83]. A number of studies have supported the importance of vein invasion as a prognostic factor. The importance of angiogenesis is further supported by the prognostic importance of tumor thrombus formation in a number of studies[39,84]. Increased numbers of platelets are also associated with a poor prognosis[85]. Microvessel density as a quantification of the status of angiogenesis is also shown to predict the clinical outcome[86,87]. However, in another study, microvessel density lacked prognostic significance[88]. Other stimu-

lators of angiogenesis such as tumor necrosis factor-α (TNF-α) and basic fibroblast growth factor (bFGF), and inhibitors such as angiostatin and tumor growth factor-β (TGF-β) might also be factors with prognostic impact in renal cell carcinoma but remain to be further evaluated.

Patient-related factors and symptoms

A number of patient-related factors, including disease presentation, performance status, weight loss and other clinical symptoms are of prognostic importance, although strongly associated with disease stage[89]. In contrast, age, sex and race are factors with no independent prognostic value[90]. Differences in survival by age and sex are mostly related to differences in stage and grade. Patients with incidentally diagnosed renal cell carcinoma who have a disease presentation without symptoms, generally have smaller tumors, less advanced stage and better survival. In renal cell carcinoma there is no specific tumor marker available but a number of variables in the serum are predictive for tumor progression. In a recent study, erythrocyte sedimentation rate (ESR) and five acute-phase reactants, haptoglobin, ferritin, C-reactive protein, orosomucoid and α-1-antitypsin, were studied and, in another study, interleukin–6 (IL–6) was also included. Each of these parameters had significant prognostic value but only ESR was an independent prognostic parameter[59,91]. Citterio and co-workers[92] reported that anemia, hypercalcemia, hypoalbuminemia and elevated serum alkaline phosphatase predicted outcome in metastatic renal cell carcinoma. Other studies have demonstrated that a number of prognostic markers have been identified in serum including chromogranin A, neuron-specific enolase (NSE), cancer antigen 125 (CA–125), tumor-associated trypsin inhibitor (TATI) and erythropoietin[93,94]. At present, genetic markers can also be monitored in serum and in urine that may possibly improve the prediction of progression in renal cell carcinoma can also be monitored in serum and urine[95,96].

Treatment decisions in patients without metastatic disease

As indicated above, prognostic factors are useful for treatment decisions in patients with small tumors confined to the kidney[97]. Patients presenting with factors that indicate a possible adverse impact might benefit more from radical surgery than nephron-sparing surgery which leaves an increased risk for local recurrence[98]. Since tumor thrombus formation itself, and not the upper level of the thrombus, indicates poorer survival, aggressive surgery with complete resection of the thrombus extension into the right atrium is as justified as nephrectomy, in patients with invasion into the renal vein alone[39].

Treatment decisions in patients with metastases

One controversy in the management of renal cell carcinomas is the role of nephrectomy in patients with metastatic disease. Nephrectomy is indicated for the relief of intractable local symptoms that are caused by the tumor, such as pain, hemorrhage or local tumor mass effects. Other systemic manifestations such as hyper-calcemia, hypertension, gastrointestinal tract dysfunction and heart failure secondary to blood shunting in the tumor, if proved refractory to other treatments, might be managed by nephrectomy. Furthermore, as Barnley and Churchill first reported in 1939, nephrectomy is also indicated in conjunction with resection of a solitary metastasis[99]. The role of nephrectomy as an adjunct to systemic immunotherapy is less clear. A randomized trial with interferon-α therapy on patients with lung metastases showed a higher response rate in nephrectomized patients than in those not treated[100].

Nurmi and Nikkanen[101] found that survival after nephrectomy was not dependent on tumor site in patients with metastases. A disease-free interval of less than 6 months was associated with an adverse prognosis. In a recent study undertaken in our department,

we found that nephrectomy gave a survival advantage[35]. The selection of patients for surgery might be one reason for this advantage since these patients had a better performance status, significantly smaller tumor size and, more frequently, metastases were limited to one single site. The survival advantage of nephrectomy was supported in a randomized EORTC study of patients with distant-stage metastases and with a good performance status, demonstrating that combined treatment with nephrectomy and interferon resulted in a significantly longer survival time than treatment with interferon only[102]. In contrast, other authors have found no improvement in survival after palliative nephrectomy[103,104].

A number of significant factors, valuable for deciding on the treatment of patients with metastatic renal cell carcinoma can be identified. Factors having no association with survival time are metastatic site, tumor size and nuclear grade[35]. In contrast, other authors have found that improved survival was correlated to lung or bone metastases[55,105] while Uygur and co-workers[106] demonstrated that histopathological grade and tumor size < 7 cm were associated with better survival. Neves and colleagues had previously found that patients with solitary metastases had significantly better survival[107]. In the study by Ljungberg and co-workers[35], serum albumin, DNA ploidy and solitary versus multiple metastases were significant predictors of survival in univariate analysis but not after multivariate analysis[35]. Instead, after multi-variate analysis, only performance status, number of metastatic sites, ESR, serum calcium levels and vein invasion remained as independent predictive variables. Thus, a careful clinical examination of the patient with routine laboratory analyses and adequate radiological investigations is important in order to obtain data useful for the recommendation of therapy in these patients.

By using multiple prognostic factors, considerable information can be obtained for the clinical management of renal cell carcinoma. Patients with a high risk for progressive disease who might benefit from adjuvant treatment strategies can be identified. Also, those with a low risk, as, for example, suitable candidates for nephron-sparing surgery can be identified. Furthermore, prognostic factors can be used for determining patients eligible for entering and stratifying studies and therapy trials. Refinements of the staging system and the developing knowledge on biomarkers and molecular genetics may possibly improve further the ability to predict accurately the prognosis in renal cell carcinoma.

References

1. Thrasher JB, Paulson DF. Prognostic factors in renal cancer. *Urol Clin North Am* 1993;20:247–62
2. Kovacs G, Akhtar M, Beckwith BJ, *et al.* The Heidelberg classification of renal cell tumours. *J Pathol* 1997;183:131–3
3. Hoffman DM, Gitlitz BJ, Belldegrun A, *et al.* Adoptive cellular therapy. *Semin Oncol* 2000; 27:221–33
4. Favrot MC, Puisieux I. Application of gene transfer in cancer immunotherapy. From experimental data to clinical protocols. *Adv Exp Med Biol* 1998;451:539–41
5. Jonas D, Thoma B, Beckert H, *et al.* The value of morphological prognostic criteria in the assessment of renal cell carcinoma. *Urol Int* 1985;40:148–54
6. Thönes W, Störkel S, Rumpelt HJ. Histopathology and classification of renal cell tumors (adenomas, oncocytomas and carcinomas): the basic cytological and histopathological elements and their use for diagnostics. *Pathol Res Pract* 1986;181:125–43
7. Kovacs G, Wilkens L, Papp T, *et al.* Differentiation between papillary and non-papillary renal cell carcinomas by DNA analysis. *J Natl Cancer Inst* 1989;81:527–30
8. Kovacs G. Molecular cytogenetics of renal cell tumors. *Adv Cancer Res* 1993;62:89–124
9. Gnarra JR, Lerman MI, Zbar B, *et al.* Genetics of renal-cell carcinoma and evidence for a critical role for von Hippel-Lindau in renal tumorigenesis. *Semin Oncol* 1995;22:3–8
10. Schullerus D, Herbes J, Chudek J, *et al.* Loss of heterozygosity at chromosomes 8p, 9p and 14q is associated with stage and grade of non-papillary renal cell carcinomas. *J Pathol* 1997; 183:151–5
11. Kovacs G, Fuzesi L, Emanual A, *et al.* Cytogenetics of papillary renal cell tumors. *Genes Chromosomes Cancer* 1991;3:249–55
12. Speicher MR, Schoell B, du Manoir S, *et al.* Specific loss of chromosomes 1, 2, 6, 10, 13, 17 and 21 in chromophobe renal cell carcinomas revealed by comparative genomic hybridization. *Am J Pathol* 1994;145:356–64
13. Bugert P, Gaul C, Weber K, *et al.* Specific genetic changes of diagnostic importance in chromophobe renal cell carcinomas. *Lab Invest* 1997;76:203–8
14. Akhtar M, Kardar H, Linjawi T, *et al.* Chromophobe cell carcinoma of the kidney. A clinicopathologic study of 21 cases. *Am J Surg Pathol* 1995;19:145–56
15. Verdorfer I, Culig Z, Hobisch A, *et al.* Characterisation of a collecting duct carcinoma by cytogenetic analysis and comparative genomic hybridisation. *Int J Oncol* 1998;13: 461–4
16. Steiner G, Cairns P, Polascik TJ, *et al.* High-density mapping of chromosomal arm 1q in renal collecting duct carcinoma: region of minimal deletion at 1q32.1–32.2. *Cancer Res* 1996;56:5044–6
17. Ljungberg B, Iranparvar Alamdari F, Stenling R, *et al.* Prognostic significance of the Heidelberg Classification of renal cell carcinoma. *Eur Urol* 1999;36:565–9
18. Moch H, Gasser T, Amin MB, *et al.* Prognostic utility of the recently recommended histologic classification and revised TNM staging system for renal cell carcinoma: a Swiss experience with 588 tumors. *Cancer* 2000;89:604–14
19. Sene AP, Hunt L, McMahon RF, *et al.* Renal carcinoma in patients undergoing nephrectomy: analysis of survival and prognostic factors. *Br J Urol* 1992;70:125–34
20. Amin MB, Corless CL, Renshaw AA, *et al.* Papillary (chromophil) renal cell carcinoma: histomorphologic characteristics and evaluation of conventional pathologic prognostic

parameters in 62 cases. *Am J Surg Pathol* 1997;21:621–35

21. Crotty TB, Farrow GM, Lieber MM. Chromophobe cell renal carcinoma: clinico-pathological features of 50 cases. *J Urol* 1995;154:964–7

22. Beroud C, Fournet JC, Droz JPC, *et al.* Correlations of allelic imbalance of chromosome 14 with adverse prognostic parameters in 148 renal cell carcinomas. *Genes Chromosom Cancer* 1996;17:215–24

23. Jiang F, Richter J, Schrami P, *et al.* Chromosomal inbalances in papillary renal cell carcinoma differences between histological subtypes. *Am J Pathol* 1998;153:1467–73

24. Schraml P, Muller D, Bednar R, *et al.* Allelic loss at the D9S171 locus on chromosome 9p13 is associated with progression of papillary renal cell carcinoma. *J Pathol* 2000;190:457–61

25. Reiter RE, Anglard P, Liu S, *et al.* Chromosome 17p deletions and p53 mutations in renal cell carcinoma. *Cancer Res* 1993;53:3092–7

26. Uchida T, Wada C, Wang C, *et al.* Genomic instability of microsatellite repeats and mutations of H-, K-, and N-ras, and p53 genes in renal cell carcinoma. *Cancer Res* 1994;54:3682–5

27. Kamel D, Turpeenniemi-Hujanen T, Vahakangas K, *et al.* Proliferating cell nuclear antigen but not p53 or human papillomavirus DNA correlates with advanced clinical stage in renal cell carcinoma. *Histopathology* 1994;25:339–47

28. Moch H, Sauter G, Gasser TC, *et al.* p53 protein expression but not mdm-2 protein expression is associated with rapid tumor cell proliferation and prognosis in renal cell carcinoma. *Urol Res* 1997;25(Suppl 1):25–30

29. Shiina H, Igawa M, Urakami S, *et al.* Clinical significance of immunohistochemically detectable p53 protein in renal cell carcinoma. *Eur Urol* 1997;31:3–80

30. Cairns P, Tokino K, Eby Y, *et al.* Localization of tumor suppressor loci on chromosome 9 in primary human renal cell carcinomas. *Cancer Res* 1995;55:224–7

31. Skinner DG, Colvin RB, Vermillion CD, *et al.* Diagnosis and management of renal cell carcinoma. A clinical and pathological study of 309 cases. *Cancer* 1971;28:1165–77

32. Ljungberg B, Mehle C, Stenling R, *et al.* Heterogeneity in renal cell carcinoma and its impact on prognosis – a flow cytometric study. *Br J Cancer* 1996;74:123–7

33. Hatcher PA, Anderson EE, Paulson DF, *et al.* Surgical management and prognosis of renal cell carcinoma invading the vena cava. *J Urol* 1992;20–3

34. Ljungberg B, Larsson P, Stenling R, *et al.* Flow cytometric deoxyribonucleic acid analysis in

stage I renal cell carcinoma. *J Urol* 1991; 146:697–9

35. Ljungberg B, Landberg G, Alamdari FI. Factors of importance for prediction of survival in patients with metastatic renal cell carcinoma, treated with or without nephrectomy. *Scand J Urol Nephrol* 2000;34:246–51

36. Minervini R, Minervini A, Fontana N, *et al.* Evaluation of the 1997 tumour, nodes and metastases classification of renal cell carcinoma: experience in 172 patients. *Br J Urol* 2000;86:199–202

37. Giuliani L, Giberti C, Martorana G. *et al.* Radical extensive surgery for renal cell carcinoma: long term results and prognostic factors. *J Urol* 1990; 143:468–73

38. Sánchez de la Muela P, Zudaire JJ, Robles JE, *et al.* Renal cell carcinoma: vena caval invasion and prognostic factors. *Eur Urol* 1991;19:284–90

39. Ljungberg B, Stenling R, Österdahl B, *et al.* Vein invasion in renal cell carcinoma: impact on metastatic behaviour and survival. *J Urol* 1995;154:1681–4

40. Montie JE, El Ammar R, Pontes JE, *et al.* Renal cell carcinoma with inferior vena cava thrombi. *Surgery* 1991;173:107–15

41. Sosa RE, Muecke EC, Vaughan DTr, *et al.* Renal cell carcinoma extending into the inferior vena cava: the prognostic significance of the level of vena caval involvement. *J Urol* 1984:132:1097–100

42. Mrstik CH, Salamon J, Weber R, *et al.* Microscopic venous infiltration as predictor of relapse in renal cell carcinoma. *J Urol* 1992;148:271–4

43. Yoshino S, Kato M, Okada K. Prognostic significance of microvessel count in low stage renal cell carcinoma, *Int J Urol* 1995;2:156–60

44. Selli C, Hinshaw WM, Woodard BH, *et al.* Stratification of risk factors in renal cell carcinoma. *Cancer* 1983;52:899–903

45. Golimbu M, Joshi P, Sperber A, *et al.* Renal cell carcinoma: survival and prognostic factors. *Urology* 1986;27:291–301

46. Nurmi MJ. Prognostic factors in renal carcinoma. An evaluation of operative findings. *Br J Urol* 1984;56:270–5

47. Johnsen JA, Hellsten S. Lymphatogenous spread of renal cell carcinoma: an autopsy study. *J Urol* 1997;157:450–3

48. Schafhauser W, Ebert A, Brod J, *et al.* Lymph node involvement in renal cell carcinoma and survival chance by systematic lymphadenectomy. *Anticancer Res* 1999;19:1573–8

49. Blom JH, van Poppel H, Marechal JM, *et al.* Radical nephrectomy with and without lymph node dissection: preliminary results of the EORTC randomized phase III protocol 30881.

EORTC Genitourinary Group. *Eur Urol* 1999;36: 570–5

50. Wunderlich H, Schlichter A, Reichelt O, *et al.* Real indications for adrenalectomy in renal cell carcinoma. *Eur Urol* 1999;35:272–6

51. Sandock DS, Seftel AD, Resnick MI. Adrenal metastases from renal cell carcinoma: role of ipsilateral adrenalectomy and definition of stage. *Urology* 1997;49:28–31

52. Motzer RJ, Mazumdar M, Bacik J, *et al.* Survival and prognostic stratification of 670 patients with advanced renal cell carcinoma. *J Clin Oncol* 1999;17:2530–40

53. Cerfolio RJ, Allen MS, Deschamps C, *et al.* Pulmonary resection of metastatic renal cell carcinoma. *Ann Thorac Surg* 1994;57:339–44

54. O'Dea MJ, Zincke H, Utz DC, *et al.* The treatment of renal cell carcinoma with solitary metastasis. *J Urol* 1978;120:540–2

55. Montie JE, Stewart BH, Straffon RA, *et al.* The role of adjunctive nephrectomy in patients with metastatic renal cell carcinoma. *J Urol* 1977; 117:272–5

56. Pomer S, Klopp M, Steiner HH, *et al.* Hirnmetasierung beim nierenzellkarzinom. Behandlungsergebnisse und prognose. *Urologe A* 1997;36:117–25

57. Fourquier P, Regnard JF, Rea S, *et al.* Lung metastases of renal cell carcinoma: results of surgical resection. *Eur J Cardiothorac Surg* 1997;11:17–21

58. Fuhrman SA, Lasky LC, Limas C. Prognostic significance of morphologic parameters in renal cell carcinoma. *Am J Surg Pathol* 1982;6:655–63

59. Ljungberg B, Grankvist K, Rasmuson T. Serum interleukin-6 in relation to acute-phase reactants and survival in patients with renal cell carcinoma. *Eur J Cancer* 1997;33:1794–8

60. Onodera Y, Matsuda N, Ohta M, *et al.* Prognostic significance of tumor grade for renal cell carcinoma. *Int J Urol* 2000;7:4–9

61. Bertoni F, Ferri C, Benati A, *et al.* Sarcomatoid carcinoma of the kidney. *J Urol* 1987;137:25–8

62. Tomera KM, Farrow GM, Lieber MM. Sarcomatoid renal carcinoma. *J Urol* 1983; 130:657–9

63. Carducci MA, Piantadosi S, Pound CR, *et al.* Nuclear morphometry adds significant prognostic information to stage and grade for renal cell carcinoma. *Urology* 1999;53:44–9

64. Gutierrez JL, Val-Bernal JF, Garijo MF. Nuclear morphometry in prognosis of renal adenocarcinoma. *Urology* 1992:39:130–4

65. Eschwege P, Saussine C, Steichen G, *et al.* Radical nephrectomy for renal cell carcinoma 30 mm or less: long-term follow-up results. *J Urol* 1996;155:1196–9

66. Polascik TJ, Proud CR, Meng MV, *et al.* Partial nephrectomy: technique, complications, and pathological findings. *J Urol* 1995;154:1312–18

67. Nativ O, Sabo E, Raviv G, *et al.* The impact of tumor size on clinical outcome in patients with localized renal cell carcinoma treated by radical nephrectomy. *J Urol* 1997;158:729–32

68. Di Silverio F, Casale P, Colella D, *et al.* Independent value of tumor size and DNA ploidy for the prediction of disease progression in patients with organ-confined renal cell carcinoma. *Cancer* 2000;88:835–43

69. Ruiz-Cerda JL, Hernandez M, Sempere A, *et al.* Intratumoral heterogeneity of DNA content in renal cell carcinoma and its prognostic significance. *Cancer* 1999;86:664–71

70. del Vecchio MT, Lazzi S, Bruni A, *et al.* DNA ploidy pattern in papillary renal cell carcinoma. Correlation with clinicopathological parameters and survival. *Pathol Res Pract* 1998;194:325–33

71. Currin SM, Lee SE, Walther PJ. Flow cytometric assessment of deoxyribonucleic acid content in renal adenocarcinoma: does ploidy status enhance prognostic stratification over stage alone? *J Urol* 1990;143:458–63

72. Rainwater LM, Hosaka Y, Farrow GM, *et al.* Well differentiated clear cell renal carcinoma: significance of nuclear deoxyribonucleic acid patterns studied by flow cytometry. *J Urol* 1987;137:15–20

73. Barretton G, Kuhlman B, Krech R, *et al.* Intratumoral heterogeneity of nuclear DNA-content and proliferation in clear cell type carcinomas of the kidney. *Virchows Arch B Cell Pathol* 1991;61:57–63

74. Larsson P, Roos G, Stenling R, *et al.* Proliferating cell nuclear antigen expression in renal cell carcinoma – prognostic implications. *Scand J Urol Nephrol* 1996;30:445–50

75. Ljungberg B, Larsson P, Roos G, *et al.* Cell kinetics of renal cell carcinoma studied with *in vivo* iododeoxyuridine incorporation and flow cytometry. *J Urol* 1994;151:1509–13

76. Renshaw AA, Loughlin KR, Dutta A. Cyclin A and M1B1 (Ki67) as markers of proliferative activity in primary renal neoplasms. *Mod Pathol* 1998;11:963–6

77. Larsson P, Roos G, Stenling R, *et al.* Cell proliferation in renal cell carcinoma – a comparative study of cell kinetic methods. *Urol Res* 1996;24:291–5

78. Aaltoma S, Lipponen P, Ala-Opas M, *et al.* Expression of cyclins A and D and p21 (waf1/cip1) proteins in renal cell cancer and their relation to clinicopathological variables and patients' survival *Br J Cancer* 1999; 80:2001–7

79. Hunter T, Pines J. Cyclins and cancer II: cyclin D and CDK inhibitors come of age. *Cell* 1994;79:573–82

80. Graña X, Reddy P. Cell cycle control in mammalian cells: role of cyclins, cyclin dependent kinases (CDKs), growth suppressor genes and cyclin-dependent kinase inhibitors (CKIs). *Oncogene* 1995;11:211–19

81. Hedberg Y, Davoodi E, Roos G, *et al.* Cyclin D1 expression in renal cell carcinoma. *Int J Cancer* 1999;84:268–72

82. Jacobsen J, Rasmuson T, Grankvist K, *et al.* Vascular endothelial growth factor as prognostic factor in renal cell carcinoma. *J Urol* 2000;163:343–7.

83. Baccala AA, Zhong H, Clift SM, *et al.* Serum vascular endothelial growth factor is a candidate biomarker of metastatic tumor response to *ex vivo* gene therapy of renal cell cancer. *Urology* 1998;51:327–32

84. Van Poppel H, Vandendriessche H, Boel K, *et al.* Microscopic vascular invasion is the most relevant prognosticator after radical nephrectomy for clinically nonmetastatic renal cell carcinoma. *J Urol* 1997;58:45–9

85. Symbas NP, Townsend MF, El-Galley R, *et al.* Poor prognosis associated with thrombocytosis in patients with renal cell carcinoma. *BJU Int* 2000;86:203–7

86. Yoshino S, Kato M, Okada K. Clinical significance of angiogenenesis, proliferation and apoptosis in renal cell carcinoma. *Anticancer Res* 2000;20:591–4

87. Nativ O, Sabo E, Reiss A, *et al.* Clinical significance of tumor angiogenesis in patients with localized renal cell carcinoma. *Urology* 1998;51:693–6

88. MacLennan GT, Bostwick DG. Microvessel density in renal cell carcinoma: lack of prognostic significance. *Urology* 1995;46:27–30

89. Elson PJ, Witte RS, Trump DL. Prognostic factors for survival in patients with recurrent or metastatic renal cell carcinoma. *Cancer Res* 1988;48:7310–11

90. Nurmi M, Puntala P, Touminen J, *et al.* Prognostic significance of symptoms and findings in renal adenocarcinoma. *Strahlentherapie* 1985;161:632–6

91. Ljungberg B, Grankvist K, Rasmuson T. Serum acute phase reactants and prognosis in renal cell carcinoma. *Cancer* 1995;76:1435–9

92. Citterio G, Bertuzzi A, Tresoldi M, *et al.* Prognostic factors for survival in metastatic renal cell carcinoma: retrospective analysis from 109 consecutive patients. *Eur Urol* 1997;31:286–91

93. Lukkonen A, Lintula S, von Boguslawski K, *et al.* Tumor-associated trypsin inhibitor in normal and malignant renal tissue and in serum of renal-cell carcinoma patients. *Int J Cancer* 1999;83:486–90

94. Ljungberg B, Rasmuson T, Grankvist K. Erythropoietin in renal cell carcinoma: evaluation of its usefulness as a tumor marker. *Eur Urol* 1992;21:160–3

95. Eisenberger CF, Schoenberg M, Enger C, *et al.* Diagnosis of renal cancer by molecular urinalysis. *J Natl Cancer Inst* 1999;91:2028–32

96. Kim YS, Kim KH, Choi JA, *et al.* Fas (APO-1/CD95) ligand and Fas expression in renal cell carcinomas: correlation with the prognostic factors. *Arch Pathol Lab Med* 2000;124:687–93

97. Butler BP, Novick AC, Miller DP, *et al.* Management of small unilateral renal cell carcinomas: radical versus nephron-sparing surgery. *Urology* 1995;45:34–40

98. Ljungberg B. Nephron sparing surgery or radical nephrectomy in the treatment of small renal cell carcinoma. *Rev Ser Urol* 1999;1:2–5

99. Barnley JD, Churchill EJ. Adenocarcinoma of the kidney with metastases to the lung: cured by nephrectomy and lobectomy. *J Urol* 1939;42:269–71

100. Minasian LM, Motzer RJ, Gluck L. Interferon alfa-2a in advanced renal cell carcinoma: treatment results and survival in 159 patients with long term follow-up. *J Clin Oncol* 1993;11:1368–75

101. Nurmi M, Nikkanen TAV. Prognosis of metastatic renal adenocarcinoma. *Strahlentherapie* 1984;160:411–15

102. Mickisch GH, Garin A, Madej M, *et al.* Value of cytoreductive tumour nephrectomy in conjunction with immunotherapy in metastatic renal cell carcinoma (RCC). Results of a randomised phase III trial (EORTC 30947). *Eur Urol* 2000;37(Suppl 2):55

103. Johnson DE, Kaesler KB, Samuels ML. Is nephrectomy justified in patients with metastatic renal carcinoma. *J Urol* 1975;114:27–9

104. DeKernion JB, Ramming KP, Smith RB. The natural history of metastatic renal cell carcinoma: a computer analysis. *J Urol* 1978;120:148–52

105. Maldazys JD, deKernion JB. Prognostic factors in metastatic renal carcinoma. *J Urol* 1986;136:376–9

106. Uygur MC, Usubutun A, Ozen H, *et al.* Prognostic factors and the role of nephrectomy in metastatic renal cell carcinoma. *Int Urol Nephrol* 1998;7:681–7

107. Neves RJ, Zincke H, Taylor WF. Metastatic renal cell cancer and radical nephrectomy: identification of prognostic factors and patients survival. *J Urol* 1988;139:1173–6

Laparoscopic radical nephrectomy and nephroureterectomy for treatment of renal cell and transitional cell carcinoma – own experience and review of the literature

5

J. Rassweiler and T. Frede

Introduction

At the beginning of the decade, Clayman and colleagues pioneered laparoscopic nephrectomy, when they removed a renal oncocytoma in 1990[1]. Almost 1 year later, Coptcoat and associates used the same technique for radical extirpation of a T_2 renal cell carcinoma[2]. In 1992, Chiu and co-workers reported the use of laparoscopic nephroureterectomy for malignant disease[3]. Our first personal experience with radical nephrectomy was reported in 1993 for both renal cell and transitional cell carcinoma[4].

Despite the enthusiasm of the pioneering surgeons, laparoscopic surgery, especially laparoscopic nephrectomy has not become a widespread procedure, but expertise has been concentrated in centers that are now becoming increasingly active throughout the entire world[5–11]. However, even among laparoscopic surgeons, radical nephrectomy is still under debate. Only 37 of the 482 nephrectomies carried out in a recently published German multicenter study were performed for renal malignancy[12]. Nevertheless, during the last 3 years there has been an increasing number of reports of laparoscopic radical nephrectomy using different technical approaches, such as transperitoneal laparoscopy, retroperitoneoscopy and hand-assisted and gasless laparoscopy[13–19].

In this chapter, we describe the technical alternatives used for laparoscopic radical nephrectomy and nephroureterectomy and carry out a critical analysis of our own long-term results and the recent literature.

Technique

Transperitoneal laparoscopic radical nephrectomy

Patient preparation All patients received a similar preoperative preparation to that performed prior to open surgery (including informed consent and bowel preparation with 10 mg bisacodyl taken orally). Prior to the procedure, a nasogastric tube and a bladder catheter were inserted. Under general anesthesia, the patient was placed in the lateral traditional flank position with the table broken to extend the uppermost flank.

Trocar placement After a pneumoperitoneum had been attained with the inserted Veress needle, placed laterally to the rectus abdominis muscle on line with the umbilicus, trocars were inserted through the ventral abdominal wall as follows:

> Port I: 10 mm periumbilical (lateral edge of musculus rectus abdominis);
>
> Port II: 12 mm subcostal (mamillary line) for right kidney, 5 mm for left side;

Port III: 12 mm above spina iliaca superior (mamillary line) for left kidney, 5 mm for right side.

The laparoscope was passed through port I and used to inspect intra-abdominally the trocar insertion for ports II and III. The ports were 'secured' with sterile adhesive tape and sutured to the skin. After complete inspection of the intra-abdominal situs, either the ascending (right kidney) or descending (left kidney) colon was mobilized by laterocolic incision of the peritoneum (line of Toldt). Since the respective colon was free to fall away medially, one or two further ports could be inserted through the newly exposed retroperitoneum.

Port IV: 5 mm along the lateral abdominal wall parallel to Port II;

Port V: 5 mm along the lateral abdominal wall parallel to Port III.

These two ports are mainly used to grasp the kidney during dissection and kidney retrieval[4,19].

Clipping the ureter   The ovarian/spermatic vein was identified in proximity to the sacral promontory, clipped and dissected, as was the ureter. Retraction of the ureter can be established with an Endo bowel clamp inserted through port IV or V and can be helpful during dissection of the renal hilum. The lower pole of the kidney including the fatty capsule was isolated.

Renal vessel clipping   The main renal artery and vein were stapled with the Endo GIA 30 (Tyco, Autosuture, Toenisvorst, Germany) while smaller vessels were clipped in the normal way. For cost reduction, the main renal artery can be dissected between large double clips at each side; however, the main renal vein should be stapled in almost every case. Dissection of the renal vessels was carried out bimanually with Endo shears, an Endo dissector and an Endo right angle clamp, quite similar to the way it is carried out in open surgery.

Organ retrieval   The upper pole of the kidney, including the fatty capsule, was then dissected free of the respective adrenal gland and the relevant peritoneum. Next, the organ was grasped in the hilar region and moved down into the pelvic area preventing any interference with intra-abdominal introduction of the organ bag. In selected cases (i.e. upper pole renal cell carcinoma) we also removed the adrenal gland using clips or the Endo GIA stapler. The LapSac® (Cook Europe, Paris, France) was twirled around on a previously placed 4.5 mm converter-reduced Endo Grasp and passed through port III. The organ bag unfolded intra-abdominally and was held open by three Endo clamps (via ports II, IV and V) while the kidney was maneuvered into the LapSac[21].

Digital fragmentation   After the Endo dissector had pulled the drawstring, thereby closing the bag, the trocar sleeve was removed and the neck of the bag was pulled out over the surface of the abdomen (subcostal port II for right kidney, suprailiacal port for the left side). The port wound was further incised (20 mm) making possible the removal of fatty tissue using forceps and the digital fragmentation of the kidney into 3–5 pieces. This was carried out very carefully in order to be able to distinguish between the fatty capsule, normal renal tissue and the renal tumor, which was sent separately for histopathological analysis. We have never used a mechanical liquidizer, aspirator or morcellator device[1,22].

Complete organ removal   In some cases we have used a 8–10 cm muscle-splitting lower abdominal incision for complete organ removal[8,9]. This access has also been used for a hand-assisted laparoscopic approach towards the end of the procedure.

Before all trocar sleeves were removed under direct vision, the nephrectomy situs was inspected to rule out any active bleeding. Similar to the procedure in open surgery, a drainage tube was placed routinely through ports IV or V. This permits drainage of blood and irrigation fluid and may reveal postoperative bleeding. The enlargened incision(s) were closed with fascia and skin suture. All other port incisions were sutured intracutaneously or covered with adhesive strips.

Retroperitoneal laparoscopic radical nephrectomy

Patient preparation All patients received a similar preoperative preparation to that performed prior to open surgery or trans-peritoneal laparoscopic nephrectomy.

Access to the retroperitoneum Under general anesthesia, the patient was placed in the typical kidney position – the Trendelenburg position is unnecessary. Then a 15–18 mm incision was made in the 'muscle-free' triangle between the 12th rib and the anterior iliac spine (between the lateral edges of the musculus latissimus dorsi and the musculus obliquus externus). Then, by blunt dissection with an Overhold forceps a canal was created as far as the retroperitoneal space. The canal was then dilated so that the index finger could be introduced in order to push forward the peritoneum, thus creating a retroperitoneal cavity for correct placement of the secondary trocars.

Placement of secondary tocars We then placed the next two secondary trocars directly under palpation beside the index finger introduced via the primary access[23]. To avoid any injury to the surgeon's finger, the canal must be dilated using forceps: port II (10–11 mm) for the right hand of the surgeon (use of Endo shears and Endo clip applicator); port III (5 mm) for the left hand of the surgeon (use of Endo dissector).

Then the trocar wound was closed around the sheath to avoid gas leakage (matress suture) and the trocar was connected to the CO_2 insufflator to establish a pneumoretro-peritoneum (15 mmHg, 3.5 l/min) and retro-peritoneoscopy was performed.

Finally, where necessary, another 5-mm trocar was inserted (port IV) medially to rim of the peritoneum under endoscopic view, for retraction of the kidney during the dissection. After placement of all the trocars the maximal insufflation pressure was decreased to 12 mmHg. As in the open procedure, the surgeon and the camera assistant stand on the dorsal side of the patient.

Laparoscopic nephroureterectomy

In our series, ureterectomy was performed by two different techniques. A completely endoscopic ureterectomy was realized by transurethral circumcision of the orifice prior to laparoscopy using a Turner–Warwick hook[4,24,25] after stenting the ureter. The intra-mural part of the ureter was completely isolated until it retracted into the extraperitoneal space. Then the patient was positioned as for radical nephrectomy and the ureter was primarily dissected and clipped to prevent tumor cell spillage alongside the stent. After the radical nephrectomy was accomplished, the ureter was antegradely dissected towards the bladder and subsequently extracted *in toto*.

In most of our recent patients, we preferred the retrieval of the entire kidney specimen to avoid morcellation via a suprainguinal incision. This access was then used for open dissection of the distal ureter including a bladder cuff. Another reason for this approach was the fact that in four out of our last six patients with upper tract transitional cell carcinoma, the tumor was located in the distal ureter.

Patients

Since 1992, we have treated 24 patients (21 male, three female) with 26 renal cell carcinomas and 12 patients (eight male, four female) with transitional cell carcinoma of the kidney and ureter. Stage and grade are listed in Table 1. The majority have been pT_a–pT_1 tumors and there have been two bilateral renal cell carcinomas in patients under dialysis. All relevant perioperative data have been recorded, including operative time, complications, conversion and reintervention rates as well as

Table 1 Laparoscopic radical nephrectomy: pathological classification

Tumor	Stage	Grade	n
Renal cell carcinoma	pT_1	G_2	14
	pT_2	G_2	8
	pT_2	G_3	2
	pT_3	G_2	1
Transitional cell carcinoma	pT_a	G_2	5
	pT_1	G_2	1
	pT_2	G_2	2
	pT_2	G_3	3
	pT_3	G_3	1

Table 2 Laparoscopic radical nephrectomy: perioperative data

Criteria	Nephrectomy (RCC)	Nephroureterectomy (TCC)
Total number	26	12
Access		
transperitoneal	18	3
retroperitoneal	8	9
Specimen retrieval		
morcellation	17	3
by incision	9	9
Mean operating time (min)	235	220
with manual assistance (min)	185	n.a.
Mean blood loss (cc)	400	300
Conversion to open surgery	0	1
Complications (%)	13	25
bleeding	1	3
pulmonary embolism	1	—
ileal stenosis	1	—
Reintervention	1	1
Hospital stay (days)	7.4	8.4
Back to normal activity (days)	21	n.a.

RCC, renal cell carcinoma; TCC, transitional cell carcinoma; n.a., not available

length of hospital stay. The follow-up time averaged 54 months (7–80 months). We focused on local recurrence, regional progression, development of metastases and disease-specific survival.

Results

Laparoscopic radical nephrectomy

Perioperative data The operating time averaged 235 min (140–350 min), there was no difference according to whether a transperitoneal ($n = 18$) or a retroperitoneal ($n = 8$) approach was used (Table 2). In 17 cases, the specimen was entrapped in an organ bag (LapSac) and retrieved after digital morcellation, whereas, in nine instances, the intact organ was removed via a 8–10-cm incision in the lower abdomen. This incision was used for manual assistance during the procedure. The mean estimated blood loss was 400 cc (200–1000 cc). There were no conversions to open surgery. We observed one bleeding episode from the surface of the spleen which was managed by laparoscopic tamponading using a hemostyptic gauze (Tachotamp®, Ethicon, Norderstedt, Germany). Another patient developed bleeding from one of the trocar sites 6 h after the operation; this was controlled by a transcutaneous suture. Two months later the same patient suffered from ileus due to a stenosis of the terminal ileum most probably induced by the aforementioned suture. The patient was successfully treated by a

segmental ileal resection. One patient had a pulmonary embolism which was managed conservatively. The mean postoperative hospital stay was 7.4 days.

Follow-up data The mean observation time was 60 months (36–80 months). There was no recurrence at the site of the trocars. One patient with a pT_2G_2 tumor developed a local recurrence and bone metastases 4 years after laparoscopic radical nephrectomy. He died 56 months after the procedure. Another patient with a pT_2G_3 tumor developed pulmonary and bone metastases 31 months after the procedure and died 34 months after surgery. The cumulative overall disease-free survival rate after 5 years is 91%, but is 100% for pT_1 tumors and 82% for pT_2/T_3 tumors.

Laparoscopic radical nephroureterectomy

Perioperative data The operating time averaged 220 min (190–300 min), there was no difference according to whether a transperitoneal ($n = 3$) or a retroperitoneal ($n = 9$) approach was used (Table 2). In three cases the specimen was entrapped in an organ bag (LapSac) and retrieved after digital morcellation, whereas, in nine instances, the intact organ was removed via a suprainguinal incision of 8–10 cm. This incision was used for open dissection of the distal ureter including a bladder cuff. The mean estimated blood loss was 300 cc (100–900 cc). There was one conversion to open surgery due to laceration of the renal vein. One patient developed an extraperitoneal hematoma in the region of the circumcised orifice. Another patient suffered from acute bleeding on the second postoperative day following a left, manually assisted, nephro-ureterectomy originating from the duodenal artery. The bleeding was stopped during open surgery, but recurred 1 week later. Again, surgical intervention was successful for hemostasis; however, the patient died on the 32nd postoperative day from multiple organ failure. There was no direct explanation for the primary bleeding site. Possibly, it was induced by monopolar coagulation in the retroperitoneal space. The mean postoperative hospital stay for the remaining 11 patients was 8.4 days.

Follow-up data Mean follow-up time was 48 months (7–78 months). There was no recurrence at the site of the trocars. Four of six patients with $pT_{2/3}G_3$ tumors of the distal ureter ($n = 5$) and pelvis ($n = 1$) developed regional progression ($n = 2$, lymph nodes) or distant metastases in bone and lungs ($n = 2$), 5–7 months after laparoscopic nephro-ureterectomy. In three of these cases, the ureterectomy was performed via the suprainguinal incision. One patient died 7 months after surgery; another after 30 months. All five patients with $pT_{a/1}G_2$ tumors showed no evidence of disease; however, two developed a superficial bladder tumor after 4 and 15 months. One patient died 31 months after surgery due to a carcinoma of the prostate. The cumulative overall disease-free survival rate after 5 years is 60%; however, it is 100% for pT_a/T_1 tumors and 33% for pT_2/T_3 tumors. Four of the 11 patients (36%) who left hospital after surgery subsequently developed bladder tumors.

Table 3 Laparoscopic radical nephrectomy: follow-up data

Criteria	Radical nephrectomy (RCC)	Radical nephro-ureterectomy (TCC)
Total number	26	12
Mean observation time (months)	60	48
Number of deaths from disease	2	3
Number of deaths from other causes	—	2
Overall survival (%)	91	58
Disease-free survival (5 years) (%)		
overall	91	60
pT_a/T_1	100	100
pT_2/T_3	82	33
Subsequent bladder tumors (%)	n.a.	36

RCC, renal cell carcinoma; TCC, transitional cell carcinoma; n.a., not available

Discussion

The role of laparoscopic radical nephrectomy and nephroureterectomy in patients with malignancies of the kidney and ureter remains controversial. Primary concerns have centered around the safety of the procedure, the reproducibility of the open technique by laparoscopy, the risk of tumor cell spillage and port-site metastases. Further concerns have been related to cost-effectiveness and the steep learning curve involved in the procedure. Finally, until now, long-term follow-up has not been available.

In the meantime, more than 7 years after its first description[2], the technique of trans-peritoneal laparoscopic radical nephrectomy has been standardized, fulfilling the principles of non-touch uro-oncological surgery. Recently, some authors have proposed a retroperitoneal approach[13,18,23], advocating the advantage of earlier control of the renal artery and the reduced need for dissection (i.e. deflection of the colon). These authors report significantly shorter operative times compared to the initial reports (Table 4). However, we feel that, as in open surgery, the access should be of secondary interest only. Nevertheless, the reproducibility of the procedure has been documented in two multicenter studies[12,17], as well as in a review of the literature (Table 4). The complication rate is acceptable and still decreasing; the operative time exceeds that of open surgery (140–150 min) by about 60–100 min. The retrieval of the specimen is accomplished most often by a small incision following entrapment in an organ bag rather than by morcellation.

Some authors have used this incision earlier in the procedure to perform hand-assisted laparoscopy. They emphasize that this speeds up the procedure and reduces the learning curve[8,9,15,19]. According to our experience, we were able to reduce the operative time by about 60 min (Table 2); however, standardization of the use of the hand proved to be very difficult, in particular, because the surgeon has to insert different hands for left- and right-sided radical nephrectomies. Considering the interest in a standard training program for laparoscopy and retroperitoneoscopy in urology, we feel that hand assistance should be limited to problematic situations. In contrast, the increasing expertise of the first-generation laparoscopists offers a variety of dissecting techniques and retraction standards to future generations who will be able to perform the operation much more easily and with less complications than the pioneers[12,23]. Of course, if radical nephrectomy represents an accepted indication, the workload at the different centers will increase significantly as has been shown by Gill and colleagues at the Cleveland Clinic Foundation[13].

With regard to the cost–benefit analysis of laparoscopic radical nephrectomy, the situation in the USA differs significantly from that in Europe: the operating times reported by the different groups are mostly longer, the charges for the theater are higher and the postoperative hospital stay is shorter, for both open and laparoscopic surgery in the USA than in Europe[10,11,19]. The higher perioperative costs of laparoscopy cannot be completely compensated for by the reduction in hospital stay. At our center, we have replaced almost all of our disposable instruments by a re-usable armamentarium (i.e. metal trocars, Endo shears, Endo graspers, clip appliers). For radical laparoscopic nephrectomy only, the use of an endoscopic stapler (i.e. the Endo GIA)

Table 4 Laparoscopic radical nephrectomy: world-wide experience

Author	n	Stage	Access	OR time (min)	Hospital stay (days)	Complications (%)	5-year survival rate (%)
McDougall et al., 1996[11]	17	pT_1–pT_3	transperitoneal	400	4.5	18	n.a.
Cicco et al., 1998[18]	21	pT_1–pT_2	retroperitoneal	131	4.6	n.a	n.a.
Gill et al., 1998[13]	42	pT_1–pT_2	retroperitoneal	199	2.1	10	n.a.
Ono et al., 1998[14]	60	pT_1–pT_2	transperitoneal/ retroperitoneal	330	5.2	n.a.	96
Caddedu et al., 1998[17]	157	pT_1–pT_3	transperitoneal/ retroperitoneal	n.a.	n.a.	6	89
Present study	26	pT_1–pT_3	transperitoneal/ retroperitoneal	235	7.4	13	91

OR, operating time; n.a., not available

contributes to the higher costs when compared to open surgery[20]. The operative time is still 60–90 min longer for laparoscopy; however, these costs can be mostly compensated for by the reduced postoperative hospital stay. Based on this, a significant benefit for the social security system can be obtained by a shorter convalescence time of about 2–3 weeks compared to that for open surgery[10,11] (Table 2).

In summary, despite some technical modifications by the different groups, laparoscopic radical nephrectomy can be regarded as a standardized and safe procedure, which allows transmission and reproduction of the surgical principles of the open procedure. In addition, the perioperative morbidity of the patients can be reduced significantly by use of laparoscopy.

In contrast, reports on laparoscopic radical nephroureterectomy are limited (Table 5). In principle, three modifications to ureterectomy have been applied: first, antegrade extraction following transurethral circumcision of the orifice[3,4,6,16], second, antegrade dissection including a bladder cuff by using an Endo stapler[11,26,27], and, third, retrieval of the kidney specimen via a suprainguinal incision which facilitates open dissection of the ureter including a bladder cuff[15]. The major advantage of the latter is that it represents a significant reduction in the operating time (Tables 2 and 5). Moreover, the incison does not have a significant impact on postoperative morbidity. It must be noted that, depending on the aggressiveness of transitional cell carcinoma, we recommend retrieval of the complete specimen, despite the proven safety of entrapment and morcellation of the specimen in the LapSac[28,29]. Therefore, it is only logical to use the incision for open dissection of the distal ureter.

Much more important than the technical feasibility of laparoscopic radical nephrectomy is the long-term outcome as shown in the studies available (Table 4). It must be noted that all the authors in these studies limited their range of indications to small-sized renal tumors (3–6 cm) of clinical stage T_{1-2}. However, as in our series, histopathology also showed evidence of pT_3 tumors among the treated cases[10,14,17]. This has to be taken into consideration when discussing the long-term results. The overall 5-year disease-free survival rates are excellent, ranging between 89 and 96% (Table 4). This corresponds to the recently published experience of the M.D. Anderson Hospital following open radical nephrectomy with 86% 5-year disease-free survival rates for $pT_{1/2}$ tumors[30]. Even after open surgery of clinical T_{1-2} tumors, local recurrence, as well as distant metastases, have been observed[30–33]. It must be emphasized that, until now, after more than 250 documented cases, no port-site metastases have been documented following laparoscopic radical nephrectomy for renal cell cancer.

Again, when considering laparoscopic radical nephroureterectomy, the situtation is different. In several instances regional and distant progression including one port-site recurrence[15] have been documented (Table 5); however, these concerned only high-grade

Table 5 Laparoscopic radical nephroureterectomy: world-wide experience

Author	n	Stage	OR time (min)	Hospital stay (days)	Complications (%)	Bladder recurrence (%)	5-year survival rate (%)
McDougall et al., 1995[10]	10	pT_a–pT_3*	500	5.0	10	37.5	87.5†
Keeley et al., 1998[16]	22	pT_a–pT_3‡	156	5.5	27	n.a.	95
Barrett et al., 1998[15]	21	pT_a–pT_3	200	8.5	14	23	81**
Present study	12	pT_a–pT_3	220	8.4	25	37	60††

OR, operating time; *one pT_2, one pT_3; †only 2-year follow-up; ‡one pT_3 tumor, no tumors of distal ureter; **one port-site metastasis; ††50% pT2/3 tumors

pT_{2-3} tumors. Conclusively, the 5-year disease-free survival rates ranged between 60% and 95%, depending on the different patient population in the series (Table 5).

Recently, Andersen and Steven reported a case of implantation metastasis in the abdominal trocar channel following laparoscopic biopsy of a transitional cell bladder tumor[34]. Bangma and co-workers reported a cutaneous metastasis following laparoscopic pelvic lymphadenectomy. In this case, the nodes were not entrapped in an organ bag[35]. The port-site recurrence in the series of Barrett and colleagues occurred after an uncomplicated laparoscopic assisted nephroureterectomy for a pT_1G_2 tumor with removal of the intact specimen[15]. Interestingly, this did not develop at the suprainguinal incision. At present, the development of trocar metastases cannot be explained completely, but they seem to occur more frequently in aggressive tumors[11].

In our series, we did not observe any port-site metastases, but the 5-year disease-free survival rate of patients with pT_{2-3} tumors was only 33%. However, these data correspond to the experience with open surgery, as recently reported by Corrado and colleagues[36] who found a 27% survival rate for this specific high-risk group of patients. In contrast, the disease-free 5-year survival rate for $pT_{a/1}$ tumors is 100%, which is consistent for all laparoscopic groups. The survival rates for patients with bladder tumors (25–37.5%) did not differ from those reported after open nephroureterectomy (Table 5)[24].

In conclusion, despite some technical modifications regarding access, laparoscopic radical nephrectomy has become a well-standardized and, thus, reproducible but technically demanding, procedure. Ideal indications are small tumors (T_{1-2}) which are not candidates for nephron-sparing surgery. The complication rates are acceptable and still decreasing. The long-term results are excellent and correspond to the results obtained with open surgery. The data base is now sufficiently large to initiate a multicenter prospective phase III study in comparison with open radical nephrectomy.

Radical nephroureterectomy can be performed very time efficiently when the suprainguinal incision is used for open extraction of the distal ureter including a bladder cuff. According to the aggressiveness of the transitional cell carcinoma, the procedure can be recommended only for $pT_{a/1}$ tumors. All other patients should be treated only in specially designed multicenter studies.

References

1. Clayman RV, Kavoussi LR, Soper NJ, et al. Laparoscopic nephrectomy: initial case report. J Urol 1991;146:278–82
2. Coptcoat MJ, Rassweiler J, Wickham JEA, et al. Laparoscopic radical nephrectomy for renal cell carcinoma. In Proceedings of the Third International Congress for Minimal Invasive Therapy. 1991: abstr D-66
3. Chiu AW, Chen MT, Huang WJS, et al. Laparoscopic nephroureterectomy and endoscopic incision of bladder cuff. Min Invas Ther 1992;1:299–303
4. Rassweiler JJ, Henkel TO, Potempa DM, et al. The technique of transperitoneal laparoscopic nephrectomy, adrenalectomy and nephroureterectomy. Eur Urol 1993;22:425–30
5. Coptcoat MJ, Joyce A, Rassweiler J, et al. Laparoscopic nephrectomy: the Kings and Mannheim clinical experience. J Urol 1992;147:433A abstr 881
6. Chirpaz A, Petibon E. Nephro-ureterectomie gauche sous control coelioscopique. J Coeliochir 1992;2:32–4
7. Ono Y, Sahashi M, Yamada S, Ohshima S. Laparoscopic nephrectomy without morcellation

for renal cell carcinoma: report of initial 2 cases. *J Urol* 1993;150:222–4

8. Tschada RK, Henkel TO, Seemann O, *et al.* First experiences with laparoscopic radical nephrectomy. *J Endourol* 1994;8:S80 abstr P1–68

9. Tschada RK, Rassweiler JJ, Schmeller N, *et al.* Laparoscopic radical nephrectomy – the German experience. *J Urol* 1995;153:479A abstr 1003

10. McDougall EM, Clayman RV, Elashry OM. Laparoscopic nephroureterectomy for upper tract transitional cell cancer: Washington University experience. *J Urol* 1995;154:975–80

11. McDougall EM, Clayman RV, Elashry OM. Laparoscopic radical nephrectomy for renal tumor: the Washington University experience. *J Urol* 1996;155:1180–5

12. Rassweiler J, Fornara P, Weber M, *et al.* Laparoscopic nephrectomy: the experience of the laparoscopic working group of the German Urological Association. *J Urol* 1998;160: 18–21

13. Gill IS, Soble J, Gyung TS, *et al.* Retroperitoneoscopic radical nephrectomy in 41 patients: expanding indications and impact of specimen size. *J Endourol* 1998;12:S103 abstr F1–1

14. Ono Y, Kinukawa T, Hattori R, *et al.* Long-term result of laparoscopic radical nephrectomy. *J Endourol* 1998;12:S103 abstr F1–2

15. Barrett PH, Fentie DD, Taranger LA, *et al.* Laparoscopic assisted nephroureterectomy (TCC). *J Endourol* 1998;12:S103 abstr F1–3

16. Keeley FX, Tolley DA. Laparoscopic nephro-ureterectomy: making management of upper tract transitional-cell carcinoma entirely minimally invasive. *J Endourol* 1998;12:139–41

17. Cadeddu JA, Moore RG, Nelson JB, *et al.* Laparoscopic nephrectomy for renal cell cancer: a multi-center evaluation of efficacy. *J Urol* 1998; 159:147A abstr 557

18. Cicco A, Joual A, Hoznek A, *et al.* Radical nephrectomy by retroperitoneal laparoscopic approach versus open surgery. *J Urol* 1998;159:154A abstr 585

19. Wolf S, Moon TD, Madisom WI, *et al.* Hand-assisted laparoscopic nephrectomy: comparison to standard laparoscopic nephrectomy. *J Urol* 1998;160:22–7

20. Rassweiler J, Coptcoat MJ. Laparoscopic surgery of the kidney and adrenal gland. In Janetschek G, Rassweiler J, Griffith D, eds. *Laparoscopic Surgery in Urology*. New York: Thieme Stuttgart, 1996:139–55

21. Rassweiler J, Stock C, Frede T, *et al.* Organ retrieval systems for endoscopic nephrectomy: a comparative study. *J Endourol* 1998;12:325–33

22. Coptcoat MJ, Ison KT, Wickham JEA. Endoscopic tissue liquidization and surgical aspiration. *J Endourol* 1988;2:321–9

23. Rassweiler JJ, Seemann O, Frede T, *et al.* Retroperitoneoscopy: experience with 200 cases. *J Urol* 1998;160:1265–9

24. Abercrombie GF, Eardley I, Payne SR, *et al.* Modified nephro-ureterectomy. Long-term follow-up with particular reference to subsequent bladder tumours. *Br J Urol* 1988; 61:198–200

25. Bub P, Rassweiler J, Eisenberger F. Harnleiterstripping nach transurethraler Ostiumumschneidung – eine Alternative zur Ureterektomie. *Akt Urol* 1989;20:67–9

26. Figenshau RS, Albala DM, Clayman RV, *et al.* Laparoscopic nephrourectomy: initial laboratory experience. *Min Invas Ther* 1991;1:93–7

27. Shalhav AL, Elbahnasy AM, McDougall EM, *et al.* Laparoscopic nephroureterectomy for upper tract transitional-cell cancer: technical aspects. *J Endourol* 1998;12:345–53

28. Rassweiler J, Stock C, Frede T, *et al.* Organ retrieval systems for endoscopic nephrectomy: a comparative study. *J Endourol* 1998;12:325–33

29. Shalhav AL, Leibovitch I, Lev R, *et al.* Is laparoscopic radical nephrectomy with specimen morcellation acceptable cancer surgery. *J Endourol* 1998;12:255–7

30. Levy DA, Slaton JW, Swanson DA, *et al.* Stage specific guidelines for survival after radical nephrectomy for local renal cell carcinoma. *J Urol* 1998;159:1163–7

31. Mickisch G, Tschada R, Rassweiler J, *et al.* Das lokale Rezidiv nach Nierentumoroperation. *Akt Urol* 1990;21:77–81

32. Moch H, Gasser TC, Urrejola C, *et al.* Metastastic behaviour of renal cell cancer: an analysis of 871 autopsies. *J Urol* 1997;157:66A abstr 254

33. Johnsen JA, Hellsten S. Lymphatogenous spread of renal cell carcinoma: an autopsy study. *J Urol* 1997;157:450–3

34. Andersen JR, Steven K. Implantation metastasis after laparoscopic biopsy of bladder cancer. *J Urol* 1995;153:1047–8

35. Bangma CH, Kirkels WJ, Chada S. Cutaneous metastasis following laparoscopic lymphadenectomy for prostatic carcinoma. *J Urol* 1995;153:1635–6

36. Corrado F, Ferri C, Mannini D, *et al.* Transitional cell carcinoma of the upper urinary tract: evaluation of prognostic factors by histopathology and flow cytometric analysis. *J Urol* 1991;145:1159–63

Modern management of advanced renal cell carcinoma

6

G. H. J. Mickisch

Introduction and objective

Approximately 2–3% of all malignant tumors in adults develop in the kidney. In 85% of them, the tumor originates from cells of the proximal tubules and is known as a Grawitz tumor, a hypernephroma or a renal cell carcinoma. In the Netherlands, the annual incidence of the third most common urological tumor is about 11 per 100 000. Men are twice as often afflicted as women, most often in the 5th to 6th decade. At the time of diagnosis, about 20% of the patients have disseminated disease and another 25% will have locally advanced disease. The incidence of renal cell carcinoma has gradually increased over the years and approximately 40% of all patients with this disease will die of it in contemporary series.

Traditionally, the classic presentation of a patient with kidney carcinoma consisted of a flank pain, macroscopic hematuria and a palpable abdominal mass. Nowadays, more than half of all tumors are incidental findings during the investigation of other symptoms, such as high blood pressure, low-grade pyrexia, weight loss and increased erythrocyte sedimentation rate[1]. Another 25% are diagnosed during routine ultrasound examinations. Undoubtedly, with the increasing availability of ultrasonography or computer tomography (CT) scanning, incidental renal tumors are more frequently diagnosed. Therefore, the cohort of patients that seeks treatment for renal cell carcinoma has dramatically changed over the last 25 years, and the question arises whether this alteration should also translate into different approaches to surgical treatment strategies. This is the topic of the present paper.

Approaches to organ-sparing kidney tumor excision

An organ-sparing resection, sometimes called 'partial nephrectomy' of a malignant tumor is the most flagrant violation of Robson's concepts of a 'radical' tumor nephrectomy[2,3]. Here, the surgeon deliberately opens Gerota's fascia, frees the kidney from surrounding fatty tissue and resects the tumor only. The techniques applied in various series[4] range from tumor excision over truly 'partial' nephrectomy to *ex vivo* (bench) surgery. Nevertheless, from a theoretical point of view, the tumor dissection must be performed within a safe rim of healthy parenchyma, guided by intraoperative frozen-section analysis to avoid margin positivity responsible for local recurrence.

Indications for nephron-sparing surgery evolved out of necessity when malignancy was detected in a solitary kidney, or in the setting of bilateral cancer or diminished renal function. Results were reasonable, with a mean recurrence rate of 7.5%[5]. More recently, in a review article about a single-center study with 500 patients[6], preservation of kidney function was achieved in 489 patients (98%), exhibiting a cancer-specific 5-year survival rate of 93%. Recurrent renal cell carcinoma developed postoperatively in 39 of 473 patients (8.2%); 13 of these patients (2.7%) were diagnosed with a local recurrence in the remnant kidney, while 26 developed metastatic disease.

Several investigators have now expanded the indication for organ-sparing resections to include patients with a normal contralateral unit, termed 'elective' nephron-sparing surgery. The argumentation against an elective nephron-sparing operation is derived from the potentially incomplete or inadequate dissection of the primary tumor, resulting in local recurrence and presumably diminished disease-free and cause-specific survivals. In addition, distinct features of a 'radical' tumor nephrectomy, such as adrenalectomy or local regional lymph node dissection, are not routinely performed during elective nephron-sparing techniques. However, the therapeutic value of lymphadenectomy remains highly controversial[7] and the incidence of tumor extension to, or metastatic deposits in, the adrenals in the context of small, organ-confined renal cell carcinomas is minute[8]. Hence, there is no authoritative evidence urging these procedures to be included into a nephron-sparing approach.

Local recurrence was reported in three cases of a review article[5] incorporating 388 cases of elective nephron-sparing operations from 11 centers, which comprised two local recurrences in two cases and metachronous recurrence elsewhere in the kidney in one case. At a mean follow-up of 31–75 months, the local recurrence rate amounted to 0.8%, which is 10 times lower than after a mandatory indication for kidney-sparing operations. Suffice it to say that appropriate patient selection is partly responsible for this excellent outcome. There is consensus that, in addition to the size of the primary tumor, the feasibility of a radical resection in terms of the anatomical localization of the cancerous mass is critical[9]. In most series, elective indications are reserved for tumors less than 4 cm in diameter.

The risk of local recurrence, which can occur many years after the procedure, remains the major point of concern. It may be difficult to distinguish recurrences due to incomplete resection (true local recurrence) from those secondary to the presence of occult satellite lesions and which are related to the multifocal behavior of renal cell carcinoma.

The incidence of tumor multifocalities has been reported to be as high as 25% (reviewed in reference 10). Further retrospective studies demonstrated an incidence of any small nodules of only 13%, and that the incidence of multifocality decreased to 7% in kidneys with a primary tumor diameter of less than 80 mm.

Furthermore, only 3% of these cancers were not readily visible and, thus, not amenable to removal at the time of operation of the larger primary tumor. A prospective analysis of step-sectioned (3-mm intervals) radical nephrectomy specimens confirmed the low incidence of unsuspected multifocal renal cell carcinoma. The overall incidence of multifocal lesions was 16% (16 out of 100 kidneys), but only six cases were not detected by preoperative imaging or at exploration. Therefore, the true incidence of occult multifocality in a surgical setting was only 6%, which is still higher than the documented low incidence in series compiling nephron-sparing operations. Hence, the real clinical relevance and natural history of a small secondary renal cell carcinoma remain unknown at present and its biological potential is not yet established.

Direct comparisons of nephron-sparing surgery versus radical nephrectomy with respect to the disease-free and cause-specific survivals have been few and comprise two retrospective studies matching for patients' age and sex, renal function, diabetes, hypertension, tumor size (< 4 cm), tumor localization and tumor stage. In the Cleveland series[11], 88 patients with single, small (< 4 cm), localized, unilateral, sporadic renal cell carcinoma were matched for radical ($n = 42$) and nephron-sparing ($n = 46$) surgical groups. There was one recurrence in each group, and the 5-year cancer-specific survival rates were 97% and 100%, respectively. The Mayo Clinic[12] reported on 185 patients with nephron-sparing surgery matched to 209 patients undergoing tumor nephrectomy with the same low pathological stage as well as similar patient characteristics. There was no difference with respect to disease-specific mortality or cancer progression. Respective 5- and 10-year cause-specific survival rates were 89 and 77% in the nephron-sparing group, and 89 and 87% in the radical nephrectomy group ($p = 0.16$). Hence, both studies appear to affirm that both approaches provide equally effective curative treatment for patients with single, small, unilateral, localized renal cell carcinoma.

To address this issue in a more systematic way, the European Organization for Research and Treatment of Cancer Genitourinary (EORTC-GU) group embarked in 1990 on a prospective study randomizing between tumor nephrectomy and nephron-sparing tumor excision in small unilateral renal cell carcinoma with a normal contralateral kidney (EORTC 30904, coordinator H.v. Poppel, Louvain). The study was originally designed to detect a survival difference of 15%, and 350 patients were entered until 1998, when the study stopped recruitment. There was no reason for a premature closure of the study, but results were never published, because the EORTC redesigned the protocol to accommodate for a study of true equivalence (< 5% difference) requiring more than 1000 randomized patients. Until results of this worldwide intergroup study are peer-reviewed and made public, one still has to consider elective nephron-sparing surgery as an experimental surgical approach. Patients undergoing the procedure must be adequately counselled and need to agree after informed consent. Preferably, patients should be enrolled in controlled clinical trials, such as Intergroup 30904.

Lymphadenectomy for renal cell cancer

It is a well-known fact that nodal involvement is one of the major factors influencing the prognosis of cancer patients, including carcinoma of the kidney. In the various series reported in the literature, the overall 5-year survival rates for stage I renal cell carcinoma (tumor confined to the kidney) range from 56 to 82% and, for stage II renal cell carcinoma (extension to perirenal fat but within Gerota's fascia), from 43 to 100%[1]. These survival rates decrease considerably when lymph node metastases are present. In a reported series, the overall 5-year survival rates for lymph node-positive disease range from 8 to 35%[13].

In older series, the incidence of lymph node metastases in renal cancer ranges from 13 to more than 32%[14,15]. The incidence of lymph node involvement increases with the stage of the tumor. Giuliani and associates[16] found a 6% incidence of lymph node metastases in tumors confined to the kidney, a 46.4% incidence in

locally advanced tumors, a 61.9% incidence in patients with distant metastases and a 66.6% incidence of lymph node metastases in patients with both vascular infiltration and distant metastases.

Lymph node dissection has resulted in the finding of lymphatic metastases in 7.5–22.5% of patients who have no other evidence of meta-static disease[8,14], and there is little doubt about the value of regional lymph node dissection as a staging procedure.

Since renal carcinoma metastasizes by both blood-borne and lymphatic routes, regional lymphadenectomy has been proposed as a method of improving the results of surgical therapy. However, the therapeutic value of lymphadenectomy for renal cell carcinoma is still controversial. Lymph node dissection may improve the prognosis of renal cell carcinoma, but factors, such as distribution of lymph node metastases, the extent of the lymph node dissection, the possibly increased operative morbidity and mortality, and the relation between histological type, and the incidence of nodal metastases should be investigated in a well-planned prospective study (EORTC 30881, coordinator J. Blom, Rotterdam). Preliminary results of this study have been published[17].

From May until September 1991, 772 patients with a clinically locally confined adenocarcinoma of the kidney were entered into the study. A total of 389 patients were randomized to have a radical nephrectomy without a lymph node dissection. The remaining 383 patients were randomized to undergo a radical nephrectomy with a complete lymph node dissection. Forty-one patients were not eligible, mainly due to an incorrect disease stage or histopathology, thus leaving 731 eligible patients, 369 in the group not receiving a lymph node resection and 362 in the group having a lymph node dissection. Patients who had clinically detectable lymph node metastases or distant metastases before surgery were ineligible and excluded from the study.

There was virtually no difference between the two treatment groups in the number of complications. There was a slightly larger number of patients with blood loss during operation among the patients who had a lymph node dissection, but the differences are not statistically significant (χ^2 test). Thus the extension of the operation caused by the lymph node dissection had no real impact on the complication rate.

In 336 patients, information is available on the lymph node status. Of these patients, 43 had palpable lymph nodes during surgery. Almost 97% of the patients had no lymph node metastases on pathological examination of the resected lymph nodes. Of the patients who underwent a nephrectomy without lymph node dissection, 29 of 346 patients (8.4%) had palpable lymph nodes during surgery. Only six of these 29 patients had lymph node metastases at biopsy of the glands.

As only 17% of the patients entered have progressed or died, based on a median follow-up of 5 years, it is too early to consider treatment efficacy.

There are some points that might have contributed to the differences in survival found in older, non-randomized series[15,16,18,19] and that may be arguments against lymphadenectomy. First, the number and location of the involved nodes were not specified in any of the reported series. It is possible that the survivors were the patients with only one or several microscopically involved lymph nodes in the renal hilum. These nodes would also have been removed by a standard radical nephrectomy without an extensive lymphadenectomy. Second, one has to take into account the potentially increased morbidity and mortality from the extended operation in the light of the small improvement in survival reported in most series. Third, many patients with negative lymph nodes may die of disseminated tumor, indicating that blood-borne metastases are perhaps more common causes of death from renal carcinoma than are lymphatic metastases. So, lymphadenectomy can only be justified if lymphatic metastases are the only extent of tumor dissemination.

In summary, it can be concluded from the present study that a lymph node dissection combined with a radical nephrectomy does not increase morbidity or mortality, but a longer follow-up is needed to make conclusions on its efficacy in terms of prolonged tumor-free survival. EORTC protocol 30881 may give an answer to most of the pending questions once a sufficiently long period of follow-up has been achieved.

Approaches to tumor nephrectomy

Radical nephrectomy is the treatment of choice for patients with tumors confined to Gerota's fascia (stage $\leq pT_{3a}$) or growing intraluminally below the level of the diaphragm (stage pT_{3b}) (Table 1). Whether surgical extirpation of a caval thrombus exceeding the level of the diaphragm (stage pT_{3c}) or regional nodal involvement (stage pN_2) may lead to prolongation of survival in more than anecdotal cases is still a matter of scientific debate. The technique of radical nephrectomy in the treatment of renal cell carcinoma has traditionally encompassed primary ligation of the renal artery, subsequent ligation of the renal vein, and ultimate dissection and excision of the kidney within the confines of Gerota's fascia. The rationale for this approach is to avoid potential tumor cell dissemination that might occur during mobilization of the kidney, and to remove *en bloc* a tumor that may have extended into perinephric fat[2]. In taking these considerations into account, the transperitoneal approach has generally been preferred, since this approach tends to permit the securement of the renal vessels before proceeding to dissection of the kidney[3].

Occasionally, ileus may occur following the transperitoneal approach to nephrectomy, presumably because of the manipulation of small bowel that accompanies this dissection. Some authors[20], therefore, began to consider

Table 1 Surgical incisions for advanced renal cell carcinoma

(1) Chevron (semi-, c.q. Mercedes extension)
(2) Midline
(3) Thoraco-abdominal (5–7th rib)
(4) Semi-Chevron + intracostal extension
(5) Lumbar (obsolete)
(6) Muscle-sparing (obsolete)

applying a purely extraperitoneal approach in patients who required radical nephrectomy, in order to determine whether ileus could be avoided and recovery hastened. Since the approach implied the need for some mobilization of the kidney within Gerota's fascia before the renal vessels could be secured, it also became important to document that dissemination of greater numbers of tumor cells did not occur during such a dissection.

This approach has been documented in 24 patients with renal cell carcinomas, both on the right and the left sides, involving both upper and lower poles. The length of hospital stay has averaged 7 days (range 6–8 days), with most patients having begun to eat after passage of flatus by days 3–4.

In three cases, kidneys were removed and then perfused with normal saline both without and with direct manipulation of the tumor mass. The effluent from the renal vein was collected and analyzed cytologically. Manipulation did not appear to cause an increased number of tumor cells to appear, suggesting that the minimal intraoperative handling of the kidney during an extraperitoneal approach that might be required for renal vessel control would not necessarily be expected to result in an increased risk of tumor cell dissemination. These authors have also not seen a burst of distant metastasis suddenly developing in patients undergoing extraperitoneal tumor nephrectomy as long as 36 months after surgery. However, it remains to be seen in further studies whether or not this is a risk of the approach with clinical relevance.

There are two other retrospective studies and one preliminary report on a prospective trial comparing extra- with transperitoneal approaches. Fifty-six or 35 patients were operated for renal cell carcinoma through lumbar or transperitoneal approaches, respectively[21]. Both groups exhibited the same patient and tumor characteristics (retrospectively), and the 5-year survival rates for Robson's stage 1, 2 or 3 were 93.1, 70.4 and 60%, or 90.5, 72.2 and 25%, respectively. In this study, there was no difference in survival rates for either surgical procedure, and the authors

suggested that lumbar incision had fewer complications than transperitoneal exploration.

Similar results were reported for 29 or 22 patients undergoing tumor nephrectomy through translumbar versus transabdominal approaches, respectively, for T_1–T_3 N_0M_0 renal cell carcinoma[22]. Again, retrospectively, there was no significant difference in actuarial or disease-free survival period between the two groups. In this study, statistical analysis appeared to reveal shortened operating time, decreased blood loss and quickened postoperative recovery in the translumbar group, as compared with those in the transperitoneal group.

Finally, 49 or 45 patients were randomized to undergo translumbar or transperitoneal tumor nephrectomy for renal cell carcinoma < 15 cm without involvement of the upper pole or the vena cava[23]. Kaplan–Meier curves detected no difference in survival rate after a median follow-up of nearly 3 years, and parameters, such as mean blood loss, hospital stay, or the overall complication rate, were significantly in favor of the translumbar resection. The technique of radical nephrectomy is based on two primary concepts: the first is to excise all of the tissue contained within Gerota's fascia to maximize the likelihood of removing the renal cancer, even if it has extended through the renal capsule into the perinephric fat; the second is to gain early control of the renal vessels prior to manipulation of the kidney, to minimize the likelihood of dissemination of tumor cells during the course of the procedure. The authors favoring a translumbar approach claim to take both of these considerations into account and attempt to provide a means whereby both patient recovery and hospital stay are shortened without compromising the primary principles of the procedure.

The thrust of this approach is that the entire dissection be performed extraperitoneally. This is based on several considerations. The first involves the observation that patients appear to recover more quickly when the peritoneum has not been violated. Presumably, this is because of the decreased postoperative ileus that is seen because bowel manipulation is avoided. The second concerns the minimization of intra-peritoneal adhesion formation, which could conceivably produce postoperative obstructive problems in the short term and could possibly make subsequent intraperitoneal exploration more difficult.

To analyze this intriguing question in a more systematic way, the EORTC has decided to embark on a prospective, randomized study of translumbar versus transperitoneal approaches involving more than 1000 patients with renal cell carcinoma stage pT_1–pT_3 that would normally undergo 'radical' nephrectomy (study coordinator: D. Jacqmin, Strasbourg). This large number is necessary to make it a true study of equivalence between the two treatment arms, with less than 5% difference to be detected. Additional important study endpoints include a thorough assessment of quality of life, the determination of the time to return to normal activity after the operation, and the evaluation of perioperative morbidity associated with either one of the surgical approaches.

Adjuvant immunotherapy

In the case of a macroscopically radical tumor resection for renal cell carcinoma, adjuvant immunotherapies have been advocated to reduce the recurrence rate. Current reviews on this topic concluded, however, that this approach must be considered as experimental therapy[24,25], since all six randomized trials so far, including the large Delta-P-protocol, were negative and did not demonstrate a survival benefit. Nevertheless, all these trials were not statistically powerful enough to detect small differences at a low event rate so as not to permit firm conclusions. In this situation, the EORTC went on to develop a protocol randomizing between one cycle of adjuvant triple drug (interferon-β, interleukin-2, 5-fluorouracil) therapy versus watchful waiting in a group of patients considered to be at higher risk for a relapse after a potentially curative tumor resection (such as positive lymph nodes, positive surgical margins or macroscopic/microscopic venous tumor invasion). Until results from EORTC 30955 become available, adjuvant immunotherapy should only be applied in the context of controlled clinical trials.

Conclusion

For many years, the textbook belief was to advocate 'radical' nephrectomy via a trans-peritoneal approach as the standard procedure for renal cell carcinoma. This philosophy was based on retrospective data[2,3] which were never confirmed in a controlled trial. Since then, evidence has kept accumulating that some patients may be better served by an extra-peritoneal approach, providing similar oncological efficacy, but reduced morbidity. However, these results are either retrospective again[20–22] or statistically not significant[23], and, therefore, do not permit firm conclusions. Nevertheless, it is clear that, if there is a difference at all with respect to a possible intraoperative tumor dissemination, depending on the type of surgical approach performed, this difference will be small, awaiting analysis in a large, randomized, multicenter trial.

Until reliable data from this EORTC trial become available, it is advisable to remain careful. It is most probable that small (< 7 cm) unilateral renal cell carcinomas may safely be approached via a translumbar (intercostal) incision. In patients with a large tumor mass, involvement of the vena cava, or where local regional lymph node dissection is desired, the author still prefers to perform a transperitoneal tumor nephrectomy.

References

1. Mickisch GH. New trends in the treatment of renal cancer. *Akt Urol* 1994;25:77–83

2. Robson CJ. Radical nephrectomy for renal cell carcinoma. *J Urol* 1963;89:37–42

3. Robson CJ. The results of radical nephrectomy for renal cell carcinoma. *J Urol* 1969;101:297–301

4. Hafez KS, Novick AC, Butler B. Management of small, solitary, unilateral renal cell carcinomas: impact of central versus peripheral tumor location. *J Urol* 1998;159:1156–60

5. Poppel v H, Baert L. Elective conservative surgery for renal cell carcinoma. *AUA Update Series* 1994; 13:246–58

6. Novick AC. Nephron-sparing surgery for renal cell carcinoma. *Br J Urol* 1998;82:321–4

7. Mickisch GHJ. Lymph node dissection for renal cell carcinoma – the value of operation and adjuvant therapy. *Urologe (A)* 1999;38:326–31

8. Wunderlich H, Schlichter A, Reichelt O, *et al.* Real indications for adrenalectomy in renal cell carcinoma. *Eur Urol* 1999;35:272–6

9. Poppel v H, Bamelis B, Oyen R, Baert L. Partial nephrectomy for renal cell carcinoma can achieve long-term tumor control. *J Urol* 1998;160: 674–8

10. Poppel v HP, Bamelis BF, Baert LV. Non-metastatic renal cell carcinoma. *Curr Opin Urol* 1996;6:241–6

11. Butler BP, Novick AC, Miller DP, Campbell SA, Licht MR. Management of small unilateral renal cell carcinomas: radical versus nephron-sparing surgery. *Urology* 1995;45:34–40

12. Lemer SE, Hawkins CA, Blute ML, *et al.* Disease outcome in patients with low stage renal cell carcinoma treated with nephron sparing or radical surgery. *J Urol* 1996;155:1868–73

13. Pizzocaro G. Lymphadenectomy in renal adeno-carcinoma. In deKemion JB, Pavone-Macaluso M, eds. *Tumors of the kidney.* Baltimore: Williams & Wilkins, 1986:75–86

14. Waters WB, Richie JP. Aggressive surgical approach to renal cell carcinoma: review of 130 cases. *J Urol* 1979;122:306–9

15. Herrlinger A, Schrott KM, Sigel A, Giedl J. Results of 381 transabdominal radical nephrectomies for renal cell carcinoma with partial and complete en-bloc lymph-node dissection. *World J Urol* 1984;2:114–21

16. Giuliani L, Martorana G, Giberti C, Pescatore D, Magnani G. Results of radical nephrectomy with extensive lymphadenectomy for renal cell carcinoma. *J Urol* 1983;130:664–8

17. Blom JHM, van Poppel H, Marechal JM, *et al.* Radical nephrectomy with and without lymph node dissection; preliminary results of the EORTC randomised phase III protocol 30881. *Eur Urol* 1999;36:570–5

18. Peters PC, Brown GL. The role of lymph-adenectomy in the management of renal cell carcinoma. *Urol Clin North Am* 1980;7:705–9

19. Guiliani L, Gilberti C, Martorana G, Rovida S. Radical extensive surgery for renal cell carcinoma: long-term results and prognostic factors. *J Urol* 1990;143:468–77

20. Droller MJ. Anatomic considerations in extra-peritoneal approach to radical nephrectomy. *Urology* 1990;36:118–23

21. Sugao H, Matsuda M, Nakano E, Seguchi T, Sonoda T. Comparison of lumbar flank approach and transperitoneal approach for radical nephrectomy. *Urol Int* 1991;46:43–5

22. Kageyama Y, Fukiu I, Goto S, *et al.* Treatment results of radical nephrectomy for relatively confined small renal cell carcinoma. Translumbar versus transabdominal approach. *Jpn J Urol* 1994;85:599–603

23. Ditonno P, Saracino GA, Macchia M, Battaglia M, Selvaggi FP. Prospective randomized trial comparing lombotomic versus laparotomic access in the surgery of renal cell carcinoma. *Br J Urol* 1997;80(Suppl 2):119

24. Bukowsky RM. Natural history and therapy of metastatic renal cell carcinoma. *Cancer* 1997; 80:1198–220

25. Novick AC. Current surgical approaches, nephron-sparing surgery, and the role of surgery in the integrated immunologic approach to renal cell carcinoma. *Semin Oncol* 1995; 22:29–33

New applications of cytokines: inhalation of interleukin-2 to control pulmonary metastases

7

E. Huland, H. Heinzer, M. Aalamian and H. Huland

Introduction

The rationale for local cytokine therapy is to expose tumor tissue and surrounding lymph nodes to therapeutic – immunomodulatory – levels of the cytokine in question, without the toxicity associated with systemic administration. Michael Lotze highlighted this strategy in a recent Editorial[1] stating that 'delivery of high local concentrations of IL-2 [interleukin-2] may more closely mirror the normal physiological production of IL-2, which is normally produced at high concentration in a localized milieu'.

Local IL-2 application without intravascular IL-2 produces objective local tumor responses, induces local and systemic immunomodulation, and, most importantly, is much less toxic than systemic therapy. Patients at risk or in poor general condition can be treated and long-term treatment to maintain partial responses or stabilization becomes possible.

In addition, it has been demonstrated, that soluble products from renal cell carcinoma explants induce immune dysfunction in normal T cells by loss of IL-2 and interferon (IFN)-γ production and reduced proliferative capacity. This effect is dose-dependent and influences immune responses significantly, especially at local sites[2]. Local IL-2 administration may restore local immune dysfunction.

Local administration can be accomplished via continuous infusion, continuous perfusion or repeated injection of a tumor, via inhalation, intravesical instillation, intrasplenic or intrahepatic infusion or perfusion. Delivery systems such as portable infusion pumps, transdermal carriers, biodegradable hydrogels and gene modulation can be used to provide continuous low-level exposure of local tissues to cytokines. The diversity of administration routes and schedules indicates that we are still in the early process of defining optimum strategies for local cytokine therapy and there may be individual advantages and disadvantages as discussed at a recent meeting in Hamburg[3]. Local cytokine tumor necrosis factor (TNF)-α treatment is already approved. Isolated limb perfusion using TNF-α in combination with melphalan has been demonstrated to induce high local response rates in melanoma and sarcoma patients and prevent amputation[4–6]. As TNF-α by itself has no, or only minimal, effect on tumor growth, an increase in local concentrations of chemotherapeutic drugs might well be the main mechanism for the synergistic antitumor effects[7].

The use of pulmonary IL-2 delivery to perform local cytokine therapy and control pulmonary metastatic growth has been reported from different groups and for different cancers. Several hundred patients have been treated with inhalation of IL-2, exclusively, or in addition to systemic therapy, operation and/or radiation[8]. Good tolerance has been confirmed. Inhaled IL-2 is reported to induce dose-dependent local and systemic immunomodulation with minimal toxicity, seen mainly as World Health Organization (WHO) grade I and II cough, and to prevent progression of pulmonary and mediastinal metastases of renal cell carcinoma and other primary tumors, such as melanoma, mammary carcinoma and gynecological tumors in first- and second-line therapy. Dosage and schedule may influence treatment outcome.

In bronchoalveolar lavage a dose-dependent, significant increase in lymphocyte and eosinophils has been described in patients as well as in animals.

This report summarizes the experience with local inhaled IL-2 application in advanced tumor disease. Most patients had renal cell carcinoma but gynecological tumors, breast carcinoma, melanoma and primary lung tumors have also been reported. Use of local inhaled IL-2 may serve as a model for providing relevant information concerning the advantages and problems of local application in general.

Biological activity

Using cytokines in new applications requires the evaluation of preserved biological activity under the specific conditions in use and with the cytokine in question. It has been shown that nebulized IL-2 is biologically active. A jet nebulizer (Salvia Lifetec, Kronberg, Germany), of the same type used clinically, was adapted for laboratory needs to allow sterile recovery after *in vitro* nebulization. Natural IL-2, recombinant glycosylated IL-2 and recombinant non-glycosylated IL-2 were each nebulized under sterile conditions in doses and schedules comparable with those used in patients. The mean quantitative re-detection rate of IL-2 using the enzyme-linked immunosorbent assay (ELISA) was 15–22 %, but this rigid system might produce substantial losses not directly comparable with *in vivo* use. More importantly, the biological activity of nebulized solutions was tested in a cytotoxic T lymphocyte line (CTLL) proliferation assay and was proved after *in vitro* nebulization in all IL-2 preparations. The CTLL cell number increased by 1.41–1.98 times 5 days after incubation, well in the range of stimulation with the rat IL-2 used as a control[9].

Exclusive local therapy

Phase I trial

Treatment with inhaled IL-2 was found to be safe and to induce significant local immuno-modulatory and antitumor effects.

Study design A phase I trial in which three doses of IL-2, given as five inhalations per day for 6 weeks were used, was carried out at the University of Mainz[10]. The study was performed according to 'Good Clinical Practice' guidelines. Inhalation of IL-2 was the only treatment given to 16 patients with proven progressive disease – 14 with metastatic renal cell carcinoma and two with non-small-lung carcinoma – who were treated as outpatients. Five of the 16 patients had undergone unsuccessful pre-treatment with one or more immunotherapies. Five times a day the patients inhaled 200 000, 600 000 and 1 200 000 BRMP U (biologic response modifier units) of natural IL-2. According to our *in vitro* nebulization, those numbers have to be multiplied by about a factor of 15–20 to compare with international units (IU) of IL-2 (data not published). Compliance with treatment was close to 100% (as counted by empty vials).

Bronchoalveolar lavage was performed before treatment and at 2 weeks of treatment. This allowed measurement of total broncho-alveolar lavage cell recovery, absolute counts of different immune cells, and analysis of a huge series of cell-surface antigens by fluorescent activated-cell sorting (FACS) in both blood and bronchoalveolar lavage fluid. Serum IL-2 and soluble CD25 were also determined. Detailed lung function analysis – including spirography, flow-volume analysis, body plethysmography and blood-gas analysis – was performed once a week.

Tumor response was evaluated at week 6 and treatment was continued in the event of partial or complete response (according to WHO criteria). In the event of stable or progressive disease, treatment was stopped.

Side-effects and feasibility All but three of the 16 patients completed the trial according to the protocol. Treatment was stopped in two patients because of progression of non-pulmonary metastases to the brain and bone.

The only adverse event related to the study medication was a rib fracture caused by severe coughing and occurred in a patient receiving the highest dose of IL-2 – 5 × 1 200 000 BRMP U per day.

Toxicity consisted of a non-productive cough and was dose-dependent. Only one of the five patients receiving the lowest dose, but all of the five patients receiving the highest dose, experienced coughing. Local irritation of the upper respiratory tract was observed in two of the patients on the highest dose and no one else. All other events were sporadic. No patient experienced a flu-like syndrome. Severe side-effects and signs of capillary leak syndrome were absent.

Lung function disturbances were mild to moderate, with a tendency to be dose-dependent, and showed a restrictive pattern. They were influenced by throat irritation, partly because spirography maneuvers were difficult to perform. Severe or life-threatening lung function disturbances followed by pronounced oxygen desaturation were not observed throughout the trial. All respiratory symptoms disappeared rapidly after treatment was stopped.

Clinical response   Three of the 14 patients with renal cell carcinoma experienced regression of pulmonary metastases. One patient, with multiple small-lung metastases, experienced a durable complete remission (33+ months); one experienced a partial remission but died after 9 months from brain metastases and one showed complete regression of pulmonary metastases, but progression at non-pulmonary sites of the disease. According to the authors, the mixed response in the third patient is of particular interest because this patient was heavily pretreated with systemic IL-2 and IFN-α[10].

Local immune response by bronchoalveolar lavage
Two weeks after the start of treatment with aerosolized IL-2, bronchoalveolar lavage fluid showed a significant dose-dependent increase in cell concentration, that was due mainly to lymphocytes and eosinophil granulocytes. Lymphocyte numbers increase by a factor of more than eight 14 days after the beginning of treatment at the highest dose. Inhalation of IL-2 affected not only the number, but also the phenotype of lymphocytes. Bronchoalveolar lavage lymphocytes showed an activated lymphocyte phenotype, with a significant dose-dependent increase in expression of human leukocyte antigen (HLA)-DR and CD11b[10].

Further detailed functional analysis of alveolar macrophages has been based on measuring the accessory cell function as mediated by cell–cell interaction. Accessory signals are considered to be a prerequisite for an optimal stimulation of T cells. Before IL-2 inhalation, alveolar macrophages of patients showed a lower accessory index than those of the controls. However, combining the results of the patients with those of the controls revealed a significant negative correlation between the accessory index of alveolar macrophages and peripheral blood monocytes and patient age. The accessory index of alveolar macrophages increases after IL-2 inhalation in a dose-dependent manner, and this abrogates the negative correlation with patient age and suggests an activation of accessory cells regardless of the age of the cell donor[11].

Alveolar macrophage cytokine release was not altered in analyses for TNF-α, IL-6, IL-8 and macrophage inflammatory protein-1α[12].

Systemic immune response in peripheral blood   In all patients, an increase in serum soluble CD25 could be detected, peaking on day 7 after the start of treatment with the highest dose level of IL-2. No changes were observed in the lower-dose groups. Peripheral blood monocytes also responded to IL-2 inhalation; the rise was not as pronounced as that of the accessory index for alveolar macrophages, but was significant at the highest dose[10,11].

Phase II trial: clinical, multicenter study

Seven investigative centers in Germany participated in a multicenter study according to 'Good Clinical Practice' guidelines in order to evaluate tolerance to, and efficacy of, inhaled natural IL-2 in patients with pulmonary metastases of renal cell carcinoma[13]. The study was terminated prematurely after inclusion of 24 of the projected 47 patients, because the company (Biotest, Dreieich, Germany) expected recombinant IL-2 to be more cost-effective than natural IL-2, a possibly infectious natural blood product. The treatment achieved a response rate of 29%, including two patients with partial response and five patients with stable disease for at least 6 months. Every patient had to have proven progressive disease prior to inclusion. Adverse events most frequently reported concerned the respiratory tract. No serious adverse event was directly related to the study medication. Of ten episodes of serious adverse events reported during the study, nine were not related to the medication and the tenth was probably not related. Inhaled IL-2 in this study appeared to combine good efficacy and improved tolerance.

Inhaled IL-2 in combination with systemic immunotherapy and immunochemotherapy

Several hundred patients with metastatic renal cell carcinoma have been treated with inhaled IL-2 in combination with systemic therapy, and long-term data on safety and efficacy are available. Early results are also available on the use of inhaled IL-2 in a variety of different diseases and in combination with various systemic therapies.

Renal cell carcinoma

The most advanced information on the benefits of and risks posed by inhalation of IL-2 is related to metastatic renal cell carcinoma involving the lung or mediastinum. Inhaled IL-2 is therapeutically effective and has low toxicity[14–22]. The Hamburg database includes long-term experience with inhaled IL-2 in 208 patients (151 men, 57 women) who had pulmonary or mediastinal metastatic renal cell carcinoma. To receive treatment, patients had to have proven progressive pulmonary metastases. Most patients were referred to our clinic for inhalation immunotherapy because it has been the standard procedure at our clinic for

outpatient treatment of pulmonary metastatic renal cell carcinoma since 1996 and has been analyzed in studies since 1989.

The mean age of the patients was 58.6 (19–76) years; the performance status of the patients according to the Eastern Cooperative Oncology Group (ECOG) was as follows: 24 had an ECOG of 0, 150 had an ECOG of 1, 33 had an ECOG of 2 and one had an ECOG of 3. Overall median expected survival according to risk criteria[23] prospectively assigned, was 5.3 months. High-dose inhaled IL-2 application was used exclusively in 11% of the patients, low-dose systemic IL-2 in 58% of the patients and low-dose systemic IL-2 with IFN-α in 31% of the patients.

Out of the patients, 42% had only pulmonary metastases and 58% had other metastases in addition. Some 44 patients (21%) had received prior systemic immunotherapy with IL-2, IFN-α or a combination of the two. At least 80–90% of the dose of IL-2 was applied by inhalation and 10–20% by subcutaneous injection. A total of 36×10^6 IU of IL-2 were divided into six parts, five parts given as five inhalations per day and one part given as a subcutaneous injection 6 days per week. Treatment was continued as long as at least stabilization of pulmonary metastases was present. Pulmonary metastatic tumor growth was influenced in 68% of all patients: complete response was achieved in 3% and partial response in 10% for a median duration of 16.8 and 10.3 months, respectively, (range 4.1–43.9 months) and stabilization was achieved in 55% of the patients for a median of 18, 10.7 and 8.5 months in complete response, partial response and stable disease, respectively. A total of 32% had progressive disease. Overall median actual survival time in patients was significantly prolonged to 17.2 months (range 0.9–67.3 months).

Maximum toxicity, analyzed weekly during the mean treatment time of 12.6 months, was WHO grade I in 11% of patients, grade II in 65% and grade III in 24% of patients. No patient experienced grade IV toxicity.

Pulmonary and mediastinal progression can be prevented by inhaled IL-2 without major toxicity in 68% of patients. Risk analysis gives evidence of a significant survival benefit. Interestingly, subgroup analysis shows benefit not only for 'good-risk' groups but also for high-risk groups, according also to Elson and colleagues[23] (Table 1). Quality of life during outpatient treatment was good and allowed performance of social activities and professional roles. In addition, patients for whom systemic IL-2 was not suitable could still be treated with inhaled IL-2.

Heidenreich and Neubauer[20] treated 16 patients with metastatic renal cell carcinoma after radical nephrectomy as the first-line therapy with mainly inhaled IL-2, according to a published schedule[16]. Mean treatment duration was 12 months, and 13 patients were evaluable with regard to response (follow-up over 3 months). Two patients (15.4%) developed a partial response and nine patients (69.3%) were stable. The mean duration of response was 9 months (range 3–22 months). Patients developed cough, nausea and fatigue not exceeding WHO grade II, except in one patient, whose therapy had to be discontinued.

In Marburg, 14 patients with pulmonary metastases of renal cell carcinoma underwent IL-2 inhalation (18×10^6 IU given as three inhalations per day for 5 days per week) in combination with systemic IFN-α and vinblastine as reported by Varga and Knobloch[19]. Twelve weeks after the initiation of therapy, patients with responding and stable disease received a maintenance treatment of inhalation of IL-2 only. Two patients were not evaluable (unrelated death and poor compliance), two patients had complete response (36 and 6 months), six patients partial response (16, 8, 7,

6, 6 and 5 months) and two patients stable disease (4 and 3 months). Two patients had disease progression. Except for moderate irritative coughing, no side-effects were reported.

In Hanover, Atzpodien initiated a multi-center randomized trial[24], to evaluate the safety and efficacy of adding short-term inhaled IL-2 to a protocol using systemic subcutaneous IL-2, IFN-α and 13-cis-retinoic acid. The first patient in Hamburg treated according to this protocol with additional inhalation showed significant tumor reduction (Figure 1).

Nakamoto and co-workers[21] report the use of inhalation of IL-2 in combination with the subcutaneous administration of IFN-α-2a in seven patients treated in Hiroshima, Japan. Six patients received therapy for at least 3 months, five of these six responded to treatment, two had partial response and three had stable disease. One patient progressed and one had to stop

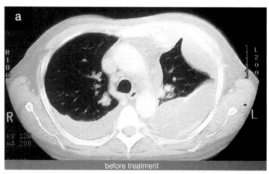
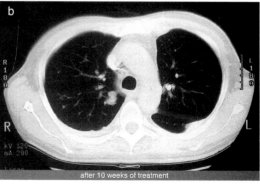

Figure 1 Patient before (a) and after 3 months (b) of combination therapy using high-dose inhalation of IL–2 and systemic subcutaneous IL–2, interferon-α and 13-cis-retinoic acid according to a multicenter protocol initiated by Atzpodien[24]

Table 1 Observed versus expected survival in pulmonary metastatic renal cell carcinoma patients treated mainly with inhaled IL-2 immunotherapy[23]

Elson risk group	Number of patients	Expected median survival (months)	Observed median survival (months)
1	25	12.8	26.7
2	62	7.7	24.4
3	67	5.3	16.1
4	38	3.4	11.8
5	16	2.3	3.8

treatment early because of poor performance status. No serious side-effects were reported, except dyspnea, described as 'pulmonary fibrosis', which occurred 4 months after treatment started and which was immediately reversible on stopping treatment.

Inhalation as second-line immunotherapy Seven patients who had progressive disease after treatment with a combination of IL-2, IFN-α and 5-fluorouracil who presented with a high pulmonary tumor burden received high-dose $(36 \times 10^6 \text{ IU})$ inhalation of IL-2 in combination with low doses of subcutaneous IL-2 according to the protocol used in Hamburg, as a second-line option[22]. Partial response was observed in four patients, two remained stable and one progressed under therapy. Partial responses and stable disease had a median response time of 8 months. Home-based therapy was well-tolerated and toxicity did not exceed WHO grades I–II, except for a cough at grade III. Two patients were able to continue their professions.

Atzpodien has reported second-line treatment using inhaled IL-2 therapy in addition to immunochemotherapy (rIFN-α, rIL-2, 13-*cis*-retinoic acid and intravenous vinblastine)[25]. He describes safety, good tolerance, reduction in pulmonary tumor load and long-term pulmonary disease stabilization in up to 30% of patients. Inhaled IL-2 was given in four inhalations per day for a total daily dose of $36 \times 10^6 \text{ IU}$. Treatment was performed 5 days per week.

Inhaled IL-2 in combination with systemic chemotherapy

Melanoma (second-line)

High-dose $(36 \times 10^6 \text{ IU})$ IL-2 given as five inhalations per day was used by Enk and colleagues in 27 patients suffering from stage IV metastatic melanoma[26]. All patients were pretreated with dacarbazine (DTIC) chemotherapy, all except one with systemic immunotherapy and four with cisplatin. Inhalation therapy was combined with a bolus infusion of chemotherapy consisting of DTIC at a dose of $850 \text{ mg}/\text{m}^2$ of body surface once every 4 weeks. Five patients had complete response, eight partial response, five stable disease and eight progression; one patient was not evaluable. Side-effects of treatment were minimal and quality of life during treatment was good[26].

Breast carcinoma and ovarian cancer (second-line)

Petzoldt and colleagues reported eight patients with pulmonary metastases of breast carcinoma and two with ovarian cancer who received, in addition to chemotherapy, inhaled IL-2 $(15–36 \times 10^6 \text{ IU}$ divided into five inhalations per day) for 5 days per week during the interval of cytotoxic treatment. All patients were pretreated with one or several kinds of chemotherapy $(4 \times \text{high dose}, 3 \times \text{taxane}, 3 \times \text{cyclophosphamide})$ after the operation. In addition, four patients received prior hormone treatment, one antibody therapy and one intrapleural interferon instillation. The two patients with ovarian carcinoma were pretreated with six cycles of gemcitabine and cisplatin. Progressive pulmonary metastases responded in seven of the ten patients with partial response (mean duration 6.4 months), two of the ten had no change (mean duration 7.5 months) and one had progression under therapy. Toxicity was limited to WHO grades I–II and consisted mainly of cough[27].

Inhaled IL-2 as cyclic therapy

Bronchioloalveolar carcinoma

This rare malignant lung tumor is a disease mainly of elderly patients without clear correlation to tobacco smoking. The tumor is characterized by its growth, spreading along the alveolar septa. It shows clinical behavior that differs from classical pulmonary adeno-carcinoma. Eight patients were treated with $3 \times 6 \times 10^6 \text{ IU}$ IL-2 daily by inhalation in cycles consisting of 2 weeks of inhalation therapy with 1 week pause, repeated 3 times.

All but one patient progressed after the first cycle (3 × weeks). No adverse effects except for a mild cough were reported. According to the authors, the study design was not sufficient to answer the question of whether higher dosages or combination therapies might improve the results[28]. Using a non-cyclic schedule, the same group has reported the induction of an objective response in one of three patients and stable disease (dose-dependent) in another[29].

Quality of life

A subjective and objective prospective quality-of-life analysis during high-dose IL-2 inhalation treatment (mean treatment times of 13.4 months) in 15 patients who had metastatic renal cell carcinoma showed a modest but statistically significant decrease 1 month after the beginning of treatment. However, at 3, 6, 9 and 12 months, the scores did not differ significantly from pretreatment scores. Inhaled IL-2 stabilized the quality of life for a median of 13.4 months in these patients. In comparison, patients receiving low-dose intravenous IL-2 (9×10^6 IU/m^2) had a more marked statistically significant decrease in subjective quality of life, and three of ten were not evaluable, because they felt too functionally impaired[30].

Comparison of systemic versus inhalative therapy

We compared two databases, that included patients with metastatic renal cell carcinoma treated in different protocols with subcutaneous IL-2 and inhaled IL-2. Except for the ECOG performance status (45% had an ECOG status of 0, 55% of 1 and 4% of 2 in the subcutaneous IL-2 group, while 5% had an ECOG status of 0, 86% of 1 and 9% of 2 in the inhaled IL-2 group), patients were comparable in risk factors. The two groups had about the same median survival (13.1 and 13.8 months), and the same 1-year survival (56% and 55%) and 2-year survival rates (26% and 28%, respectively). However, toxicity was clearly different, the inhalation group had no grade IV and about 50% of grade III toxicity, despite less co-medication[31].

Liposomal IL-2 for inhalation

In animal therapy, inhaled liposomal IL-2 has been reported to be effective and to induce local lung immunomodulation[32]. Seven dogs with pulmonary metastases and two dogs with primary lung carcinomas were treated with aerosols of IL-2 liposomes. Two of four dogs with pulmonary metastatic osteosarcoma had complete regression of disease for more than 12 and 20 months. One of two dogs with lung carcinoma experienced stabilization for more than 8 months. Toxicity was minimal. Broncho-alveolar lavage cell numbers increased more than four-fold ($p = 0.01$) and included significantly greater proportions and numbers of eosinophils ($p = 0.006$) and lymphocytes ($p = 0.008$). Canine antibodies against human IL-2 and human serum albumin were detected in all dogs.

Conclusions

Inhaled IL-2 has minimal toxicity and is effective in preventing pulmonary progressive disease in metastatic renal cell carcinoma, melanoma and possibly in other diseases such as breast carcinoma and gynecological tumors. Inhaled IL-2 therapy may serve as a model for the use of new cytokine applications.

Local application is useful if local control of metastases induces better quality of life and/or prolongation of survival. Avoiding amputation through limb perfusion clearly has an impact on the quality of life as has the control of pulmonary tumor growth to avoid choking. Analysis of survival benefits may help to identify subgroups who would also benefit in terms of survival, e.g. patients with lung metastases, only or predominantly.

One major advantage of such a well-tolerated application of IL-2 is the inclusion of patients who would be untreatable using toxic systemic immunotherapy because of their co-morbidity or advanced disease. According to risk analysis, these patients also seem to benefit significantly in survival from inhaled IL-2. Another advantage for all patients is that a good quality of life during therapy makes outpatient treatment possible and permits the performance of social activities[30] and various groups report that patients can stay in their profession during therapy. All groups using inhaled IL-2 reported good tolerance to treatment. Cost-effectiveness and acceptance of expensive cytokine therapy must be discussed in the light of such findings. The American Society of Clinical Oncology (ASCO) guidelines[33] state that 'patient outcomes (e.g. survival and quality of life) should receive a higher priority than cancer outcome (e.g. response rate)'. Another advantage is the possibility of long-term treatment, which might contribute to long-term stabilization of proven progressive disease. Comparison of the Chiron and Hamburg databases[31] provides evidence that, despite different ECOG and response rates, the survival of patients in the inhalation group can be as good as that of systemically treated patients.

The success of inhaled IL-2 seems to be dose-dependent and schedule-dependent. Higher doses lead to significant increases in local immunomodulation, but also to increased local toxicity, such as cough. Frequent daily applications have been reported to be effective; single daily inhalations have not shown significant effects so far. Frequently repeated exposure of immune cells to IL-2 may be necessary to induce immunomodulation. Bronchoalveolar lavage fluid in patients receiving exclusive inhalation of IL-2, using five inhalations per day, showed a significant and dose-dependent increase in lymphocytes and eosinophils[10,11]. This effect has been confirmed in animals treated with IL-2 liposome inhalation[32]. Three of seven dogs responded to treatment.

A special concern with inhalation of IL-2 is long-term safety. In patients using inhaled IL-2, no chronic inflammation or irreversible fibrotic tissue reactions in the lung have been reported. Long-term safety of additives especially in combination with IL-2 must be confirmed before clinical use since IL-2 changes the immunological reaction pattern and is able to

break tolerance to possible antigens. Liposomes in combination with IL-2 and antigen are reported to induce a significant secondary immune response against liposomal vesicles[32]. Long-term safety of liposome IL-2 inhalation is unclear since animal numbers are small and follow-up and treatment times are short. In patients, no additives to buffer solutions have been used except human serum albumen. Median treatment times of 12.6 months and individual treatment times of more than 60 months have been safe in short-term and long-term evaluations.

Several groups report tumor responses in all or individual patients using inhaled IL-2 as a second-line treatment after systemic immunotherapy or after systemic chemotherapy, and a response to inhaled IL-2 in patients pretreated with chemotherapy, immunotherapy and, in particular, with systemic IL-2 has been reported repeatedly.

Metastatic tumor spread is a systemic disease most probably requiring systemic treatment. Local use of IL-2 has therapeutic efficacy, avoids vascular leakage, and, thus, allows the use of the full potential of cytokines with little or no toxicity. A combination of local and systemic IL-2 tailored individually to the patient's ECOG and acceptance may be a future approach for optimizing treatment for the individual patient. In a recently started multicenter protocol at our Institute, a combination of systemic immunotherapy and inhalation is being evaluated and has already led to significant tumor reduction in the first patient treated with this schedule (Figure 1). Regional IL-2 application is not in competition with, but complementary to, systemic treatment.

Regional application of IL-2 may change treatment options not only for metastatic melanoma and renal cell carcinoma, but also for a variety of other different tumors. Efficacy has been reported and life-threatening toxicity is of no concern in local treatment. This might lead to a favorable outcome in many patients.

References

1. Lotze MT. The future role of interleukin-2 in cancer therapy [Editorial]. *Cancer J Sci Am* 2000; 6(Suppl 1):S58–60
2. Rayman P, Uzzo RG, Kolenko V, *et al.* Tumor-induced dysfunction in interleukin-2 production and interleukin-2 receptor signaling: a mechanism of immune escape. *Cancer J Sci Am* 2000;6(Suppl 1): S81–7
3. Bubenik J, Den Otter W, Huland E. Local cytokine therapy of cancer: interleukin-2, interferons and related cytokines. *Cancer Immunol Immunother* 2000;49:116–22
4. Bickels J, Manusama ER, Gutman M, *et al.* Isolated limb perfusion with tumour necrosis factor-alpha and melphalan for unresectable bone sarcomas of the lower extremity. *Eur J Surg Oncol* 1999;25:509–14
5. Lienard D, Eggermont AM, Koops HS, *et al.* Isolated limb perfusion with tumour necrosis factor-alpha and melphalan with or without interferon-gamma for the treatment of in-transit melanoma metastases: a multicentre randomized phase II study. *Melanoma Res* 1999;9:491–502
6. Rauthe G, Sistermanns J. Recombinant tumour necrosis factor in the local therapy of malignant pleural effusion. *Eur J Cancer* 1997;33:226–31
7. van der Veen AH, de Wilt JH, Eggermont AM, *et al.* TNF-alpha augments intratumoural concentrations of doxorubicin in TNF-alpha-based isolated limb perfusion in rat sarcoma models and enhances anti-tumour effects. *Br J Cancer* 2000;82:973–80
8. Huland E, Heinzer H, Huland H, *et al.* Overview of interleukin-2 inhalation therapy. *Cancer J Sci Am* 2000; 6(Suppl 1):S104–12
9. Kelling S, Heinzer H, Huland E, *et al.* In-vitro model for nebulizing interleukin-2: quantitative evaluation and biological activity of three different preparations of nebulized interleukin-2 (Abstract). *Immunobiology* 1996;196:110–11
10. Lorenz J, Wilhelm K, Kessler M, *et al.* Phase I trial of inhaled natural interleukin 2 for treatment of pulmonary malignancy: toxicity, pharmacokinetics, and biological effects. *Clin Cancer Res* 1996;2:1115–22
11. Zissel G, Aulitzky WE, Lorenz J, *et al.* Induction of accessory cell function of human alveolar macrophages by inhalation of human natural interleukin-2. *Cancer Immunol Immunother* 1996; 42:122–6
12. Gaede KI, Zissel G, Schwulera U, *et al.* Spontaneous and interleukin-2-modulated cytokine release by bronchoalveolar cells in pulmonary malignancy. *Eur Cytokine Netw* 1997;8:395–400
13. Huland E, Heinzer H, Falk B, Huland H. Exklusive Inhalation von Interleukin-2 bei Patienten mit pulmonal metastasiertem Nierenzellkarzinom: erste Ergebnisse einer multizentrischen Studie (Abstract). *Urologe A* 1994;1/94:S72
14. Huland E, Huland H, Heinzer H. Interleukin-2 by inhalation: local therapy for metastatic renal cell carcinoma. *J Urol* 1992;147:344–8
15. Heinzer H, Huland E, Alamian M, *et al.* Treatment of pulmonary metastases from kidney cell carcinoma with inhalational interleukin-2. 10-year experience Hamburger Unicenter. *Urologe A* 1999;38:466–73
16. Huland E, Heinzer H, Huland H. Inhaled interleukin-2 in combination with low-dose systemic interleukin-2 and interferon alpha in patients with pulmonary metastatic renal-cell carcinoma: effectiveness and toxicity of mainly local treatment. *J Cancer Res Clin Oncol* 1994; 120:221–8
17. Huland E, Heinzer H, Mir TS, *et al.* Inhaled interleukin-2 therapy in pulmonary metastatic renal cell carcinoma: six years of experience. *Cancer J Sci Am* 1997;3 (Suppl 1):S98–105
18. Huland E, Heinzer H, Huland H. Immunotherapy of pulmonary metastatic renal cell carcinoma: success dependent on risk factors? *Hepatogastroenterology* 1999;46(Suppl):1257–62
19. Varga Z, von Knobloch R. Interleukin-2 inhalation in combination with systemic alfa-interferon and vinblastine in pulmonary metastatic renal cell cancer: the Marburg experience (Abstract). *Anticancer Res* 1999;19: 2014
20. Heidenreich A, Neubauer S. Interleukin-2 inhalation therapy in pulmonary metastases of renal cell cancer – Cologne experience (Abstract). *Anticancer Res* 1999;19:2003
21. Nakamoto T, Kasaoka Y, Mitani S, *et al.* Inhaled interleukin-2 combined with subcutaneous administration of interferon for the treatment of pulmonary metastases from renal cell carcinoma. *Int J Urol* 1997;4:343–8
22. Roigas J. Inhalation of interleukin-2 as second line treatment: the Charite experience (Abstract). *Anticancer Res* 1999;19:2010–11
23. Elson PJ, Witte RS, Trump DL. Prognostic factors for survival in patients with recurrent or metastatic renal cell carcinoma. *Cancer Res* 1988;48:7310–13

24. Atzpodien J. Konsensusprotokoll Chemo-Immuntherapie des metastasiertten Nierenzell-karzinoms: subkutan Interferon alfa 2a, subkutan Interleukin-2 und peroral Isotretinoin mit inhalativem Interleukin-2, intravenösem 5-Fluoruracil oder peroral Capecitabine. *Ein Therapieoptimierungsvergleich der Deutschen Urologisch-Internistischen Multicentergruppe*, 1998

25. Atzpodien J. Immunotherapy in combination with inhalatory interleukin-2 therapy: first results. *Anticancer Res* 1999;19:1997

26. Enk AH, Nashan D, Rubben A, *et al*. High dose inhalation interleukin-2 therapy for lung metastases in patients with malignant melanoma. *Cancer* 2000;88:2042–6

27. Petzoldt B, PG, Kupka M, Köhler S, *et al*. Additive Immuntherapie bei pulmonal metastasierten gynäkologischen Karzinomen mit inhalativem Interleukin-2. *Geburtshilfe Frauenheilkd* 1999;59:157–62

28. Kullmer J, Kaiser UFK, Wolf M. Interleukin-2 inhalation in advanced bronchio-alveolar carcinoma. *Anticancer Res* 1999;19:2007

29. Kaiser U, Pflüger K, Havemann K. Inhalation therapy with interleukin-2 in broncho-alveolar carcinoma. *Onkologie* 1995;18:94

30. Heinzer H, Mir TS, Huland E, *et al*. Subjective and objective prospective, long-term analysis of quality of life during inhaled interleukin-2 immunotherapy. *J Clin Oncol* 1999;17:3612–20

31. Huland E, Heinzer H, Huland H. A comparison of systemic versus inhaled recombinant IL-2 administration for the treatment of metastatic renal cell carcinoma. *Folia Biologica* 2000;in press

32. Khanna C, Anderson PM, Hasz DE, *et al*. Interleukin-2 liposome inhalation therapy is safe and effective for dogs with spontaneous pulmonary metastases. *Cancer* 1997;79:1409–21

33. American Society of Clinical Oncology. Outcomes of cancer treatment for technology assessment and cancer treatment guidelines. *J Clin Oncol* 1996;14:671–9

Management of advanced renal cell carcinoma

8

R. O. Northway, C. W. M. Ritenour and F. F. Marshall

Renal cell carcinoma may present as a serendipitous finding on a routine radiological evaluation for vague abdominal symptoms. Relatively few patients present with the classic triad of hematuria, flank pain and a flank mass. They may also present with unusual metastases, ranging from the thyroid gland to the vagina[1]. Paraneoplastic syndromes may be quite common with renal cell carcinoma. Hypercalcemia, hepatic dysfunction, anemia, hypertension, cachexia, pyrexia, erythrocytosis and amyloidosis have all been reported with renal cell carcinoma[2]. Serum ferritin, erythropoietin, calcium and renin[3] levels have all been elevated in some patients. More recently, even thrombocytosis has been associated with a poor prognosis compared to a normal platelet count in patients with metastatic disease[4]. The aggressiveness of tumors can be measured with tests such a proliferating cell nuclear antigen[5]. Metastasis may involve more than proliferation. Cellular adhesion molecules (CAMs) and angiogenesis factors undoubtedly play a role. Cadherins are a large family of transmembrane proteins responsible for mediating cell-to-cell adhesion. Lack of E-cadherin correlates with aggressiveness from tumors[6]. Cadherin-6 is expressed primarily in the proximal renal tubule and tumors. Aberrant expression of cadherin-6 is associated with poor survival[7,8].

Standard radiological evaluations with sonography, intravenous pyelography, computerized tomographic (CT) scans and magnetic resonance imaging (MRI) have all been refined. More recently, three-dimensional helical CT has been very accurate in predicting the pathological stage of tumors and the delineation of renal arteries and renal veins[9,10]. It can also delineate tumor in the vena cava, although MRI is the preferred radiological investigation when there is apparent intracaval tumor.

The therapy for advanced renal cell carcinoma remains varied. Therapy can include surgery, radiation, chemotherapy and immunotherapy. Frequently, patients undergo combination therapy. Very large tumors are not necessarily contraindications for surgical removal. Associated regional lymphadenectomy remains controversial. The regional lymphatic drainage of the kidney is periaortic on the left and perivenacaval on the right[11]. In addition, on the right there is interaortocaval drainage. As a result, a left-sided lymphadenectomy may be more efficacious than a right-sided one where an interaortocaval dissection is rarely performed. Although the efficacy of regional lymphadenectomy has been questioned, an occasional patient with microscopic disease can be cured. In the future, pathological staging and subsequent adjuvant therapy may continue to mandate regional lymphadenectomy.

Extension of renal cell carcinoma can occur into the vena cava. Extensive vena caval involvement to the right atrium was often thought to be inoperable; however, surgical advances, including cardiopulmonary bypass, hypothermia and circulatory arrest, have allowed the surgical excision of even intracardiac disease[12].

Chemotherapy for metastatic disease has generally been disappointing. Vinblastin was thought to be a more effective agent. However, when Yagoda and colleagues[13] performed an extensive review of over 83 published trials from 1983 to 1993, the overall response rate was 6%, in more than 4000 treated patients with advanced renal cell carcinoma. The most efficacious agents included continuously infused 5-fluorouracil and floxuridine, with remissions in 10–12% of patients. Other attempts to block multi-drug resistance to these tumors, using medications such as cyclosporin A, tamoxifen and calcium channel blockers[14], have largely been unsuccessful.

Radiotherapy has been used primarily in the setting of locally advanced or metastatic disease in the treatment of renal cell carcinoma. In general, radiation of a large renal tumor has not been effective. These tumors tend to be radioresistant. Bowel and surrounding structures may not tolerate a higher radiotherapeutic dose. Prolonged survival has not been improved with perioperative treatment[15]. On the other hand, intracranial lesions have been treated with stereotactically guided high-precision irradiation, which has been somewhat effective[16]. Radiotherapy can alleviate bone pain in as high as 77% of treated sites when osseous metastases are observed[17]. Novel phase I trials are utilizing the therapeutic potential of a radiolabelled (I-131) monoclonal antibody (G250) in the treatment of metastatic renal cell carcinoma[18]. Previously, this monoclonal antibody was identified in metastatic sites for renal cell carcinoma, even when they were not clear on CT scan.

Immunotherapy has become a recognized form of treatment for metastatic renal cell carcinoma. Through the years, as many as 100 cases of spontaneous regression have been reported[19]. Many approaches have been used, including biological response modifiers (cytokines, vaccinations and gene therapy). Interferon (IFN) has a recognized anti-tumor activity. Multiple studies have shown a reproducible response rate of 10–20%[20]. The patients who appear most likely to respond are those patients with good performance status who have undergone a prior nephrectomy. In general, patients with predominantly pulmonary metastases appeared to fare better[21]. Randomized trials have demonstrated only a modest increase in survival time, typically measured in months[22].

Interleukin-2 (IL-2) has been approved for the treatment of metastatic renal cell carcinoma by the US Food and Drug Administration since 1992. A 15–19% objective response rate with intravenous administration has been demonstrated[23]. In addition, the complete responders appear to have a durable response and most complete responders remain disease-free for more than 3 years. Toxicity can be severe, particularly with the higher dose intravenous therapy. Not only can there be gastrointestinal symptoms, but also capillary leak syndrome can produce hypotension, acute respiratory distress, confusion and renal failure. Modifying the dose may improve toxicity without changing efficacy[24]. Adding lymphokine-activated killer cells[25], tumor infiltrating lymphocytes[26], or interferon-α[27] does not appear to significantly improve survival over interleukin-2 alone.

Gene therapy is another new form of therapy that has generated much interest. Gene therapy involves the introduction of therapeutic DNA into cells with the use of a vector. The process of carcinogenesis may be reversed or prevented.

There are different kinds of treatment strategies. Corrective gene therapy involves the replacement or inactivation of defective genes so that cancer can be prevented or reversed. A number of years ago, the introduction of a normal 3p chromosome was shown to change the tumor growth rate in a renal cell carcinoma cell line[28]. On the other hand, significant limitations exist for corrective therapy, including the targeting efficacy and efficiency of vector transfer.

Cytoreductive gene therapy is a different approach, which utilizes recombinant DNA to selectively enhance the destruction of malignant cells. More than 80 clinical trials have been approved worldwide[29]. Extensive research investigating multiple cytokine genes has demonstrated that granulocyte macrophage colony-stimulating factor (GM-CSF) is one of the most effective single cytokines. Gene-transduced vaccines produce the most vigorous and durable tumor-specific immunity[30]. In patients with metastatic renal cell carcinoma, genetically transduced irradiated tumor vaccines induced a potent T-cell-mediated anti-tumor activity with minimal toxicity[31]. In this study, a paracrine, or local response, from the tumor vaccine was demonstrated to become systemic. Many other immunotherapies are being investigated. The mode of delivery, dose of cytokine, number of tumor cells for vaccine, and duration of treatment are all factors that will require significant additional study. Novel approaches using tumor-specific vaccination[32] or monoclonal antibodies may also be utilized[18].

Deficiencies in the immune system may influence tumor growth and metastasis. Immune suppression is a known characteristic of malignancy. Lymphocytes obtained from patients with metastatic renal cell carcinoma may have gene defects or defective T-cell receptor complexes[33]. Immune dysfunction may be present in more than one-half of patients with renal cell carcinoma[34]. More recently, several studies have indicated the benefit of a nephrectomy prior to systemic and interferon-α treatment, with prolongation of survival[35,36]. Most recently, a different

approach has yielded encouraging results. A non-myeloablative, allogeneic, peripheral blood stem cell transplantation has induced a graft versus tumor effect in patients with metastatic renal cell carcinoma[37]. A 53% response rate was seen in 19 patients (three complete responses, seven partial responses).

The normal kidney is exposed to many toxic elements during its normal existence and efficiently detoxifies or excretes these agents. As a result, it is not surprising that toxic chemotherapeutic agents do not exhibit a beneficial therapeutic effect in the treatment of renal cell carcinoma compared to many other cancers. As we obtain a greater understanding of the genetic basis of renal carcinogenesis, diagnosis and therapy of this tumor may change significantly. Surgical management for large tumors will remain, but molecular diagnosis and treatment will increase.

References

1. Belldegrun A, deKernion JB. Renal tumors. In Walsh P, Retik A, Vaughn ED, Wein A, eds. *Campbell's Urology*, 7th edn. Philadelphia: WB Saunders, 1998:ch 76

2. Marshall FF, Walsh PC. Extrarenal manifestations of renal cell carcinoma. *J Urol* 1977; 117:439–40

3. Sufrin G, Chasan S, Golio A, Murphy GP. Paraneoplastic and serologic syndromes of renal adenocarcinoma. *Semin Urol* 1989;7: 158–71

4. Sufrin G, Mirand EA, Moore RH. Hormones in renal cancer. *J Urol* 1977;117:433–8

5. Delahunt B, Bethwaite P, Nacey J, Ribas J. Proliferating cell nuclear antigen (PCNA) expression as a prognostic indicator for renal cell carcinoma: comparison with tumor grade, mitotic index and siver staining nucleolar organizer region numbers. *J Pathol* 1993;170: 471–7

6. Katagiri A, Wantanabe R, Tomita Y. E-cadherin expression in renal cell cancer and its significance in metastasis and survival. *Br J Urol* 1995;71:376–9

7. Shimazui T, Oosterwijk E, Akaza H, *et al.* Expression of cadherin-6 as a novel diagnostic tool to predict prognosis of patients with E-cadherin-absent renal cell carcinoma. *Clin Cancer Res* 1998;4:2419–24

8. Paul R, Ewing C, Robinson J, *et al.* Cadherin 6, a cell adhesion molecule specifically expressed in the proximal renal tubule and renal cell carcinoma. *Cancer Res* 1997;57:2741–8

9. Coll D, Usso R, Herts B, *et al.* Three-dimensional volume rendered computerized tomography for preoperative evaluation and intraoperative treatment of patients undergoing nephron-sparing surgery. *J Urol* 1999;161:1097–102

10. Smith P, Marshall F, Corl F, Fishman E. Planning nephron-sparing surgery using 3D helical CT angiography. *J Comp Assist Tomogr* 1999;23: 649–54

11. Marshall FF, Powell KC. Lymphadenectomy for renal cell carcinoma: anatomical and therapeutic considerations. *J Urol* 1982;128: 677–81

12. Marshall FF, Dietrick DD, Baumgartner WA, Rietz BA. Surgical management of renal cell

carcinoma with intracaval neoplastic extension above the hepatic veins. *J Urol* 1988;139:1166–72

13. Yagoda A, Abi-Rached B, Petrylak, D. Chemotherapy for advanced renal cell carcinoma 1983–1993. *Semin Oncol* 1995;22:42–62

14. Overmayer B, Fox B, Tomaszewski J, *et al.* A phase II trial of R-verapamil and infusional vinblastine (Velban) in advanced renal cell carcinoma (RCC). *Proc Am Soc Clin Oncol* 1993;12:251(792A)

15. Van der Werf-Messing B. Carcinoma of the kidney. *Cancer* 1973;32:1056–106

16. Mori Y, Kondziolka D, Flickinger J, *et al.* Stereotactic radiosurgery for brain metastasis from renal cell carcinoma. *Cancer* 1999;83: 344–53

17. Halperin E, Harisiadis L. The role of radiation therapy in the management of metastatic renal cell carcinoma. *Cancer* 1983;51:614–17

18. Divgi C, Bander N, Scott A, *et al.* Phase I/II radioimmunotherapy trial with iodine-131-labeled monoclonal antibody G250 in metastatic renal cell carcinoma. *Clin Cancer Res* 1998; 4:2729–39

19. Fairlamb D. Spontaneous regression of metastases of renal cancer. *Cancer* 1981;47:2102–6

20. Figlin R, deKernion J, Mukamel E, *et al.* Recombinant interferon alfa-2a in metastatic renal cell carcinoma: assessment of antitumor activity and anti-interferon antibody formation. *J Clin Oncol* 1988;6:1604–10

21. Mani S, Tood M, Katz K, Poo W. Prognostic factors for survival in patients with metastatic renal cancer treated with biologic response modifiers. *J Urol* 1995;154:35–40

22. Solchok J, Motzer R. Management of renal cell carcinoma. *Oncology* 2000;14:29–39

23. Rosenberg S, Yang J, White D, Steinberg S. Durability of complete responses in patients with metastatic cancer treated with high-dose interleukin-2. Identification of the antigens mediating response. *Ann Surg* 1998;228:307–19

24. Stadler W, Vogelzang N. Low-dose interleukin-2 in the treatment of metastatic renal cell carcinoma. *Semin Oncol* 1995;22:67–73

25. Law T, Motzer R, Mazumdar M, *et al.* Phase III randomized trial of interleukin-2 with or without lymphokine-activated killer cells in the treatment of patients with advanced renal cell carcinoma. *Cancer* 1995;76:824–32

26. Bukowski R, Sharfman, W, Murthy S, *et al.* Clinical results and characterization of tumor-infiltrating lymphocytes with or without recombinant interleukin-2 in human metastatic renal cell carcinoma. *Cancer Res* 1991;51: 4199–205

27. Negrier S, Escudier B, Lasset C, *et al.* Recombinant human interleukin-2, recombinant human interferon alfa-2a, or both in metastatic renal cell carcinoma. *N Engl J Med* 1998;338:1272–8

28. Shimizu M, Yokota J, Mori N, *et al.* Introduction of normal chromosome 3p modulates the tumorigenicity of human renal cell carcinoma cell line YCR. *Oncogene* 1990;5:185–94

29. Simons J, Marshall F. The future of gene therapy in the treatment of urologic malignancies. *Urol Clin North Am* 1998;25:23–38

30. Dranoff G, Jaffee E, Lazenby A, *et al.* Vaccination with irradiated tumor cell engineered to secrete murine GM-CSF stimulates potent specific and long lasting tumor immunity. *Proc Natl Acad Sci USA* 1993;90:3539–43

31. Simons J, Jaffe E, Weber C, *et al.* Bioactivity of autologous irradiated renal cell carcinoma vaccines generated by *ex vivo* granulocyte-macrophage colony-stimulating factor gene transfer. *Cancer Res* 1997;57:1537–46

32. Holti L, Rieser C, Papesh C, *et al.* Cellular and humoral immune responses in patients with metastatic renal cell carcinoma after vaccination with antigen pulsed dendritic cells. *J Urol* 1999;161:777–82

33. Finke J, Zeal A, Stanley J, *et al.* Loss of T-cell receptor zeta chain and p561ck in T-cells infiltrating human renal cell carcinoma. *Cancer Res* 1993;53:5613–16

34. Bukowski R. Immunotherapy in renal cell carcinoma. *Oncology* 1999;13:801–13

35. Flanigan RC, Blumenstein BA, Salmon S, *et al.* Cytoreduction in nephrectomy in metastatic renal cancer. The results of Southwest Oncology Group trial 8949. *J Urol* 2000;163(Suppl 4): 685

36. Mickisch GH, Garin A, Madej M, *et al.* Tumor nephrectomy plus interferon alpha is superior to interferon alpha alone in metastatic renal cell carcinoma. *J Urol* 2000;156(Suppl 4):778

37. Childs R, Chernoff A, Contentin N, *et al.* Regression of metastatic renal cell carcinoma after nonmyeloablative allogeneic peripheral blood stem-cell transplantation. *N Engl J Med* 2000;343:750–8

Section III

Prostate cancer: early diagnosis and natural history

Molecular markers (PSA, hK2, RT-PCR of PSA and hK2 mRNA): recent progress and perspectives

H. Lilja

Introduction

Measurements in serum or plasma of prostate-specific antigen (PSA or hK3) provide unique opportunities in urological oncology compared to other areas of oncology where tumor markers of equal power in early detection and monitoring of disease stage and therapeutic responses are not yet available. However, testing for conventional total PSA still lacks both sufficient sensitivity and specificity to be ideal. Efforts to improve PSA-testing performance have been mostly focused on enhanced specificity as false-positive tests create patient anxiety and are expensive as they result in additional laboratory testing, transrectal ultrasound, antibiotics, biopsy and pathology charges. False-negative testing may be less harmful, although it needs to be emphasized that no means exists at present for reliably discriminating between the men with indolent slow-growing cancers that may not require curative treatment, and those who are likely to die from the fast and aggressive growth of the prostate cancer if they are left untreated. The discovery that PSA circulates bound to protease inhibitors was the most significant advance in enhancing the performance of the conventional PSA testing mainly because it increased the specificity for a very moderate loss in sensitivity. Other attempts to enhance the results of conventional PSA testing have not been successful. These include:

(1) The age-referenced PSA levels that suggested a lower cut-off in younger men and a higher cut-off in older men (due to the increase of PSA levels with advancing age);

(2) PSA density, which is a volume normalization obtained by calculating the quotient of serum PSA divided by the volume of the prostate;

(3) The transition zone PSA density; and

(4) PSA velocity which is the change in PSA over time that in men with cancer will have a more rapid increase in total PSA levels than in men who do not have cancer.

Occurrence of different complexed PSA forms in the blood

About 10 years ago, it was first reported by two separate research groups – those of Stenman and colleagues[1] and Lilja and co-workers[2] – that PSA occurs both in a free, non-complexed form and also linked in very stable covalent complexes to different proteinase inhibitors in the serum. These findings were based on the earlier discoveries that PSA is a catalytically active kallikrein-like serine protease[3] that becomes inactivated by several of the major extracellular protease inhibitors[4], such as α_2-macroglobulin (AMG), α_1-antichymotrypsin (ACT), α_1-proteinase inhibitor (API), and that is mainly linked in a complex to ACT (PSA–ACT complex) in serum. PSA–AMG is not detected by commercial immunoassays because of steric hindrance of the PSA epitopes by the huge size and conformation of AMG[2,4]. Specific methods that have been developed to measure PSA–AMG levels in patient samples suggest that PSA–AMG occurs at low and non-detectable levels in freshly collected anticoagulated plasma samples from men with clinically localized prostate cancer *in vivo*[5]. This is despite the fact that enzymatically active PSA becomes mainly bound to AMG (and not to ACT) when it is added to serum *in vitro*[4]. This is in very sharp contrast to the non-detectable levels *in vivo* that are very likely due to the rapid elimination kinetics in the blood of PSA–AMG which can be explained by the efficient low-density lipoprotein (LDL) receptor-like mechanisms with an estimated half-life of < 10 min that were proposed in a rat model system[6]. Other groups have reported higher levels of PSA–AMG complexes in sera exposed to long storage at –20 °C[7]. This discrepancy could partly be explained by a more sensitive assay procedure but it is probably mainly due to pre-analytical *in vitro* changes that occur during the non-ideal storage of the samples. Hence, the majority of PSA in blood, about 55–95%, is complexed to ACT[1,2,8]. This may be due to the fact that the complex is unusually stable during physiologically relevant storage conditions *in vitro*[9,10] but, in particular, it might also be due to the fact that the 90-kDa PSA–ACT complex may not be eliminated by the kidneys and, instead, is cleared in a capacity-limited non-exponential and very slow manner at estimated rates of < 1.0 ng/ml[11]. The mechanism of PSA–ACT complex formation and structure has been studied in detail by epitope mapping and computer-based three-dimensional homology modelling[12,13]. It has been suggested that, to involve a two-step mechanism, an initial reversible Michaelis–Menten intermediary form is transferred into a very stable acyl–enzyme complex which renders the part of the kallikrein loop structure that surrounds the active site cleft on one side completely inaccessible to interaction with the vast majority of the 'free-specific' monoclonal antibodies against PSA[13]. There are also several reports from Stenman's group on the presence of the PSA–API complex in serum[14,15] although the immunodetection of this complex is complicated by variable non-specific background signals[15]. According to the most recently reported data from Stenman's group,

PSA linked to API (PSA–API) accounts for no more than 0.9–1.6% of the total PSA in serum[15], and the proportion of PSA–API to total PSA is significantly lower in cancer than in benign prostatic conditions.

Characteristics of free PSA subfractions in the blood

Free, non-complexed PSA forms comprise about 5–45% of the total PSA in blood. Free PSA in the blood is enzymatically inert, i.e. it does not form inhibitor complexes with ACT or AMG which occur in large amount compared to PSA[10]. The approximately 28-kDa size of the free PSA in blood allows rapid clearance by the kidneys with a half-life of 12–18 h[11]. The composition of the free PSA in serum is presently unclear as some data have been reported that show that free PSA may consist of internally cleaved two- or multichain forms often referred to as 'nicked PSA'[16]. One such example is the internal cleavage between Lys_{182} and Ser_{183} called BPSA[17]. By contrast, other reports have suggested that free PSA may consist of proPSA[18,19]. However, these contradictory data could also result from substantial heterogeneity of the free, non-complexed PSA fraction(s) in blood; a disease-specific variation has not yet been shown by analysis of the composition of free PSA subfractions. However, the LNCaP tumor cell line secretes about 50% of PSA as zymogen (proPSA) whereas it does not secrete any internally cleaved ('nicked') two- or multichain forms of PSA[20–22]. By contrast, no zymogen is present in PSA isolated from benign tissue or seminal fluid, whereas > 30% of the PSA in seminal fluid consists of internally cleaved ('nicked') two- or multichain forms[4,23]. Such data suggest that differences in the extent of post-translational processing could exist for free PSA released from benign prostatic tissue compared to the free PSA that is released from prostate cancer cells. The detailed nature of free PSA forms is now being clarified, e.g. by contributions made by the generation of specific antibodies which either react with the N-terminal residues in the activation peptide of the PSA-zymogen (i.e. proPSA), or antibodies that selectively bind to the BPSA neo-epitope which is formed when PSA is internally cleaved between Lys_{182} and Ser_{183}[17,19]. We recently generated antibodies that bind only to single-chain forms of PSA, and lose binding capacity when free PSA is internally cleaved between Lys_{145} and Lys_{146}[24]. This internal cleavage contributes the predominant inactive form of PSA in the seminal fluid[4], but so far, little is known about whether disease-specific changes occur and whether there is clinical utility to measure any of these free PSA subfractions in patient samples.

Clinical utility of free and complexed PSA measurements

Measurements of free and total PSA contribute significant enhancements over conventional total PSA testing in the early detection of prostate cancer[8]. At moderately elevated PSA levels, large-sized multicenter studies have shown that free-to-total PSA measurements contribute specificity enhancements of 20–40% over total PSA testing at the expense of moderate loss (5–10%) in sensitivity[25–29]. More than one out of five negative biopsies can be avoided if clinicians are willing to miss 5% of cancers. However, problems remain despite the advance of free-to-total PSA measurements, since significant overlap exists in free-to-total PSA ratios between men with and men without prostate cancer. Also, limited stability of free non-complexed forms in serum *in vitro* require strict pre-analytical sample handling or collection of anticoagulated EDTA or heparin plasma samples to avoid a signficant decrease in free PSA levels and, hence, falsely decreased free-to-total ratios[10,30]. Therefore, it is important to separate the blood cells from the serum or plasma within 6 h of venipuncture and to analyze the free PSA levels in less than 24 h following collection of serum in order to avoid a significant decrease in free PSA levels in serum[10]. Collection of blood as anticoagulated EDTA or heparin plasma extends the stability of free PSA in the test tube to about 3 days[10]. The original reports that PSA–ACT complex measurements contribute diagnostic enhance-ment over total PSA testing suffered from over-recovery which was later shown to be due to difficulties in eliminating non-specific signals generated by ACT linked to granulocyte-derived proteases such as cathepsin G[1,8,9]. This difficulty has been overcome by Bayer Diagnostics who have developed a complex PSA (cPSA) assay which recognizes PSA by capturing cPSA in microparticles which do not access free PSA[31]. The assay detects both PSA–ACT as well as the PSA–API complexes although PSA–ACT is by far the predominant complex since PSA–API accounts for about 1–2% of the total PSA. Complex PSA measurements offer advantages in sample stability since PSA–ACT is more stable in the test tube than free PSA[10]. Also, cPSA levels are much less elevated than total PSA following prostatic manipulation[32]. Analysis by receiver operation characteristics (ROCs) has shown that areas under the curve (AUCs) for the cPSA assay are greater, but not always significantly greater, than AUCs for total PSA in each of ten different studies evaluating samples from over 1600 men examined with ultrasound-guided sextant prostate biopsy[33]. These data suggest enhanced performance of complexed PSA compared to conventional total PSA in discriminating between men with prostate cancer and those without cancer. However, the potential of complexed PSA measurements in enhancing the specificity of total PSA testing at lower cut-offs than the conventional 4.0 ng/ml still needs to be evaluated. This has become increasingly important, e.g. in the design and validation of assay procedures for very sensitive and specific measurements of human kallikrein 2 (hK2) in different biological fluids.

Biologic function of human kallikrein 2

hK2 is a kallikrein-like serine protease with extensive similarity to PSA, both in its tissue expression pattern and in its primary structure (about 80% identical to PSA)[34,35]. hK2 is produced by prostate epithelium as zymogen (prohK2) containing a short propeptide. By contrast to PSA, the activation mechanism of hK2 may be autocatalytic as suggested by the design of several different recombinantly expressed hK2 mutants that are secreted as zymogens as a result of point mutation of the prosequence which stabilizes the zymogen[36]. This inhibits autoactivation but also results in 15–40-fold higher expression levels of hK2. This may help us to understand why there is a large discrepancy in tissue levels of hK2 relative to PSA compared to the much smaller difference between hK2-mRNA and PSA-mRNA levels. The hK2 function in the prostate is not known, apart from putative regulation of its own activity and its capacity to convert inactive proPSA to active PSA[37–39]. That hK2 is probably a PSA activator may help us to understand why more PSA is complexed to ACT in men with cancer than in men without cancer. Also, hK2 may play a role in prostate cancer invasion due to its capacity to convert single-chain urokinase to active urokinase, inactivate and form complexes with plasminogen activator inhibitor-1 (the primary uPA inhibitor), and form complexes with plasminogen activator inhibitor-3 that is more commonly called protein C inhibitor (PCI), which is the major inhibitor and complexing ligand to hK2 in seminal fluid[40,41]. hK2 also cleaves semenogelin I and II, the major gel proteins in seminal plasma *in vitro*, but it is unknown whether this occurs *in vivo*, since identified cleavage sites are in accord with PSA-generated cleavages alone[42,43]. In addition, prostatic zinc levels are the highest in the body, around 9 mmol/l, and zinc ions inhibit hK2 action (and PSA action) by sufficiently low inhibition constants to ensure that zinc may be an efficient hK2 regulator at physiologically relevant zinc levels in the prostate[43].

Clinical utility of specific hK2 measurements in patient serum

hK2 levels in the blood correspond to about 1–2% of those of total PSA and this proportion does not differ significantly in men with prostate cancer compared to those without[44]. However, earlier studies showed that measurements of hK2 levels in serum combined with those of total and free PSA levels may improve discrimination between men with benign prostatic hyperplasia (BPH) and men with prostate cancer[45–49]. In parallel, improvements in assay performance have been reported by several groups of researchers[50–52]. To follow-up on the earlier findings, we had access to serum collected in a prostate cancer screening study conducted in 1995–96 in Göteborg, Sweden where 5853/9811 randomly selected men (aged 50–66 years) accepted PSA testing, and those found with total PSA levels (PSA–T) ≥ 3.0 ng/ml were biopsied[53]. Serum from 604 biopsied men (144 men with prostate cancer) were analyzed for hK2, using a very sensitive, specific in-house research assay for hK2 with a functional detection limit of 5 pg/ml and $< 0.05\%$ (i.e. insignificant) cross-reactivity with PSA[52]. This assay for hK2 testing in blood detects free hK2 by nearly identical signal intensity (less than 6% bias) when compared to complexed hK2[52]. Data from size-separating gel-filtration chromatography suggest that most of the hK2 ($> 80\%$) in blood may occur in the free, non-complexed form[52]. Analysis of the AUC by ROCs showed that measurements of the hK2 levels combined with those of free and total PSA, using the algorithm hK2 × PSA–T/PSA–F, significantly enhanced the discrimination of men with prostate cancer from those with BPH compared to PSA–T and percent-free PSA[53]. The cancer--detection rate was significantly improved (p values < 0.05) by hK2 × PSA–T/PSA–F compared to PSA–T and percent-free PSA at specificity levels from 75 to 90%[53]. At total PSA levels of ≥ 3.0 ng/ml, analyses of hK2, free PSA and total PSA significantly reduced the number of men without cancer needing to be biopsied (reducing false-positives) while maintaining prostate cancer detection rates at the same level as when using conventional total PSA cut-off of ≥ 4.0 ng/ml[53]. Hence, the positive predictive value (PPV) increased significantly from 31% for total PSA to 45% for hK2, free PSA and total PSA. We have now generated preliminary data to show that further enhancement can be contributed by artificial neural networks and current studies show promise of an additional 15–18% gain in sensitivity at 43% PPV. This corresponds to almost every second man with prostate cancer undergoing biopsy being detected at a sensitivity which corresponds to about 10% less than the detection rate accomplished by measurements of total PSA levels using a cut-off of ≥ 3.0 ng/ml (which gives a PPV of 24% in this population). However, we still do not know whether (or not) we only detect the significant cancers, and whether (or not) the cancers we do not detect only represent insignificant cancer. Moreover, we also need to evaluate how much more enhancement may be provided by the use of artificial neural networks.

An original study of men diagnosed with clinically localized prostate cancer strongly suggested that measurement of hK2 enabled discrimination between men with pathologically organ-confined disease and those with the extraprostatic extension stages of the disease[54]. In follow-up studies after this original report, Recker and colleagues have produced supporting data[55]. In addition, we have measured the total hK2 levels using our most sensitive and specific assay procedure that significantly discriminates between stage pT_2 (organ-confined cancer) and higher stage cancers $\geq pT_{3a}$ (extraprostatic extension) in pretreatment serum from 184 consecutive patients with clinically localized prostate cancer (131 organ-confined and 53 extraprostatic extension) with total PSA values of < 10 ng/ml who underwent radical prostatectomy. Median hK2 concentration in extraprostatic extension cancers was significantly higher ($p = 0.03$) than that found in organ-confined cancers, whereas there was no significant difference in free or total PSA levels in organ-confined compared to extraprostatic extension cancers. Hence, hK2 measurements may also be important in predicting whether or not there is extraprostatic cancer growth.

Quantitative RT-PCR assays to measure PSA- and hK2-mRNA copy numbers

Reverse transcription-PCR (RT-PCR) has been used for detection of specific tumor- or tissue-associated markers to detect metastatic tumor cells in the blood, lymph nodes or other organs. PSA-mRNA is a widely studied target for detection of prostate cancer cells in blood, lymph node and bone marrow samples. Due to the large amount of conflicting data that has been reported, it is yet unproven whether RT-PCR-based PSA-mRNA assays can predict micrometastatic spread, or monitor treatment outcome[56–59]. The largely discrepant reported clinical data are based mainly on qualitative assays and differing assay protocols[60,61]. We have now developed a standardized, highly reproducible, quantitative QRT–PCR time-resolved fluorescent endpoint assay to determine PSA-mRNA copy numbers in patient samples[62]. Variation in reaction conditions is controlled by co-amplifying the specific template with an internal standard added to the sample. To obtain accurate quantification, the internal standard is amplified with the same efficiency as the sample target and the amplification products are nearly identical in size: the internal standard contained a two-base-pair deletion which is enough to distinguish the internal standard from the target product[62]. This design enables linear detection from 50 up to 1 million PSA-mRNA copies by intra-assay coefficients of variation of $< 8\%$ and interassay coefficients of variation of $< 30\%$ (interassay imprecision is mostly due to suboptimized protocols for isolation of nucleated cells and total RNA). Our technique allows detection of a single tumor cell in 2.5 million nucleated cells and the LNCaP cell line has been shown to contain a mean of about 980 PSA-mRNA copies per cell (although there was large cell-to-cell variation)[63]. This quantitative RT-PCR assay has now been simplified by homogeneous detection chemistry enabling discrimination of specific base sequences in real-time PCR using a closed-tube system that gives very precise calculation of the number of input template molecules[64]. We have also developed dual-analyte hybridization assays for quantitative detection of both RT-PCR-amplified PSA and internal standard products which mainly improves intra-assay precision and reduces labor load[63]. At present, it is also unclear whether it is better to perform these procedures by endpoint assay formats (which we have used so far) or whether there are advantages in employing the very recently developed homogeneous real-time measurements. Lastly, we have also developed a quantitative detection protocol to determine the exact input copy number of internal standard products and target RT-PCR-amplified hK2 mRNA that gives a very similar assay performance to that reported above for PSA mRNA. A first preliminary analysis of blood samples collected from a very limited number of men with clinically advanced disease stages has shown that the hK2-mRNA copy number was significantly higher compared to the PSA-mRNA copy number in pretreatment samples. This suggests that measurements of the hK2-mRNA copy numbers may possibly be more relevant

for measuring disease activity and/or spread compared to measurements of the PSA-mRNA copy numbers in advanced disease stages. However, it still remains to be diligently evaluated in large series of very carefully characterized patient groups of prostate cancer patients whether the recently developed quantitative RT-PCR procedures of PSA mRNA and/or hK2 mRNA may be found to have clinical utility based on their putative power to discriminate between men with only localized prostate cancer and those who suffer from disease that has advanced to the more advanced stages with microscopic spread of the disease to the lymph nodes and/or bone marrow.

References

1. Stenman UH, Leinonen J, Alfthan H, *et al.* A complex between prostate-specific antigen and alpha 1-antichymotrypsin is the major form of prostate-specific antigen in serum of patients with prostatic cancer: assay of the complex improves clinical sensitivity for cancer. *Cancer Res* 1991;51:222–6
2. Lilja H, Christensson A, Dahlén U, *et al.* Prostate-specific antigen in human serum occurs predominantly in complex with α_1-antichymotrypsin. *Clin Chem* 1991;37:1618–25
3. Lilja H. (1985) A kallikrein-like serine protease in prostatic fluid cleaves the predominant seminal vesicle protein. *J Clin Invest* 1985;76: 1899–903
4. Christensson A, Laurell C-B, Lilja H. Enzymatic activity of prostate-specific antigen and its reactions with extracellular serine proteinase inhibitors. *Eur J Biochem* 1990;194:755–63
5. Lilja H, Haese A, Björk T, *et al.* Significance and metabolism of complexed and non-complexed prostate-specific antigen forms and human glandular kallikrein 2 in clinically localized prostate cancer before and after radical prostatectomy. *J Urol* 1999;162: 2029–35
6. Birkenmeier G, Struck F, Gebhardt R. Clearance mechanisms of prostate specific antigen

and its complexes with alpha-2-macroglobulin and alpha-1-antichymotrypsin. *J Urol* 1999;162: 897–901
7. Zhang WM, Finne P, Leinonen J, *et al.* Determination of prostate-specific antigen complexed to alpha(2)-macroglobulin in serum increases the specificity of free to total PSA for prostate cancer. *Urology* 2000;56:267–72
8. Christensson A, Björk T, Nilsson O, *et al.* Serum prostate-specific antigen complexed to α_1-antichymotrypsin as an indicator of prostate cancer. *J Urol* 1993;150:100–5
9. Pettersson K, Piironen T, Seppälä M, *et al.* Free and complexed prostate-specific antigen (PSA): *in vitro* stability, epitope map, and development of immunofluorometric assays for specific and sensitive detection of free PSA and PSA–α_1-antichymotrypsin complex. *Clin Chem* 1995;41: 1480–8
10. Piironen T, Pettersson K, Suonpää M, *et al.* (1996) *In vitro* stability of free prostate-specific antigen (PSA) and prostate-specific antigen (PSA) complexed to α_1-antichymotrypsin in blood samples. *Urology* 1996;48:81–7
11. Björk T, Ljungberg B, Piironen T, *et al.* Rapid exponential elimination of free prostate-specific antigen (PSA) contrasts the slow, capacity-limited elimination of PSA complexed to

alpha-1-antichymotrypsin from serum. *Urology* 1998;51:57–62

12. Villoutreix BO, Lilja H, Pettersson K, *et al.* Structural investigation of the alpha-1-antichymotrypsin : prostate specific antigen complex by comparative model building. *Protein Sci* 1996;5:836–51

13. Piironen T, Villoutreix BO, Becker C, *et al.* Determination and analysis of antigenic epitopes of prostate-specific antigen (PSA) and human glandular kallikrein 2 (hK2) using synthetic peptides and computer modeling. *Protein Sci* 1998;7:259–69

14. Zhang WM, Finne P, Leinonen J, *et al.* Measurement of the complex between prostate-specific antigen and alpha 1-protease inhibitor in serum. *Clin Chem* 1999;45:814–21

15. Finne P, Zhang WM, Auvinen A, *et al.* Use of the complex between prostate specific antigen and alpha 1-protease inhibitor for screening prostate cancer. *J Urol* 2000;164:1956–60

16. Noldus J, Chen ZX, Stamey TA. Isolation and characterization of free form prostate specific antigen (f-PSA) in sera of men with prostate cancer. *J Urol* 1997;158:1606–9

17. Mikolajczyk SD, Millar LS, Marker KM, *et al.* Seminal plasma contains 'BPSA', a molecular form of prostate-specific antigen that is associated with benign prostatic hyperplasia. *Prostate* 2000;45:271–6

18. Mikolajczyk SD, Grauer LS, Millar LS, *et al.* A precursor form of PSA (pPSA) is a component of the free PSA in prostate cancer serum. *Urology* 1997;50:710–14

19. Mikolajczyk SD, Millar LS, Wang TJ, *et al.* A precursor form of prostate-specific antigen is more highly elevated in prostate cancer compared with benign transition zone prostate tissue. *Cancer Res* 2000;60:756–9

20. Corey E, Brown LG, Corey MJ, *et al.* LNCaP produces both putative zymogen and inactive, free form of prostate-specific antigen. *Prostate* 1998;35:135–43

21. Herrala A, Kurkela R, Vihinen M, *et al.* Androgen-sensitive human prostate cancer cells, LNCaP, produce both N-terminally mature and truncated prostate-specific antigen isoforms. *Eur J Biochem* 1998;255:329–35

22. Väisänen V, Lövgren J, Hellman J, *et al.* Characterization and processing of prostate-specific antigen (hK3) and human glandular kallikrein 2 (hK2) secreted by LNCaP cells. *Prostate Cancer Prostatic Dis* 1999;2:1–7

23. Zhang WM, Leinonen J, Kalkkinen N, *et al.* Purification and characterization of different molecular forms of prostate-specific antigen in human seminal fluid. *Clin Chem* 1995;41:1567–73

24. Nurmikko P, Väisänen V, Piironen T, *et al.* Production and characterization of novel anti-PSA monoclonal antibodies which do not detect internally cleaved Lys_{145}-Lys_{146} inactivated PSA. *Clin Chem* 2000;46:1610–18

25. Luderer AA, Chen Y, Thiel R, *et al.* Measurement of the proportion of free to total PSA improves diagnostic performance of PSA in the diagnostic gray zone of total PSA. *Urology* 1995;46:187–94

26. Higashihara E, Nutahara K, Kojima M, *et al.* Significance of serum free prostate-specific antigen in the screening of prostate cancer. *J Urol* 1996;156:1964–8

27. Chen Y, Luderer AA, Thiel RP, *et al.* Using proportions of free to total prostate-specific antigen, age, and total prostate-specific antigen to predict the probability of prostate cancer. *Urology* 1996;47:518–24

28. Catalona WJ, Partin AW, Slawin KM, *et al.* Use of the percentage of free prostate-specific antigen to enhance differentiation of prostate cancer from benign prostatic disease: a prospective multicenter clinical trial. *J Am Med Assoc* 1998;279:1542–7

29. Catalona WJ, Southwick PC, Slawin KM, *et al.* Comparison of percent free PSA, PSA density, and age-specific PSA cutoffs for prostate cancer detection and staging. *Urology* 2000;56:255–60

30. Leinonen J, Stenman UH. Reduced stability of prostate-specific antigen after long-term storage of serum at −20 degrees C. *Tumour Biol* 2000; 21:46–53

31. Allard WJ, Zhou Z, Yeung KK. Novel immunoassay for the measurement of complexed prostate-specific antigen in serum. *Clin Chem* 1998;44:1216–23

32. Lynn NN, Collins GN, O'Reilly PH. Prostatic manipulation has a minimal effect on complexed prostate-specific antigen levels. *BJU Int* 2000;86:65–7

33. Brawer MK, Cheli CD, Neaman IE, *et al.* Complexed prostate specific antigen provides significant enhancement of specificity compared with total prostate specific antigen for detecting prostate cancer. *J Urol* 2000;163:1476–80

34. Schedlich LJ, Bennetts B, Morris BJ. Primary structure of a human glandular kallikrein gene. *DNA* 1987;6:429–37

35. Chapdelaine P, Paradis G, Tremblay RR, *et al.* High level of expression in the prostate of a human glandular kallikrein mRNA related to prostate-specific antigen. *FEBS Lett* 1988;236:205–8

36. Lövgren J, Tian S, Lundwall Å, *et al.* Production and activation of recombinant hK2 with propeptide mutations resulting in high expression levels. *Eur J Biochem* 1999;266:1050–5

37. Lövgren J, Rajakoski K, Karp M, *et al.* Activation of the zymogen form of prostate-specific antigen

by human glandular kallikrein 2. *Biochem Biophys Res Comm* 1997;238:549–55

38. Takayama TK, Fujikawa K, Davie EW. Characterization of the precursor of prostate-specific antigen. Activation by trypsin and by human glandular kallikrein. *J Biol Chem* 1997; 272:1582–8

39. Kumar A, Mikolajczyk SD, Goel AS, *et al.* Expression of pro form of prostate-specific antigen by mammalian cells and its conversion to mature, active form by human kallikrein 2. *Cancer Res* 1997;57:3111–14

40. Frenette G, Tremblay RR, Lazure C, *et al.* Prostatic kallikrein hK2, but not prostate-specific antigen (hK3), activates single-chain urokinase-type plasminogen activator. *Int J Cancer* 1997;71: 897–9

41. Mikolajczyk SD, Millar LS, Kumar A, *et al.* Prostatic human glandular kallikrein 2 inactivates and complexes with plasminogen activator inhibitor-1. *Int J Cancer* 1999;81:438–42

42. Deperthes D, Frenette G, Brillard-Bourdet M, *et al.* Potential involvement of kallikrein hK2 in the hydrolysis of human seminal vesicle proteins after ejaculation. *J Androl* 1996;17:659–65

43. Lövgren J, Airas K, Lilja H. Enzymatic action of human glandular kallikrein 2 (hK2): substrate specificity and regulation by Zn^{2+} and extracellular protease inhibitors. *Eur J Biochem* 1999;262:781–9

44. Piironen T, Lövgren J, Karp M, *et al.* Immunofluorometric assay for sensitive and specific measurement of human prostatic glandular kallikrein (hK2) in serum. *Clin Chem* 1996;42:1034–41

45. Charlesworth MC, Young CY-F, Klee GG, *et al.* Detection of a prostate-specific protein, human glandular kallikrein (hK2), in sera of patients with elevated prostate-specific antigen levels. *Urology* 1997;49:487–93

46. Kwiatkowski MK, Recker F, Piironen T, *et al.* In prostatism patients the ratio of human glandular kallikrein to free PSA improves the discrimination between prostate cancer and benign hyperplasia within the diagnostic 'gray zone' of total PSA 4–10 ng/ml. *Urology* 1998; 52:360–5

47. Recker F, Kwiatkowski MK, Piironen T, *et al.* The importance of human glandular kallikrein and its correlation with different prostate specific antigen serum forms in the detection of prostate carcinoma. *Cancer* 1998;83:2540–7

48. Becker C, Piironen T, Pettersson K. Discrimination of men with prostate cancer from those with benign disease by measurements of human glandular kallikrein 2 (HK2) in serum. *J Urol* 2000;163:311–16

49. Partin AW, Catalona WJ, Finlay JA, *et al.* Use of human glandular kallikrein 2 for the detection of prostate cancer: preliminary analysis. *Urology* 1999;54:839–45

50. Black MH, Magklara A, Obiezu CV, *et al.* Development of an ultrasensitive immunoassay for human glandular kallikrein with no cross-reactivity from prostate-specific antigen. *Clin Chem* 1999;45:790–9

51. Klee GG, Goodmanson MK, Jacobsen SJ, *et al.* Highly sensitive automated chemiluminometric assay for measuring free human glandular kallikein-2. *Clin Chem* 1999;45:800–6

52. Becker C, Piironen T, Kiviniemi J, *et al.* Sensitive and specific immunodetection of human glandular kallikrein 2 (hK2) in serum. *Clin Chem* 2000;46:198–206

53. Becker C, Piironen T, Pettersson K, *et al.* Clinical value of human glandular kallikrein 2 and free and total prostate-specific antigen in serum from a population of men with prostate-specific antigen levels 3.0 ng/ml or greater. *Urology* 2000;55:694–9

54. Haese A, Becker C, Noldus J, *et al.* Human glandular kallikrein 2 (hK2): a potential serum marker for predicting the organ-confined versus nonorgan confined growth of prostate cancer. *J Urol* 2000;163:1491–7

55. Recker F, Kwiatkowski MK, Piironen T, *et al.* Human glandular kallikrein as a tool to improve discrimination of poorly differentiated and non-organ-confined prostate cancer compared with prostate-specific antigen. *Urology* 2000;55: 481–5

56. Moreno JG, Croce CM, Fischer R, *et al.* Detection of hematogenous micrometastasis in patients with prostate cancer. *Cancer Res* 1992;52:6110–12

57. Katz AE, Olsson CA, Raffo AJ, *et al.* Molecular staging of prostate cancer with the use of an enhanced reverse transcriptase-PCR assay. *Urology* 1994;43:765–75

58. Israeli RS, Miller WH Jr, Su SL, *et al.* Sensitive nested reverse transcription polymerase chain reaction detection of circulating prostatic tumor cells: comparison of prostate-specific membrane antigen and prostate-specific antigen-based assays. *Cancer Res* 1994;54:6306–10

59. De La Taille A, Olsson CA, Buttyan R, *et al.* Blood-based reverse transcriptase polymerase chain reaction assays for prostatic specific antigen: long term follow-up confirms the potential utility of this assay in identifying patients more likely to have biochemical recurrence (rising PSA) following radical prostatectomy. *Int J Cancer* 1999;84:360–4

60. Galvan B, Christopoulos TK, Diamandis EP. Detection of prostate-specific antigen mRNA by reverse transcription polymerase chain reaction and time-resolved fluorometry. *Clin Chem* 1995; 41:1705–9

61. Verhaegen M, Ioannou PC, Christopoulos TK. Quantification of prostate-specific antigen mRNA by coamplification with a recombinant RNA internal standard and microtiter well-based hybridization. *Clin Chem* 1998;44:1170–6

62. Ylikoski A, Sjöroos M, Lundwall Å, *et al.* Quantitative reverse transcription-PCR assay with an internal standard for the detection of prostate-specific antigen mRNA. *Clin Chem* 1999;45:1397–407

63. Ylikoski A, Karp M, Lilja H, *et al.* Dual-label detection of prostate-specific antigen and internal standard amplified in quantitative reverse transcription-PCR assay using probes labeled with different lanthanides. *Biotechniques* 2001; in press

64. Nurmi J, Lilja H, Ylikoski A. Time-resolved fluorometry in end-point and real-time PCR quantification of nucleic acids. *Luminescence* 2000;15:381–8

Early diagnosis: state of the art in clinical routine and screening studies

10

J. Hugosson

Introduction

Although the value of early diagnosis of prostate cancer is still under debate, the search for early prostate cancer has become one of the most important clinical issues for the practising urologist. Much of the controversy around early diagnosis is the fear of over-detection and over-treatment. As many as 40% of men between 60 and 70 years of age may have microscopic foci of well-differentiated carcinoma and, today, the only parameter apart from grade thought to correlate with the risk of clinical progression is tumor size[1,2]. Well-differentiated tumors smaller than 0.2–0.5 ml are accordingly thought to represent more harmless tumors and are usually called insignificant cancers[2]. The goal of early detection is thus not only to detect prostate cancer but to detect those cancers which constitute a threat to their host, i.e. if left untreated, they will lead to clinical disease and possibly death. As only 3–5% of the male population die from prostate cancer and 10% develop clinical disease, it is obvious that the majority of men with latent cancers will not develop clinical disease[3]. These facts have led to serious concerns whether it is ethical to suggest screening for prostate cancer, as it may result in enormous over-diagnosis and over-treatment[4], especially as treatments are both expensive and associated with significant side-effects[5]. However, the experience of extensive prostate-specific antigen (PSA) screening so far is that, even if over-diagnosis may be a problem, the opposite – under-diagnosis – is probably still more common[6]. Even if prostate cancers grow slowly, these cancers inherit a large malignant potential by their growth pattern. Even at a rather low cancer volume, these cancers spread outside the prostate and become incurable; almost half of cancers detected in the PSA interval 10–20 ng/ml will progress due to clinical understaging[6]. For a screening intervention to be effective, its application must change the course of the disease in a favorable direction. As the effect of screening is usually associated with eradication of the disease, it must be diagnosed while still curable. In prostate cancer, the window of opportunity for diagnosing significant but curable cancer is rather narrow. This means that, if early diagnosis is to be successful, the timing of diagnosis is critical and cancers must be found very early, but not too early; the ideal is probably to diagnose cancers in the PSA region of 2.5–10 ng/ml[6].

There is a very important distinction between testing done in asymptomatic persons not actively seeking for prostate diseases (screening) from that in persons seeking medical advice due to symptoms or other concerns of prostate cancer (diagnosing). The latter situation demands a higher degree of diagnostic accuracy, while the former needs more to take other factors under consideration such as cost efficiency[7].

Prostate-specific antigen

The cornerstones for early diagnosis are digital rectal examination (DRE) and measurement of PSA in serum. If one or both of these two investigations are abnormal, further examination with ultrasound-guided sextant biopsies is indicated. The cut-off for PSA has generally been 4 ng/ml; however, several reports have shown that this cut-off may be too high and several cancers, especially those with the greatest chance for cure, are found within the lowest PSA interval[8]. Lowering the cut-off to 3 ng/ml or even less does not seem to increase significantly the risk of detecting low-volume cancers[8,9]. The dilemma of decreasing the PSA cut-off is the low specificity of the test. Between 3 and 4 ng/ml, only one out of seven men had cancer[9]. The correlation between PSA level and risk of cancer declines with the number of tests performed (Table 1). At the first PSA testing, a high PSA level (> 10 ng/ml) is highly correlated to the presence of cancer in biopsies; however, in subsequent testing, the risk of cancer in biopsies differs much less between different PSA intervals, at least in men with a PSA > 3 ng/ml (Table 1). This is probably because most men with cancer are identified during the first screening and the remainder consists of a higher proportion of men with other causes for increases in PSA, such as benign prostatic hyperplasia (BPH). The strength of PSA testing alone is demonstrated by the Göteborg branch of the ERSPC (European Randomized Study for Prostate Cancer), since more than 20% of men with increased PSA levels at both the second and third screenings were diagnosed with cancer (Table 1). Altogether, 408 men with cancer have been detected in this study, in which 10 000 men were invited to take part and in which 6911 have participated in at least one PSA testing and 4913 in all three.

PSA density

Several ways to increase the specificity of the PSA test have been published. One of the most popular is to use the PSA density, which is simply the quotient of the PSA level and the prostate volume. Values lower than 0.12 ng/ml are often associated with BPH, while higher values are more commonly due to cancer. Only 11% of cancers in the Rotterdam screening study had a PSA density less than 0.12[10]. However, there are several problems caused by using PSA density. First, the lower detection rate in men with low values may simply be due to the fact that cancers are more easily missed in those with larger glands. Second, the tests needs transrectal ultrasound to make the measurement which is operator-dependent, time-consuming and expensive. The PSA density may play a role in investigating men with BPH, especially those who are already scheduled for a transrectal ultrasound investigation because of lower urinary tract symptoms. However, the concept seems to be not beneficial in the early diagnosis of cancer, especially not in asymptomatic men.

Percentage of free PSA

Prostate-specific antigens occur in serum in different molecular forms. The PSA leakage from BPH is mostly present as free PSA, while leakage of the antigens from cancers are complexed to α1-antichymotrypsin[11]. This difference may be put to use by calculating the percentage of free PSA [(concentration of free PSA/concentration of total PSA) × 100]. This ratio is lower in men with cancer compared to that in men with BPH[11]. Within the range 2.6–4 ng/ml, this concept may increase specificity and only slightly decrease sensitivity[8]. Clinically significant cancers may be found by

Table 1 Risk of cancer in biopsies according to PSA interval and number of PSA screenings performed. Results from the Göteborg screening study, part of the ERSPC

| PSA interval (ng/ml) | Number of cancers/number of screenings | | |
	1st screening	2nd screening	3rd screening
3–3.99	35/234 (15%)	39/228 (17%)	49/239 (20%)
4–9.99	65/296 (22%)	63/254 (25%)	53/268 (20%)
10–19.99	21/37 (57%)	5/17 (29%)	9/33 (27%)
> 20	20/26 (77%)	3/6 (50%)	4/4 (100%)
All	141/593 (24%)	110/505 (22%)	115/544 (21%)

using the ratio of free to total PSA, even within lower PSA intervals. Since it seems that the ratio of free to total PSA also selects patients with clinically significant cancers[12] and may enhance specificity by about 30%, this concept seems especially efficient combined with a lowered PSA cut-off. The optimal cut-off for total PSA and the ratio of free to total PSA remains to be set.

Digital rectal examination

While it may be debatable whether DRE should be omitted in a screening situation, there are a certain number of cancers detectable by DRE within the normal PSA range, supporting the idea that DRE should be carried out in all men subjected to early diagnosis. However, new reports from screening programs, utilizing a lower cut-off for PSA, indicate that the value of DRE may be very small and probably not cost-efficient[13]. The decision on whether to carry out DRE depends upon the situation. In the situation where an individual patient seeks urological advice, a thorough investigation is essential, including PSA, DRE and a liberal indication for biopsy. The other situation occurs in a large-scale screening for prostate cancer, in which cost efficiency also should be considered and a 100% sensitivity is not feasible. In this situation, DRE is probably not cost-effective and the value of percentage of free PSA increases.

The limitations of DRE are also demonstrated by the fact that 85% of cancers detected in the interval 3–4 ng/ml are non-palpable and two-thirds are neither palpable nor visible on transrectal ultrasound[9].

Biopsy regimen

Indications for biopsy have increased as it has become obvious that most cancers are not palpable and not seen on transrectal ultrasound[13]. The optimal cut-off for PSA and/or percentage of free PSA has not yet been set, but studies are urgently needed to characterize cancers detected at lower PSA intervals. Several studies have shown that clinically significant cancers are diagnosed in the interval below 4 ng/ml; however, data of how often such biopsy protocols are associated with diagnosis of clinically insignificant cancers are sparse[8]. Another problem with the widely adopted technique using sextant biopsies is the high rate of false-negative results. As seen in Table 2, men with a persistently elevated PSA have almost the same risk for having cancer when biopsied again after 2 years as when biopsied for the first time. Even two sets of negative biopsies result in a 10% risk for cancer at third biopsy in men with persistently increased PSA. To increase the sensitivity of the biopsy procedure, the number of biopsies taken may need to be increased or an initially negative biopsy repeated.

Screening interval

Another issue for discussion is the screening interval. The most common recommendation is for annual examinations which have been shown to result in very few interval cancers. However, the optimal screening interval is probably not determined by the frequency of interval cancers, but instead by the stage distribution of cancers detected at repeated screening. The risk of detecting incurable

Table 2 Risk of cancer in biopsies according to PSA interval and number of previous occasions with benign biopsies (due to increased PSA)

| PSA interval (ng/ml) | Number of cancers/number of screenings | | |
	No previous biopsy	One benign biopsy	Two benign biopsies
3–3.99	102/560 (18%)	19/114 (17%)	3/38 (8%)
4–9.99	113/484 (23%)	57/242 (24%)	12/106 (11%)
10–19.99	27/50 (54%)	8/28 (29%)	3/21 (14%)
> 20	20/26 (74%)	2/5 (40%)	0
All	262/1120 (23%)	86/389 (22%)	18/165 (11%)

prostate cancer at repeated screening seems very low, even with a screening interval of 2 years, and men with PSA less than 1 ng/ml may probably have an even longer testing interval[14].

Conclusions

The goal with early diagnosis of the prostate cancer is to diagnose those cancers that would become clinical if not diagnosed, and not to detect the large bulk of small insignificant cancers. For early detection to be justified, its application must change the course of the disease in a favorable direction, from that in the absence of early detection. The diagnostic algorithm may differ between large-scale screening in asymptomatic men and normal diagnostic activity in men seeking urological advice. The latter situation demands a much lower risk of false-negative results. PSA is the key in both situations and, in the screening situation, is 'good enough' to be the only screening test. One way to enhance both the sensitivity and specificity is the introduction of the percentage of free PSA combined with a lowering of the PSA cut-off value. Sextant biopsies of the prostate seem to have a too high rate of false-negative results and better biopsy regimens are needed. A time period of 2 years between PSA tests seems sufficient, and an even longer interval may probably be justified, at least in those with very low PSA values (< 1 ng/ml). The present situation with very efficacious diagnostic tools constitutes a risk for over-diagnosing and over-treatment. In order to study these risks and benefits, randomized trials, such as the ERSPC, are of vital importance, as these data are very difficult to calculate outside such studies.

References

1. Sakr WA, Haas GP, Cassin BF, et al. The frequency of carcinoma and intraepithelial neoplasia of the prostate in young male patients. J Urol 1993;150:379–85
2. Stamey TA, Freiha FS, McNeal JE, Redwine EA, Whittemore AS. Localised prostate cancer. Relationship of tumor volume to clinical significance for treatment of prostate cancer. Cancer 1993;71:933
3. Hugosson J, Aus G, Norlén L. Surveillance is not a viable option in treatment of localized prostate cancer. Urol Clin N Am 1996;23:557–73
4. Adami HO, Baron JA, Rohman KJ. Ethics of a prostate cancer screening trial. Lancet 1994;343:958–60
5. Litwin MS, Hays RD, Fink A, et al. Quality of life outcomes in men treated for localized prostate cancer. J Am Med Assoc 1995;273:129–35
6. Partin AW, Yoo J, Carter HB, et al. The use of prostate specific antigen, clinical stage and Gleason score to predict pathological stage in patients with localized prostate cancer. J Urol 1993;150:110–14
7. Denis L, Mettlin C, Carter HB, et al. Early detection and screening. In Murphy G, Khoury S, Partin A, Denis L, eds. Prostate Cancer. 2nd International Consultation on Prostate Cancer, Paris 1999. Plymouth, UK: Plymbridge Distributors Ltd.
8. Catalona WJ, Smith DS, Ornstein DK. Prostate cancer detection in men with serum PSA concentrations of 2.6 to 4.0 ng/ml and benign prostate examination. Enhancement of specificity with free PSA measurements. J Am Med Assoc 1997;277:1452–5
9. Lodding P, Aus G, Bergdahl S, et al. Characteristics of screening detected prostate cancer in men 50 to 66 years old with 3 to 4 ng/mL prostate specific antigen. J Urol 1998;159:899
10. Bangma CH, Kranse R, Blijenberg BG, Schröder FH. The value of screening tests in the detection of prostate cancer. II. Retrospective analysis of free to total prostate-specific analysis ratio, age-specific reference ranges, and PSA density. Urology 1995;46:779–84
11. Christensson A, Björk T, Nilsson O, et al. Serum prostate specific antigen complexed to alpha

1-antichymotrypsin as an indicator of prostate cancer. *J Urol* 1993;150:100

12. Catalona WJ, Ramos CG, Carvahal GF, Yan Y. Lowering PSDA cutoffs to enhance detection of curable prostate cancer. *Urology* 2000;55:791

13. Hugosson J, Aus G, Bergdahl S, *et al.* Detection of early stage prostate cancer by measurements of free and total concentrations of prostate-specific antigen (PSA) in serum in a randomly selected population of men aged 50–66 years. *Urology*, submitted

14. Hugosson J, Aus G, Bergdahl S, Lilja H, Lodding P, Pileblad E. Biannual screening with PSA and a cut off at 3 ng/mL alone is sufficient to detect almost all prostate cancers while still curable. *J Urol*, submitted

Characteristics of prostate cancer in different prostate-specific antigen ranges

11

A. N. Vis, F. H. Schröder and T. H. van der Kwast

Introduction

Screening for prostate cancer

In Western Europe and North America, prostate cancer has become the most commonly diagnosed non-skin malignancy in men beyond middle age, the second leading cause of cancer-related death and a major cause of morbidity and health-care-related costs[1,2]. When prostate cancers were largely being diagnosed on clinical symptoms alone, the cumulative life-time risk for a man of ever being diagnosed with prostate cancer was approximately 8–10%, with a life-time risk of dying from the disease of 4%[3,4]. It is reported that men with clinically diagnosed prostate cancer will lose an average of 40% of their life expectancy as compared to an age-matched control group without prostate cancer[5]. This high mortality rate for prostate cancer may be due to the frequent clinical detection in its advanced stages, since the cancer often remains asymptomatic until it spreads systemically or invades adjacent structures. Unfortunately, no curative treatment for prostate cancer in its advanced stages is possible, indicating that a reduction of prostate cancer-related morbidity and mortality can only be achieved by enhancing the detection and radical treatment of the early (and intermediate) stages of the disease. With the introduction of serum prostate-specific antigen (PSA) measurement in the late 1980s, a powerful tool for the early detection of prostate cancer became available[3,6]. Mainly due to the widespread use of PSA as a marker for prostate cancer in the following years, a dramatic increase in the prostate cancer incidence was observed and followed by a gradual rise in the incidence/mortality ratio[7,8]. The increase in prostate cancer incidence, in addition, may also be attributed to an increased detection of cancers within an increasingly aging population, an increased public awareness of the disease, and the availability and the easy and safe application of ultrasound-guided transrectal (sextant) prostate needle biopsy[9].

In addition to the rise in incidence, screening with serum PSA to detect prostate cancer resulted in an increase in the proportion of organ-confined disease in a gradually younger population[5,8,10–13], a reduction in the proportion of patients with lymph node metastatic disease[11,14,15], an increase in the relative amount of well-to-moderately differentiated tumors[12–14,16,17] and a decrease in prostate cancer volume[12,18,19]. With respect to these prognostically favorable tumor features, early detection programs with PSA as a screening tool for prostate cancer may indeed detect prostate cancer in its curable phase more often. Therefore, PSA-based screening for prostate cancer has the potential to decrease the rate of disseminated disease and to decrease prostate cancer mortality.

Despite these favorable observations of PSA-based screening, it is argued that early detection programs for prostate cancer lead to the detection and treatment of small, indolent histological cancers, which would never have posed a threat to a patient's (quality of) life[20]. In fact, it is likely that screening for prostate cancer leads to considerable overdiagnosis and subsequent overtreatment of non-progressive cancers, whereas due to the screening test performances (i.e. the sensitivity and specificity) and the screening regimen itself, aggressive cancers may not be detected early enough. Part of the ethical consideration in deciding whether or not to conduct a national screening program for prostate cancer is whether the adverse effects of the detection and subsequent treatment of men with harmless cancers weigh against the (future) benefits of the detection and treatment of men with (future) clinically relevant disease. Until a reduction of prostate cancer mortality has been proven in a randomized fashion, screening for prostate cancer remains a controversial issue and is a subject of further debate and research.

Objectives

The European Randomized Study of Screening for Prostate Cancer (ERSPC) is a large multicenter randomized screening trial in which approximately 200 000 men are (to be) randomized into a screening and control arm. The objective of the ERSPC is to demonstrate a reduction in prostate cancer mortality of at least 20% (with a statistical power of 90%) in screened participants aged 55–74 years, compared to non-screened participants in the control group.

In the current report, the observed tumor characteristics in different PSA ranges of patients diagnosed with prostate cancer within the screening arm of the ERSPC, section Rotterdam, were compared to those reported in the literature. On the basis of the experiences of others and of those of our own, we attempted to define the clinical significance of the disease and we estimated the number of these seemingly biologically insignificant cancers within the different PSA ranges. Since it is known that tumor volume[3,21], pathological tumor stage[21,22–24] and histological grade (e.g. Gleason score)[21,25] correlate with serum PSA levels, we tested the hypothesis that the absolute number and relative proportion of clinically significant disease and, conversely, the absolute number and relative proportion of clinically insignificant disease, correlate to the serum PSA level as

well. These data provide particular insight into the value of different PSA cut-off points used in prostate cancer screening trials.

Screening regimen, cancers detected and pathological tissue processing

The ERSPC screening regimen, Rotterdam section

Between June 1st 1994 and December 31st 1999, 41 925 men, aged 55–74 years, were randomized to a screening and control arm within the Rotterdam section of the ERSPC. The Rotterdam protocol provides for re-screening after 4 years, but this report concentrates on the first screening round only (prevalence screen). Until February 1997, the screening protocol determined that screened participants with a serum PSA equal to or above 4.0 ng/ml (Hybritech Tandem E Assay) and/or a suspicious digital rectal examination (DRE) and/or a transrectal ultrasound (TRUS) finding at low PSA values (0.0–3.9 ng/ml) were to undergo prostate biopsy ($n = 20$ 193). In February 1997, a major change of protocol was implemented within the ERSPC, when the European study group (section Rotterdam) decided to take a biopsy exclusively from men with a PSA level of 3.0 ng/ml or more, without performing DRE or TRUS screening tests at all ($n = 21$ 732). Sextant transrectal biopsy was performed using a Bard (C.R. Bard, Convington, GA, USA) spring-loaded biopsy gun and an 18-gauge biopsy needle. Ultrasound guidance was performed using a 7-MHz end-fire ultrasound probe. Until December 31st 1999, 21 209 men were randomized to the screening arm of the ERSPC, and 1066 participants were diagnosed with prostate cancer after histopathological examination of the ultrasound-guided sextant transrectal biopsy. All prostate cancer patients were sent back to their general practitioner to be referred for treatment to one of the regional hospitals. Of these men, 274 (27.0%) underwent pelvic lymph node dissection and, subsequently, a radical prostatectomy within the University Hospital Rotterdam.

Methods of pathological tissue processing

All radical prostatectomy specimens were fixed, totally embedded and processed according to well-established protocols[26,27]. For each cancer, a Gleason score was determined and the tumor was staged by a single pathologist (TvdK) according to the TNM 1997 classification. All cancers detected in the radical prostatectomy specimen were examined for the relative proportion of high-grade cancer (i.e. Gleason growth pattern 4 or 5), and subsequent morphometric analysis was performed to determine overall tumor volume as described in detail by Hoedemaeker and colleagues[28].

Tumor characteristics at different PSA ranges

Comparison of tumor characteristics

The radical prostatectomy specimen offers a valuable tool for investigating the characteristics of prostate cancer in detail. The knowledge of the tumor features that may be expected within different PSA ranges may more adequately determine treatment decisions of patients diagnosed with prostate cancer. In recent years, multiple centers of excellence on prostate cancer management have reported on the tumor characteristics of prostate cancer in association with serum PSA levels. However, when directly comparing the findings of different prostate cancer early detection programs with respect to the tumor characteristics, some confounding factors may limit the comparability of different screening studies and, consequently, the conversion to one's own clinical practice.

First, participants subjected to different early detection programs may differ in age distribution, race and in socioeconomic or geographical background. A particular bias may be raised by the method of enrolment of patients to be screened for prostate cancer. Participants within a randomized screening trial may not have tumor features completely similar to those who are subjected to opportunistic screening regimens (e.g. by self-referral, media advertising, reimbursement fees). Second, a reliable comparison of tumor features between study groups is hampered by the fact that the different study groups have different 'exclusion' criteria and compliance rates for screening tests (e.g. frequency of application of screening tests before enrolment, biopsy refusal rates), they may use different screening tools (e.g. method of PSA assay, rectal examination), or they may have different biopsy recommendations (e.g. PSA cut-off level, age-specific PSA reference range, indications for repeated biopsy), and have different biopsy techniques (e.g. quadrant, sextant or lesion-directed biopsies). For instance, cancers detected by transurethral resection of the prostate (TURP) may have tumor features more favorable than those cancers in which a biopsy was prompted by an elevated PSA level only. These latter tumors, again, have tumor features more favorable than cancers detected by a suspicious DRE and subsequent lesion-directed biopsy[10,22,29,30]. Moreover, it is not clear whether the criteria used to select patients for surgery or alternative curative treatments, such as external beam therapy or brachytherapy, are comparable between the different institutes. Also, the proportion of men that refrain from any treatment may differ. In addition, the technical procedure of the radical prostatectomy itself may differ slightly (e.g. extension of nerve-sparing surgery, perineal or retropubic procedure) as may the level of radicality of the procedure itself. Last, but not least, the scrutiny of processing and examining the radical prostatectomy specimen by the pathologist (e.g. thickness of prostatic slices, experience in pathological staging, method of tumor-volume measurement) may influence the findings of the study group as a whole. With regard to these confounding factors, the listed figures (Table 1) may not be representative for all men at risk for the disease and, therefore, should be interpreted with caution.

Special attention will be given to the contribution of Partin and colleagues[11], who reported on an imposing cohort of 4133 men that underwent retropubic radical prostatectomy at three major academic urological centers within the United States between 1982

Table 1 Comparison between institutions. For each group, the method of enrolment into the study was assessed (if known), the method of the initial detection of prostate cancer (transurethral resection of the prostate (TURP), biopsies or both), the biopsy recommendation (stage T$_{1c}$, suspicious digital rectal examination (DRE)+ and/or transrectal ultrasound (TRUS)+), and the tumor characteristics determined in the radical prostatectomy specimen (if known)

PSA (ng/ml)	Reference	Method of enrolment	Method of detection/biopsies	Biopsy recommendation	Number of patients	Organ-confined (%)	Gleason score 7–10 (%)	Tumor volume (ml)
≥10.0	11	unclear	TURP/unclear	diverse	1151	29	ND	ND
	20	unclear	TURP/unclear	diverse	unclear	13	ND	8.6
	10	self-referral	lesion only	DRE+ and/or TRUS +	99	45	ND	ND
	present study	randomized	sextant	PSA+	31	47	61	2.0
	31	self-referral	quadrant/sextant	PSA+	unclear	54	ND	ND
	19	unclear	sextant	PSA+	11	82	64	2.1
4.0–9.9	11	unclear	TURP/unclear	diverse	2006	50	ND	ND
	31	self-referral	quadrant/sextant	PSA+	unclear	70	12	1.8
	10	self-referral	lesion only	DRE+ and/or TRUS+	145	75	ND	ND
	18	self-referral	quadrant/sextant	PSA+	78	59	ND	1.9
	14	unclear	TURP/unclear	PSA+ and/or DRE+	754	54	53	2.0
	20	unclear	unclear	diverse	unclear	56	ND	1.3
	30	unclear	unclear	PSA+	61	67	ND	3.0
	30	unclear	unclear	DRE+	209	44	ND	4.4
	present study	randomized	sextant	PSA+	167	76	42	1.1
	19	unclear	sextant	PSA+	18	78	39	1.1
0.0–3.9	11	unclear	TURP/unclear	diverse	943	64	ND	ND
	22	self-referral	quadrant	DRE+	33	88	ND	ND
	31	self-referral	quadrant/sextant	PSA+*	unclear	82	ND	1.1
	38	unclear	TRUS/unclear	DRE+ and/or TRUS+	187	73	ND	2.3
	36	randomized	sextant	PSA+†	14	57	21	1.8
	59	unclear	unclear	unclear	28	82	ND	ND
	19	unclear	lesion only	DRE+ and/or TRUS+	68	51	40	1.0
	present study	randomized	sextant	PSA+ and/or DRE+	76	87	32	0.5

ND, no data available; PSA, prostate-specific antigen; *for PSA 2.5–4.0 ng/ml; †for PSA 3.0–4.0 ng/ml and 1996. Despite the fact that not all patients were enrolled within prostate cancer early detection programs and, as a consequence, the methods of prostate cancer detection (e.g. detection by TURP, systematic or digitally guided biopsies) and the biopsy recommendations (i.e. PSA and/or DRE and/or TRUS) were not uniform, this large cohort of patients provided us with valuable data concerning the relationship of serum PSA to the various pathological tumor features. Since this study did not particularly focus on the correlation of serum PSA to other powerful conventional pathological prognostic factors (like tumor volume and Gleason score) we performed a literature review (Table 1).

Tumor features at high PSA values (≥ 10.0 ng/ml)

The multi-institutional update from Partin and co-workers[11] demonstrated that 29% (349/1184) of cancers in the PSA range ≥10.0 ng/ml were organ-confined (pT$_{2a-c}$), 46% (549/1184) had extraprostatic extension (pT$_{3a}$), 13% (153/1184) had seminal vesicle involvement (pT$_{3b}$) and 11% (133/1184) had positive lymph node involvement (pN$_1$) as the most advanced staging category (Table 1). Our data, from a randomized screening study, showed that 45% (14/31) of cases had organ-confined disease, whereas 36% (11/31) and 19% (6/31) of cases had evidence of extraprostatic extension (pT$_{3a}$) and invasion to adjacent structures (i.e. pT$_{3b}$ and/or pT$_4$), respectively (Table 2). The mean tumor volume was 1.9 ml and 36% (11/31) had the prognostically unfavorable indicator of more than 0.5 ml of poorly differentiated cancer. Of these tumors, 61% (19/31) had a Gleason score of 7 or higher (Table 2).

In summary, irrespective of the method of detection, cancers diagnosed at PSA values equal to or above 10.0 ng/ml often have characteristics of advanced disease, i.e. invasion and fixation to adjacent organs, established capsular penetration, a high tumor volume and a relatively high frequency of poorly differentiated components. Also, the frequency of systemic disease and the frequency of positive pelvic lymph nodes before radical prostatectomy is significantly higher than in the PSA range below 10.0 ng/ml[11,31–33]. Therefore, the presence of these highly adverse prognostic factors at a PSA value of 10.0 ng/ml or higher may be associated with rapid progression, regardless of curative therapy. On the other hand, it is likely that cancers with these advanced tumor characteristics may still be curable in some cases.

Tumor features at intermediate PSA values (4.0–9.9 ng/ml)

Partin and colleagues[11] reported that organ-confined disease was present in 50% (1009/2006) of subjects in the PSA range 4.0–9.9 ng/ml, 40% (809/2006) had extraprostatic extension, 6% (122/2006) had positive seminal vesicles and 3% (66/2006) already had disease disseminated to the lymph nodes (Table 1). Our results from the screening arm of a randomized screening trial demonstrated that 76% (127/167) of cases in this PSA range had organ-confined disease. In line with data from Catalona and co-workers[22,31], we found that men in the PSA range 4.0–9.9 ng/ml were almost twice as likely to have organ-confined disease than those with higher PSA levels (76% versus 45%). Of all cases treated with radical prostatectomy in the PSA range 4.0–9.9 ng/ml, 16% (27/167) had extraprostatic extension, 8% (13/167) had highly adverse prognostic indicators (pT$_{3b}$–pT$_4$), 42% (70/167) of subjects had a Gleason score of 7 or higher and the mean tumor volume was 1.10 ml (Table 2).

In summary, using PSA as a screening tool with rectal examination as an optional additional test, approximately 60–80% of surgically treated cases within the preoperative PSA range 4.0–9.9 ng/ml will have organ-confined disease, and most of these cases lack highly adverse pathological features with respect to tumor size and Gleason scores. The moderately favorable pathological features observed in this intermediate PSA range may render patients especially amenable to curative

Table 2 Characteristics of cases with screen-detected prostate cancer diagnosed within the screening arm (prevalence screen) of the Rotterdam section of the European Randomized Study of Screening for Prostate Cancer (ERSPC) at different prostate-specific antigen (PSA) values. The figures concern 274 men who underwent a radical prostatectomy between June 1994 and March 2000. Numbers in parentheses are percentages

PSA (ng/ml)	Pathological tumor stage (pTNM 1997)			Gleason score			Tumor volume (ml)		Tumor classification model		
	Organ-confined (pT_{2a-c})	Extraprostatic extension (pT_{3a})	Invading adjacent organs (pT_{3b}–pT_4)	2–6	7	8–10	Mean	Range	Possibly harmless* disease	Clinically significant† disease	Number of tumors
0.0–1.9	2 (100.0)	0 (0.0)	0 (0.0)	2 (100.0)	0 (0.0)	0 (0.0)	0.24	0.04–0.43	2 (100.0)	0 (0.0)	2 (0.7)
1.0–2.0	16 (84.2)	3 (15.8)	0 (0.0)	15 (78.9)	4 (21.1)	0 (0.0)	0.23	0.002–0.83	14 (73.7)	5 (26.3)	19 (6.9)
2.0–2.9	12 (80.0)	3 (20.0)	0 (0.0)	8 (53.3)	7 (46.7)	0 (0.0)	0.57	0.01–1.80	6 (40.0)	9 (60.0)	15 (5.5)
3.0–3.9	36 (90.0)	3 (7.5)	1 (2.5)	27 (67.5)	13 (32.5)	0 (0.0)	0.65	0.001–3.10	13 (32.5)	27 (67.5)	40 (14.6)
4.0–9.9	127 (76.0)	27 (16.2)	13 (7.8)	97 (58.1)	66 (39.5)	4 (2.4)	1.10	0.004–13.48	33 (19.8)	134 (80.2)	167 (61.0)
10.0–19.9	14 (46.7)	11 (36.7)	5 (16.7)	12 (40.0)	15 (50.0)	3 (10.0)	1.94	0.01–4.60	2 (6.7)	28 (93.3)	30 (11.0)
≥ 20.0	0 (0.0)	0 (0.0)	1 (100.0)	0 (0.0)	1 (100.0)	0 (0.0)	2.72	2.72–2.72	0 (0.0)	1 (100.0)	1 (0.4)
Total	207 (75.5)	47 (17.2)	20 (7.3)	161 (58.8)	106 (38.7)	7 (2.6)	1.04	0.001–13.48	69 (25.2)	205 (74.8)	274 (100.0)

*As defined as small (< 0.5 ml) organ-confined tumors, without Gleason growth pattern 4/5; †as defined as all tumors with characteristics other than those of 'possibly harmless'

treatment, radical prostatectomy in particular. However, a small proportion (< 10%) of cases with prostate cancer will be beyond cure at the time of detection.

Tumor features at low PSA values (0.0–3.9 ng/ml)

Most previous screening studies used a PSA concentration of 4.0 ng/ml as the upper limit for normal, but early studies have already indicated that sizeable carcinomas of the prostate may exist at low PSA values (0.0–3.9 ng/ml)[6,21,34]. It is even argued that cancers with advanced tumor characteristics may not be detected in these PSA ranges since poorly differentiated components within these tumors produce only little PSA[21]. Depending on the biopsy recommendation (i.e. PSA and PSA cut-off level, rectal examination), the proportion of men diagnosed with prostate cancer varies between 7% and 30% in this low PSA range[11,19,22,31,35–41].

Correspondingly, it may be assumed that the tumor characteristics will also depend on the method of initial detection. From a total of 943 patients, Partin and colleagues[11] reported that 64% (599/943) of men had tumors that were organ-confined, 32% (303/943) had capsular penetration, 3% (28/943) had seminal vesicle involvement and only 1% (13/943) of men had positive lymph nodes (Table 1). According to yet unpublished data from Catalona and co-workers[31] on 676 patients in the PSA range 2.6–4.0 ng/ml, who underwent radical prostatectomy, organ-confined disease was found in 81%. In fact, Catalona's group suggested that the rate of organ-confined disease and the proportion of cancers with a Gleason score of 7 or higher detected in the PSA range 2.6–4.0 ng/ml were similar to those detected in the PSA range 4.1–9.9 ng/ml. The mean tumor volume in the PSA range 4.0–9.9 ng/ml (i.e. 1.8 ml), on the other hand, was significantly larger than that measured in the PSA range 2.6–4.0 ng/ml (i.e. 1.1 ml; $p = 0.02$). Our data (from the Rotterdam section of the ERSPC) indicate that in the PSA range 0.0–2.9 ng/ml, in which a biopsy was prompted by a suspicious rectal examination only, the mean tumor volume was 0.39 ml, 83% (30/36) of cases were organ-confined and 31% (11/36) had a Gleason score of 7. In the group of men with combined biopsy indications (PSA only and/or suspicious rectal examination) in the PSA range of 3.0–3.9 ng/ml, the mean tumor volume was 0.65 ml, 90% (36/40) were organ-confined and 33% (13/40) had a Gleason score of 7 or higher (Table 2).

To summarize, cancers detected at PSA values below 4.0 ng/ml mostly have highly favorable tumor characteristics with respect to pathological tumor stage, tumor volume and Gleason score. Tumors detected in the PSA range 2.6–4.0 ng/ml may resemble those detected in the PSA range 4.0–9.9 ng/ml, whereas those detected in the PSA range below 2.0 ng/ml will very seldom have adverse pathological features. Therefore, the vast majority of cases (≥ 90%) in the PSA range 0.0–3.9 ng/ml can be cured with radical prostatectomy, but many may not pose a risk to the patient.

Clinically insignificant disease

What is the prevalence of prostate cancer?

Based on autopsy studies and studies evaluating the cystoprostatectomy specimen, the prevalence of prostate cancer was previously estimated to lie between 30% and 50% of the elderly male population[19,42–45]. Whereas prostate cancer is often described as a silent cancer that elderly men die *with* (other illnesses) rather than *of* (metastatic disease), the reality is that the incidence rates and mortality rates of the disease, and to a lesser extent the mean age and the stage at diagnosis, may be very similar to those of breast cancer, which is not often the subject of similar concerns. However, this high reservoir of subclinical disease within a population may not be a property of prostatic adenocarcinoma only. Black and Welch[46] estimated that at a certain moment in time, the prevalence of clinically diagnosed prostate cancer within the male population is 1%, while this exact figure can also be applied to the female population with respect to breast cancer.

The prevalence of clinically apparent thyroid cancer, on the other hand, was estimated to be lower, at 0.1% of the adult population. As autopsy studies have already clarified, the microscopical prevalence of disease may be much higher, i.e. approximately 46% for prostate cancer and 39% for breast cancer[46]. For thyroid cancer, Harach and colleagues[47] reported that, by cutting the thyroid gland in 2.5-mm slices on autopsy, 36% of cases had evidence microscopically of this malignancy too. The authors suggested that the prevalence of histologically verifiable thyroid cancer may be close to, if not equal to, 100% (!) if one could look at even thinner slices of the gland. Probably, this (extrapolated) figure reflecting the actual prevalence of disease might also be true for equivalent organs and malignancies like those of the human prostate and the human breast. On the other hand, the prevalence of cancer that has not yet caused signs and symptoms, but with time will definitely do so, can be only roughly estimated. In any case, it may be expected that the prevalence of future clinically apparent disease will be a multiplicity of the prevalence of cancers that have already revealed themselves clinically.

What is clinically (in)significant disease?

By definition, clinically significant cancers are those tumors that have already caused symptoms or are expected to do so in the future. Conversely, clinically insignificant cancers are those that cause no symptoms and will never do so in the rest of a man's lifetime. Unfortunately, it can hardly be predicted whether a prostate cancer diagnosed in an asymptomatic man will ever be able to cause clinical symptoms, especially when these cancers reside in relatively young men and have tumor features of early or intermediate-stage disease. It may be assumed that the patient's life expectancy in association with the tumor characteristics at diagnosis (like tumor volume, pathological tumor stage and histological grade) determine whether a tumor will become clinically apparent in these asymptomatic men. Although there is no absolute tumor size, pathological stage or

histological grade associated with clinical complaints, the chance of prostate cancer-related morbidity and mortality increases steadily with increasing tumor volume, tumor stage and histopathological grade[3,21].

Using one or several of these tumor characteristics, different study groups have tried independently to distinguish clinically significant from clinically insignificant disease. However, since the criteria chosen were all determined on the radical prostatectomy specimen and, thus, the natural course of disease was interrupted, the definition of what is actually clinically significant disease remains a controversial issue. Only prospective, randomized clinical trials, which show no benefit of treating cancers with clinically insignificant tumor features compared to an 'observation only' control group with similar (preoperative) tumor features may prove true biological insignificance. Despite these flaws, the group from Stanford University suggested that clinically insignificant tumors may be those that have a total tumor volume of less than 0.5 ml[45]. This definition for clinical significance was partially based on an earlier study from the same study group, which found 55 (40%) unsuspected prostate cancers in 139 cystoprostatectomy specimens removed for bladder cancer. Since it was assumed that 8% of men would experience clinically evident prostate cancer in their lifetimes, it is likely that these were the men with the largest cancers, provided that the natural course of disease was not interrupted by the cystoprostatectomy. In fact, the 8% largest prostate cancers within the cystoprostatectomy group were all at least 0.5 ml in tumor volume.

The Johns Hopkins group built on these criteria to define possibly harmless prostate cancer, but a tumor volume of the largest cancer nodule of less than 0.2 ml was used as an arbitrary cut-off for true biological insignificance. Moreover, 'clinically insignificant' cancers were assumed to be confined to the prostate and to lack poorly differentiated (i.e. Gleason growth patterns 4/5) components. Men with a tumor volume between 0.2 and 0.5 ml were categorized as having 'minimal' disease, i.e. at the threshold of biological significance[29]. The cut-off tumor volume of 0.2 ml for 'clinically significant' disease was based partially on a series of 21 clinical stage T_2 cancers, in which none demonstrated capsular penetration and none showed disease recurrence after radical prostatectomy. Of cases with a tumor volume between 0.2 ml and 0.5 ml (i.e. 'minimal' disease) 13% (3/23) had extracapsular extension and none showed PSA relapse after radical prostatectomy[48]. Curable prostate cancers (both clinically significant and insignificant) were those, for which more than 75% of cases remained free of PSA progression 10 years after radical prostatectomy[29]. More or less at the same time, the group from the Methodist Hospital, Houston proposed a similarly constructed tumor classification model, which was also based on progression-free survival rates[19].

It is obvious that the prediction of clinically insignificant prostate cancer before treatment could preclude surgery, radiation therapy and their associated morbidities. Unfortunately, the preoperative prediction of insignificant disease, using clinical and biochemical parameters, as well as tumor features determined on the biopsy specimen, remains highly unreliable[29,49–55]. Several investigators have noted that, of patients with a total cancer length of less than 3 mm in one biopsy core and in whom the cancer had features of well-to-moderately differentiated disease only, a minority of cases had a tumor volume of less than 0.5 ml[29,53–55]. Cupp and colleagues[49] concluded that prostate biopsy should be regarded as a test for identifying the presence or absence of prostate cancer, rather than determining the clinical significance of the disease.

Are indolent cancers detected by screening efforts?

Considering the fact that the microscopical prevalence of disease is high (approximately 30–50% in an elderly male population) in comparison to the prevalence of clinically apparent disease (approximately 1%), it is obvious that the vast majority of cancers will never cause symptoms, morbidity or mortality. In other words, most prevalent cancers are clinically insignificant. With respect to the tumor characteristics and the estimated tumor doubling times, this may be well comprehended, since prostate cancers found on autopsy studies and, coincidentally, within the cystoprostatectomy specimens (i.e. 'indolent' cancers) show median tumor volumes mostly of less than 0.05 ml, 10–25-fold smaller than those detected in early detection programs[12,18,19,44–56]. Indolent cancers are mostly confined to the prostate and lack features of de-differentiation[19]. However, some tumors with adverse prognostic pathological features were still found in these experimental studies[19,20]. Therefore, recently performed studies have focused on the frequency of the detection of seemingly clinically insignificant disease rather than on the difference between the tumor characteristics of cancers coincidentally found on autopsy or after cystoprostatectomy and those detected in screening programs.

Terris and co-workers[51,52] estimated the detection of clinically insignificant disease (i.e. those with a tumor volume of less than 0.5 ml) to be 4% after performing systematic biopsy on 816 men with clinical stage T_{1c} disease. Using the same criteria to define clinically insignificant prostate cancer, Stamey and associates[57] reviewed a series of 896 consecutive cases that underwent radical prostatectomy for clinical stage $T_{1c–2c}$ disease and concluded that PSA testing appears to detect clinically insignificant disease in only 6.4% of cases. Catalona and colleagues[10] reported the results from a large multicenter study and noted that low volume (i.e. < 1% cancer and no evidence of capsular penetration) and low-grade (Gleason score 2–4) or moderately low-grade (Gleason score 5–7) disease occurred in 2.9% (7/244) of surgically treated cases. In these subjects, a biopsy was performed when PSA values were 4.0 ng/ml or higher in conjunction with a suspicious DRE. Epstein and associates[29] reported on a series of 134 surgically treated cases with clinical stage T_{1c} disease, in whom a biopsy was prompted by a PSA value above

4.0 ng/ml. Despite the fact that no systematic method of performing the needle biopsy was used, 11% of cases were 'clinically insignificant' (i.e. small, < 0.2 ml, organ-confined disease with no Gleason 4/5 patterns) and 8% of cases were 'minimal' (i.e. organ-confined, tumor volume between 0.2 and 0.5 ml, no Gleason 4/5). Soh and colleagues[14] evaluated a series of 754 men who underwent radical prostatectomy for prostate cancer detected by transurethral resection, a suspicious DRE/TRUS and/or a PSA equal to or above 4.0 ng/ml. They found clinically unimportant cancer (i.e. organ-confined disease with a tumor volume of less than 0.5 ml and no Gleason 4/5) in 10% of cases and noticed that this figure was constant with time for the varying frequencies of application of the diagnostic tools. According to the Epstein criteria, Carter and associates[58] used the Baltimore Longitudinal Study of Aging population to report on the frequency of detection of clinically insignificant and minimal disease. They revealed that the proportion of minimal cancers was 69% (25/36), 84% (16/19) and 53% (9/17) in stage T_{1c} patients with a PSA value in the ranges 0.0–4.0 ng/ml, 0.0–2.5 ng/ml and 2.5–4.0 ng/ml, respectively. There was also a steady decline in the proportion of cases with clinically insignificant disease with increasing PSA values, i.e. 33% (12/36) in the PSA range 4.0–5.0 ng/ml, 26% (52/197) in the PSA range 5.0–10.0 ng/ml and 15% (18/120) in the PSA range greater than 10.0 ng/ml. Babaian and colleagues[59] reported that 12% (2/17) and 29% (8/28) of prostate cancers detected in the PSA range 2.6–4.0 ng/ml and 0.0–4.0 ng/ml, respectively, were smaller than 0.5 ml and assumed to be clinically insignificant. Further, yet preliminary data from the Washington University School of Medicine, St Louis[31] appear to show that 11.9% and 11.5% of cases in the PSA range 2.6–4.0 ng/ml and 4.0–9.9 ng/ml, respectively, had minimal disease (according to the Epstein criteria) when PSA was used as the only screening tool.

In the screening arm of our randomized study population, 25% (69/274) of cases under-going retropubic radical prostatectomy for clinical stage T_{1c-2c} prostate cancer were assessed as possibly harmless on the basis of the presence of organ-confined disease, a tumor volume of less than 0.5 ml and the absence of Gleason growth patterns 4 and 5 (Table 2). The proportion of cancers with these highly favorable tumor characteristics increased steadily with decreasing PSA levels, i.e. 35% (19/55) for PSA levels of 2.0–3.9 ng/ml, 74% (14/19) for PSA values of 1.0–1.9 ng/ml and 100% (2/2) for PSA values below 1.0 ng/ml. According to the Epstein criteria, the proportion of 'clinically insignificant' disease was 15% (40/274) for all PSA ranges and decreased sharply with rising PSA values, i.e. 33% (12/36) for the PSA range 0.0–2.9 ng/ml, 20% (8/40) for the PSA range 3.0–3.9 ng/ml, 11% (18/167) for the PSA range 4.0–9.9 ng/ml and 7% (2/31) for PSA values ≥ 10.0 ng/ml[29].

Dugan and colleagues[56] from the Mayo Clinic, Rochester were the first to propose an age-related adjustment for the definition of clinically significant disease. It may be expected that, for instance, an organ-confined, 0.4-ml sized prostate cancer with a Gleason score of 6 should be looked upon differently when it is discovered in a healthy 50-year-old man than when this same cancer is discovered in a 70-year-old man with severe cardiopulmonary complaints. Despite the fact that this study has some shortcomings and limitations (as has already been stated by the authors) two important observations were made. First, even in the most optimistic tumor behavior scenario (e.g. the longest assumed tumor doubling time), no clinically insignificant cancers were detected in patients under the age of 60 years. Second, the definition of clinically insignificant disease should probably be adapted in the future since more and more men will outlive their co-morbidities, will live longer overall and will, thus, be prone to experience clinically evident prostate cancer in their lifetime.

In summary, the morphological features of prostate cancers detected within early detection programs suggest that these do not very much resemble the average of 'indolent' cancers coincidentally found on autopsy or after cystoprostatectomy. As our results indicate, screen-detected prostate cancers very rarely have tumor volumes of less than 0.2 ml, while cancers smaller than 0.05 ml are detected even less frequently. The frequency of the detection of 'clinically insignificant' and 'minimal' disease, as arbitrarily defined by Epstein and co-workers[29], was highly associated to PSA level. For instance, in the PSA ranges 0.0–2.0 ng/ml and 2.0–4.0 ng/ml, approximately 80% and 40% of surgically treated cases, respectively, will be categorized as having minimal disease. These figures steadily decline at PSA values above 4.0 ng/ml. Therefore, although screening with PSA for prostate cancer results in stage migration, grade migration and the detection of cancers with a low tumor volume, the test may not be sensitive enough to detect many of the seemingly indolent and clinically insignificant cancers.

Why are these small tumors detected?

It seems justified to state that the cancers detected as a consequence of an abnormal screening test are detected because the tumor has reached a certain tumor volume. In general, the larger the tumor, the more likely it is to be detected by a screening test. What exact size a tumor should have to be able to increase the serum PSA level above the cut-off point of 3.0 ng/ml or, alternatively, cause it to be palpable on DRE, is unclear, but it may be assumed that a prostate cancer volume of 0.5 ml, at least, is necessary. Therefore, cancers with a tumor volume equal to or above 0.5 ml at a PSA level equal to or above 3.0 ng/ml in which the DRE was suspicious (induration, nodularity, asymmetry) are assumed to be detected as a result of a 'true-positive' screening test result. Men in whom a biopsy was prompted by a suspicious DRE or an elevated PSA level and, in the end, turn out to have no cancer on the biopsy are 'false-positives'. However, cancers with a tumor volume of less than 0.5 ml, in which the diagnosis was made after the evaluation of a positive screening test, are not 'false-positives' for the simple reason that prostate cancer is present. These cancers should be considered as detected by chance or serendipity rather than as a consequence of the evaluation of an abnormal screening test result[60]. Potentially harmless prostate cancers that have tumor volumes of less than 0.5 ml (minimal disease), or even less than 0.2 ml (clinically insignificant disease), are by definition detected by serendipity ('serendipity-positive test' result)[29]. However, serendipity may not concern only small or otherwise clinically insignificant cancers. In some clinically significant cancers in which the diagnostic biopsy was prompted by a palpably suspicious lesion, the histopathological diagnosis may have been made in one or more of the cores of the sextant, rather than in the lesion-directed biopsy core. Therefore, the suspicion is justified that these cancers were not detected as a consequence of the evaluation of the abnormal screening test itself, but coincidentally. Moreover, cancers containing poorly differentiated components, but in which the tumor volume is still small (i.e. < 0.5 ml) are also clinically significant and, with respect to their tumor volumes, should also be considered as being detected by serendipity.

When serendipity is responsible for the detection of large numbers of these clinically insignificant cancers, it may be disadvantageous in prostate cancer screening programs. The relative amount of cancers detected by serendipity seems considerable and the frequency depends highly on the serum PSA level. As we have stated earlier, the proportion of minimal and clinically insignificant disease is inversely correlated to serum PSA and, as a consequence, the proportion of serendipity-detected cancers will also increase with a decreasing PSA level. In our study, in which rectal examination was the only screening tool for prostate cancer in low PSA ranges (0.0–2.9 ng/ml), at least 61% of cases (i.e. minimal cancers) were detected by serendipity and this figure steadily increased from 74% in the PSA range 1.0–1.9 ng/ml to 100% at PSA values below 1.0 ng/ml. At these low PSA values, DRE as a screening test for prostate cancer has little or no inherent predictive value for the presence of prostate cancer. It may be assumed that these cancers were detected 'by accident' within the large pool of clinically insignificant cancers. Therefore, DRE as a screening test for prostate cancer may perform no better (i.e. in the detection of clinically significant cancers) than an unequivocally invalid screening test such as, for instance, 'the presence of gray hair' or 'wearing a blue coat'.

What is the optimal screening effort?

Unfortunately, the optimal screening regimen can only be determined after the completion of randomized clinical trials, such as the ERSPC, which may or may not demonstrate a reduction of prostate cancer mortality in the future. Until a mortality reduction is proven in these screening trials, evaluation and optimization of the screening tests (i.e. the validity) should be an objective and a major investigative focus. The optimal screening regimen will be determined on the basis of a close scrutiny of the detection rates of the screening tests (separate or in combination), the positive and negative predictive values of the screening tests and the number of biopsies required to detect one cancer. Moreover, the tumor characteristics of the cancers detected in these early detection programs should be looked at closely. The observed tumor characteristics may give detailed insight into the aggressiveness of the disease and, in combination with patient-related factors (e.g. age, coexistent diseases, awaited life expectancy), into the expected course of the disease and the proper patient management. Screening programs should detect cancers that will express themselves clinically in the near future (i.e. clinically significant disease), while the detection of cancers that are silent, and that will remain so during a man's lifetime (i.e. clinically insignificant disease), should be prevented.

Our data clearly demonstrate that clinically insignificant disease is highly prevalent in patients with low PSA values (0.0–3.9 ng/ml) who underwent a radical prostatectomy. More strongly, in the PSA range 0.0–1.9 ng/ml, nearly all patients who underwent surgery are presumed to have clinically insignificant disease

on the basis of their highly favorable tumor features. We admit that the data presented were derived from a select group of patients (i.e. those who underwent a radical prostatectomy); however, it may be very unlikely that, in cases with these low PSA ranges in particular, the tumor aggressiveness features of those subjected to the different treatment modalities will differ significantly. We proved that the screening test (DRE) that is used in cases of low PSA ranges has only little or no inherent predictive value for the presence of cancer. Most cancers in the low PSA ranges are assumed to be detected by chance only. With respect to the high prevalence of clinically insignificant disease in the population and the poor performance of the screening test (rectal examination), we postulate that screening with rectal examination as a screening test in the cases of PSA range 0.0–1.9 ng/ml, in particular, and probably also in the PSA range 2.0–2.9 ng/ml, is of little use, is potentially harmful to the participants and should be omitted.

Summary

Our investigations, in association with a review of the literature, demonstrate that tumor characteristics of the prostate cancers that are detected within screening trials depend highly on serum PSA levels. Whereas adverse pathological tumor features (i.e. high pathological tumor stage, presence of poorly differentiated components, high tumor volumes) are frequently found in cases with intermediate (4.0–9.9 ng/ml) and, even more frequently, in cases with high PSA ranges (≥ 10.0 ng/ml), the presence of these adverse prognosticators is infrequent in cases with low PSA ranges (0.0–3.9 ng/ml). A major effort in early detection programs for prostate cancer should be focused on the detection of clinically significant cancers (those that will cause complaints and mortality in the future), while the detection of clinically insignificant disease (those that will never cause symptoms) should be prevented. Since clinically insignificant disease is highly associated with the PSA level, it may be expected that the vast majority (approximately 75–100%) of cancers detected in the PSA range 0.0–1.9 ng/ml and, to a lesser extent, in the PSA range 2.0–2.9 ng/ml are potentially harmless. Also, considering the fact that the performance of the screening test is poor at low PSA values and that rational, selective and ethical screening for prostate cancer is a desirable objective, screening for prostate cancer might be limited to PSA values equal to or above 3.0 ng/ml.

References

1. Visser O, Coebergh JWW, Schouten LJ, *et al.* Incidence of cancer in the Netherlands 1995. *Seventh Report of the Netherlands Cancer Registry.* Utrecht: Vereniging van Integrale Kankercentra, 1998
2. Landis SH, Murray T, Boldon S, *et al* Cancer statistics 1999. *CA Cancer J Clin* 1999;49:8–31
3. Stamey TA, Yang N, Hay AR, *et al.* Prostate-specific antigen as a serum marker for adenocarcinoma of the prostate. *N Engl J Med* 1987;317:909–16
4. Rosen MA. Impact of prostate-specific antigen on screening on the natural history of prostate cancer. *Urology* 1995;46:757–68
5. Grönberg H, Damber J, Jonsson H, *et al.* Patient age as a prognostic factor in prostate cancer. *J Urol* 1994;152:892–5
6. Catalona WJ, Smith DS, Ratliff TL, *et al.* Measurement of prostate-specific antigen in serum as a screening test for prostate cancer. *N Engl J Med* 1991;324:1156–61
7. Potosky AL, Miller BA, Albertsen PC, *et al.* The role of increasing detection in the rising incidence of prostate cancer. *J Am Med Assoc* 1995;273:548–52
8. Jacobsen SJ, Katusic SK, Bergstrahl EJ, *et al.* Incidence of prostate cancer diagnosis in the eras before and after serum prostate-specific antigen testing. *J Am Med Assoc* 1995;274:1445–9
9. Hodge KK, McNeal JE, Terris MK, *et al.* Random systematic versus directed ultrasound guided transrectal core biopsies of the prostate. *J Urol* 1989;142:71–5
10. Catalona WJ, Smith DS, Ratliff TL, *et al.* Detection of organ-confined prostate cancer is increased through prostate-specific antigen based screening. *J Am Med Assoc* 1993;270:948–54
11. Partin AW, Kattan MW, Subong ENP, *et al.* Combination of prostate-specific antigen, clinical stage, and Gleason score to predict pathological stage of localized prostate cancer. A multi-institutional update. *J Am Med Assoc* 1997; 277:1445–51
12. Hoedemaeker RF, Rietbergen JBW, Kranse R, *et al.* Histopathological prostate cancer characteristics at radical prostatectomy after population-based screening. *J Urol* 2000;164:411–15
13. Stephenson RA, Stanford JL. Population-based prostate cancer trends in the United States: patterns of change in the era of prostate-specific antigen. *World J Urol* 1997;15:331–5
14. Soh S, Kattan MW, Berkman S, *et al.* Has there been a recent shift in the pathological features and prognosis of patients treated by radical prostatectomy? *J Urol* 1997;157:2212–18
15. Petros JA, Catalona WJ. Lower incidence of unsuspected lymph node metastases in 521 consecutive patients with clinically localized prostate cancer. *J Urol* 1992;147:1574–5
16. Mettlin CJ, Murphy GP, Rosenthal DS, *et al.* The National Cancer DataBase report on prostate carcinoma after the peak in incidence rates in the U.S. The American College of Surgeons Commission on Cancer and the American Cancer Society. *Cancer* 1998;83:1679–84
17. Aihara M, Lebovitz RM, Wheeler TM, *et al.* Prostate specific antigen and Gleason grade: an immunohistochemical study of prostate cancer. *J Urol* 1994;151:1558–64
18. Humphrey PA, Keetch DW, Smith DS, *et al.* Prospective characterization of pathological features of prostatic carcinomas detected via serum prostate-specific antigen based screening. *J Urol* 1996;155:816–20
19. Ohori M, Wheeler TM, Dunn JK, *et al.* The pathological features and prognosis of prostate cancer detectable with current diagnostic tests. *J Urol* 1994;152:1714–20

20. Scardino PT, Weaver R, Hudson MA. Early detection of prostate cancer. *Hum Pathol* 1992;23:211–22

21. Partin AW, Carter HB, Chan DW, *et al.* Prostate-specific antigen in the staging of localized prostate cancer: influence on tumor differentiation, tumor volume and benign hyperplasia. *J Urol* 1990;143:747–52

22. Catalona WJ, Richie JP, Ahmann FR, *et al.* Comparison of digital rectal examination and serum prostate-specific antigen in the early detection of prostate cancer: results of a multicenter clinical trial of 6,630 men. *J Urol* 1994;151:1283–90

23. Ercole CJ, Lange PH, Mathisen M, *et al.* Prostatic specific antigen and prostatic acid phosphatase in the monitoring and staging of patients with prostate cancer. *J Urol* 1987;138:1181–4

24. Oesterling JE, Chan DW, Epstein JI, *et al.* Prostate-specific antigen in the pre-operative and post-operative evaluation of localized prostatic cancer treated with radical prostatectomy. *J Urol* 1988;139:766–72

25. Stamey TA, Kabalin JN, McNeal JE, *et al.* Prostate specific antigen in the diagnosis and treatment of adenocarcinoma of the prostate II. Radical prostatectomy treated patients. *J Urol* 1989;141:1076–83

26. Stamey TA, McNeal JE, Freiha FS, *et al.* Morphometric and clinical studies on 68 consecutive radical prostatectomies. *J Urol* 1988;139:1235–41

27. Hoedemaeker RF, Ruijter ETG, Ruizeveld-de Winter JA, *et al.* The Biomed II MPC Study group, Van der Kwast ThH. Processing radical prostatectomy specimens. *J Urol Pathol* 1998;9:211–22

28. Hoedemaeker RF, Rietbergen JBW, Kranse R, *et al.* Comparison of pathological characteristics of T1c and non-T1c cancers detected in a population-based screening study, the European Randomized Study of Screening for Prostate Cancer. *World J Urol* 1997;15:339–45

29. Epstein JI, Walsh PC, Carmichael M, *et al.* Pathological and clinical findings to predict tumor extent of nonpalpable (stage T1c) prostate cancer. *J Am Med Assoc* 1994;271:368–74

30. Geary ES, Stamey TA. Pathological characteristics and prognosis of non-palpable and palpable prostate cancers with a Hybritech prostate specific antigen of 4 to 10 ng/ml. *J Urol* 1996;156:1056–8

31. Catalona WJ, Ramos CG, Carvalhal GF, *et al.* Lowering PSA cutoffs to enhance detection of curable prostate cancer. *Urology* 2000;55:791–5

32. Narayan P, Fournier G, Gajendran V, *et al.* Utility of preoperative serum prostate-specific antigen concentration and biopsy Gleason score in predicting risk of pelvic lymph node metastases in prostate cancer. *Urology* 1994;44:519–24

33. Bluestein DL, Bostwick DG, Bergstrahl EJ, *et al.* Eliminating the need for bilateral pelvic lymphadenectomy in select patients with prostate cancer. *J Urol* 1994;151:1315–20

34. Cooner WH, Mosley BR, Rutherford CL, *et al.* Prostate cancer detection in a clinical urological practice by ultrasonography, digital-rectal examination, and prostate specific antigen. *J Urol* 1990;143:1146–52

35. Colberg JW, Smith DS, Catalona WJ. Prevalence and pathological extent of prostate cancer in men with prostate specific antigen of 2.9 to 4 ng/ml. *J Urol* 1993;149:507–9

36. Lodding P, Aus G, Bergdahl R, *et al.* Characteristics of screening detected prostate cancer in men 50 to 60 years old with 3 to 4 ng/ml prostate specific antigen. *J Urol* 1998;159:899–903

37. Smith DS, Humphrey PA, Catalona WJ. The early detection of prostatic carcinoma with prostate-specific antigen: the Washington University experience. *Cancer* 1997;80:1852–6

38. Noldus J, Stamey TA. Histological characteristics of radical prostatectomy specimens in men with a serum prostate specific antigen of 4 ng/ml or less. *J Urol* 1996;155:441–3

39. Catalona WJ, Smith DS, Ornstein DK. Prostate cancer detection in men with serum PSA concentrations of 2.6 to 4 ng/ml and benign prostate examination: enhancement of specificity with free PSA measurement. *J Am Med Assoc* 1997;277:1452–5

40. Vis AN, Hoedemaeker RF, Roobol M, *et al.* Tumor characteristics in screening for prostate cancer with and without rectal examination as an initial screening test at low PSA (0.0–3.9 ng/ml). Validation of screening with PSA as the only tool. 2000 (submitted)

41. Reissigl A, Pointner J, Horninger W, *et al.* Comparison of different prostate-specific antigen cutpoints for early detection of prostate cancer: results of a large screening study. *Urology* 1995;46:662–5

42. Franks LM. Latent carcinoma of the prostate. *J Pathol Bacteriol* 1954;68:603–6

43. Sakr WA, Grignon DJ, Crissman JD, *et al.* High-grade prostatic intraepithelial neoplasia (HGPIN) and prostatic adenocarcinoma between the age of 20–69: an autopsy study of 249 cases. *In Vivo* 1994;8:439–43

44. Kabalin JN, McNeal JE, Price HM, *et al.* Unsuspected adenocarcinoma of the prostate in patients undergoing cystoprostatectomy for other causes: incidence, histology and morphometric observations. *J Urol* 1989;141:1091–4

45. Stamey TA, Freiha FS, McNeal JE, *et al.* Localized prostate cancer. Relationship of tumor vol-

ume to clinical significance for treatment of prostate cancer. *Cancer* 1993;(Suppl 71):993–8

46. Black WC, Welch HG. Advances in diagnostic imaging and overestimations of disease prevalence and the benefits of therapy. *N Engl J Med* 1993;328:1237–43

47. Harach HR, Franssila KO, Wasenius VM. Occult papillary carcinoma of the thyroid: a 'normal' finding in Finland: a systematic autopsy study. *Cancer* 1985;56:531–8

48. Epstein JI, Carmichael M, Partin AW, *et al.* Is tumor volume an independent predictor of progression following radical prostatectomy? A multivariate analysis of 185 clinical stage B adenocarcinomas of the prostate with five years follow-up. *J Urol* 1993;149:1478–81

49. Cupp MR, Bostwick DG, Myers RP, *et al.* The volume of prostate cancer in the biopsy specimen cannot reliably predict the quantity of cancer in the radical prostatectomy specimen on an individual basis. *J Urol* 1995;153:1543–8

50. Bassler TJ, Orozco R, Bassler IC, *et al.* Most prostate cancers missed by raising the upper limit of normal prostate-specific antigen for men in their sixties are clinically significant. *Urology* 1998;52:1064–9

51. Terris MK, McNeal JE, Stamey TA. Detection of clinically significant prostate cancer by transrectal ultrasound-guided systematic biopsies. *J Urol* 1992;148:829–32

52. Terris MK, Haney DJ, Johnstone IM, *et al.* Prediction of prostate cancer volume using prostate-specific antigen levels, transrectal ultrasound, and systematic sextant biopsies. *Urology* 1995;45:75–80

53. Stamey TA. Making the most out of six systematic sextant biopsies. *Urology* 1995;45:2–12

54. Goto Y, Ohori M, Arakawa A, *et al.* Distinguishing clinically important from unimportant prostate cancers before treatment: value of systematic biopsies. *J Urol* 1996;156:1059–63

55. Dietrick DD, McNeal JE, Stamey TA. Core cancer length in ultrasound-guided systematic sextant biopsies: a preoperative evaluation of prostate cancer volume. *Urology* 1995;45:987–92

56. Dugan JA, Bostwick DG, Myers RP, *et al.* The definition and preoperative prediction of clinically insignificant prostate cancer. *J Am Med Assoc* 1996;275:288–94

57. Stamey TA, Donaldson AN, Yemoto CE, *et al.* Histological and clinical findings in 896 consecutive prostates treated only with radical retropubic prostatectomy: epidemiological significance of annual changes. *J Urol* 1998; 160:2412–17

58. Carter HB, Epstein JI, Chan DW, *et al.* Recommended prostate-specific antigen testing intervals for the detection of curable prostate cancer. *J Am Med Assoc* 1997;277:1456–60

59. Babaian RJ, Troncoso P, Steelhammer LC, *et al.* Tumor volume and prostate specific antigen: implications for early detection and defining a window of curability. *J Urol* 1995;154:1808–12

60. McNaughton Collins M, Ransohoff DF, Barry MJ. Early detection of prostate cancer. Serendipity strikes again. *J Am Med Assoc* 1997;278:1516–19

How accurately does biopsy information determine outcome?

12

V. Narain, F. Bianco, M. Heath, D. J. Grignon, W. A. Sakr, J. E. Pontes and D. P. Wood Jr

Since prostate cancer is often a slow growing tumor affecting patients in the latter decades of life, it is important to identify prognostic factors that may predict the aggressiveness of prostate cancer for an individual patient. Current known prognostic factors for prostate cancer include serum prostate-specific antigen (PSA), clinical stage, biopsy Gleason score, pathological Gleason score and the pathological stage[1–4]. Several studies suggest that the best prognostic factors include the pathological Gleason score followed closely by the pathological stage. Unfortunately, this information is not available preoperatively when discussing the treatment options with the patient. It was hoped that with improved understanding of Gleason grading by dedicated genitourinary pathologists, the biopsy Gleason score would closely mimic the pathological Gleason score.

The Gleason system recognizes five grades representing a continuum of architectural patterns of glandular or acinar formation. An important concept of the Gleason grading system is that the quantification of the different neoplastic growth patterns (primary plus secondary pattern) is significant; by adding them together to produce a Gleason score, the two major patterns represented are acknowledged. In contemporary radical prostatectomy series, Gleason score 7 cancers currently compromise 40–50% of the specimens evaluated. One important issue that arises is what Gleason scores can be lumped together to obtain more statistically reliable results. Since many investigators consider Gleason 7 prostate cancer a poorly differentiated tumor along with Gleason score 8, 9 and 10 carcinomas, they are often lumped together as 'bad' tumors, whereas

Gleason scores 2, 3, 4, 5 and 6 are lumped as good tumors in a binary model. On the other hand, many clinicians use three groupings of histological scores: 2–3–4, 5–6–7 and 8–9–10. Even Gleason recognized that though these three groups of three have an appealing symmetry, there are many shortcomings to this grouping system[5]. This is especially true of the central group (5–6–7) where each grade shows a very different behavior. Gleason score 5–6 tumors behave only slightly worse than score 2–4, but significantly better than score 7 cancers. There is increasing evidence to indicate that the separation between Gleason score groups with respect to outcome follows different stratification strategies.

In order to answer which Gleason scores can be lumped together to obtain more statistically reliable results, we evaluated the pathological characteristics and biochemical disease-free survival differences between patients with Gleason < 7, 7 and > 7 prostate cancer. Furthermore, in an attempt to understand the association between the biopsy and pathological Gleason scores and more importantly to see whether the biopsy Gleason score was predictive of disease-free survival, we reviewed our experience at the Wayne State University by performing a retrospective analysis on 1031 patients who underwent radical retropubic prostatectomy as monotherapy for clinically localized prostate cancer.

The specimen Gleason score was < 7 in 412 (40.0%) patients, 7 in 507 (49.1%) patients and > 7 in the remaining 112 (10.9%) patients. In our series, the overall mean PSA level was 10.3 ng/ml, being 7.4, 10.6 and 19.1 ng/ml for Gleason score < 7, 7 and > 7 prostate cancers, respectively. The specimen Gleason score was a strong predictor of the pathological stage. Of patients with a specimen Gleason score of < 7, 7 and > 7, pathological organ-confined disease was present in 70.1%, 44.1% and 11.6%, respectively ($p = 0.001$). A positive surgical margin was present in 26.2%, 39.8% and 58.0% of patients ($p = 0.001$); extraprostatic extension alone was present in 5.8%, 21.9% and 20.5% ($p = 0.001$); seminal vesicle invasion was present in 1.5%, 8.0% and 33.0% ($p = 0.001$); and positive lymph nodes were present in 0.5%, 3.1% and 27.6% ($p = 0.001$) of patients with specimen Gleason scores < 7, 7 and > 7, respectively (Table 1).

Overall, the disease-free survival for the 1031 patients was 82.8% with a median follow-up of 41.4 months. The specimen Gleason score correlated with disease-free survival in patients with organ-confined disease, extraprostatic extension, positive surgical margins and seminal vesicle invasion. Overall, the disease-free survival was 95.6%, 81.0% and 43.7% for patients with specimen Gleason scores < 7, 7 and > 7, respectively ($p = 0.001$). The disease-free survival for pathological organ-confined disease was 98.6%, 94.6% and 84.6% ($p = 0.001$) while for pathological extraprostatic disease ($T_{3a,b}$) it was 87.5%, 73.0% and 47.8% ($p = 0.001$) for specimen Gleason scores < 7, 7 and > 7, respectively. In patients with positive surgical margins, analyzed independently from the other pathological findings, the specimen Gleason score proved to be statistically significant regarding disease-free survival ($p = 0.001$).

In patients with seminal vesicle invasion, disease-free survival was 83.3%, 53.7% and 32.4% for a specimen Gleason score < 7, 7 and > 7, respectively ($p = 0.001$). For patients with lymph node involvement, the Gleason score ($p = 0.001$) was again a prognostic indicator of disease-free survival. When multivariate analysis of preoperative serum PSA level (≤ 10 or > 10 ng/ml), pathological stage and specimen Gleason score (< 7, 7, > 7) was performed to determine their independent prognostic significance in detecting biochemical recurrence, the specimen Gleason score was the strongest independent predictor of disease-free survival ($p = 0.0001$). The pathological stage and serum PSA value stratified for ≤ 10 or > 10 ng/ml were also independent prognostic factors ($p = 0.001$ and $p = 0.002$) (Table 2, Figure 1).

The pathological Gleason score correlated strongly with the probability of biochemical recurrence following radical prostatectomy in our series. This was true for patients with localized and extraprostatic disease. These findings are similar to those previously reported in the literature and emphasize the fact that the histological grade is one of the most powerful prognostic factors in patients with prostate cancer.

As in the contemporary radical prostatectomy series, our series also showed that Gleason score 7 has evolved as the most common Gleason score, and accounted for 51% of all the specimens evaluated. Gleason score 7 encompasses a unique spectrum of histological differentiation and pathological characteristics

Table 1 Characteristics of patients undergoing radical prostatectomy in the present series

	Gleason score < 7	Gleason score 7	Gleason score > 7	Total	p Value
Number of patients	412 (40.0%)	507 (49.1%)	112 (10.9%)	1031	—
Mean age (years)	60.8	62.3	63.3	61.8	0.01
Mean follow-up (months)	39.5	43.6	41.2	41.4	0.32
Mean PSA (ng/ml)	7.4	10.6	19.1	10.3	0.001
Pathologically organ confined	289 (70.1%)	224 (44.1%)	13 (11.6%)	526 (51.0%)	0.001
Extraprostatic extension	24 (5.8%)	111 (21.9%)	23 (20.5%)	158 (15.3%)	0.001
Seminal vesicle invasion	6 (1.5%)	41 (8.0%)	37 (33.0%)	84 (8.2%)	0.001
Positive lymph node	2 (0.5%)	16 (3.1%)	31 (27.6%)	49 (4.8%)	0.001
Positive margins	108 (26.2%)	202 (39.8%)	65 (58.0%)	375 (36.3%)	0.001
Overall disease-free survival	394 (95.6%)	411 (81.0%)	49 (43.7%)	854 (82.8%)	0.001

PSA, prostate-specific antigen

Table 2 Relationship between specimen Gleason score, pathological findings and disease-free survival

	Gleason score < 7		Gleason score 7		Gleason score > 7		Total		
	n	%	n	%	n	%	n	%	p Value
Organ confined	285/289	98.6	212/224	94.6	11/13	84.6	508/526	96.6	0.001
Positive margin	81/91	89.0	92/115	80.0	6/8	75.0	179/214	83.6	0.001
Extraprostatic extension	21/24	87.5	81/111	73.0	11/23	47.8	113/158	71.5	0.001
Seminal vesicle invasion	5/6	83.3	22/41	53.7	12/37	32.4	39/84	46.4	0.001
Positive lymph node	2/2	100	4/16	25.0	9/31	29.0	15/49	30.6	0.001

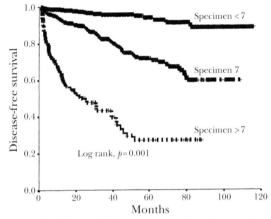

Figure 1 Kaplan–Meier curve for disease-free survival comparing specimen Gleason score < 7, 7, > 7

in this series. The proportion of patients with Gleason score 7 prostate cancer undergoing radical prostatectomy appears to be an important determinant of the biological aggressiveness of the disease. Likewise, Epstein and colleagues have also indicated that Gleason score 7 prostate cancers appear to represent a distinct prognostic group[6].

If Gleason score 7 cancers are considered a specific category, further classification by primary Gleason grade (4 + 3 or 3 + 4) might define patients who behave similarly to those with Gleason score > 7 or < 7 prostate cancer. We designed a study to correlate the occurrence of Gleason grades 3 and 4 with clinico-pathological parameters and determined the influence of the major grade component on cancer control among patients with Gleason score 7 cancer treated by radical prostatectomy. We hypothesized that further subclassification of the Gleason score 7 tumors might improve the ability to identify the subgroup of patients at higher risk of early disease relapse.

Correlating the major grade proportion (3 + 4 versus 4 + 3) to preoperative parameters of age, race, clinical stage and serum PSA levels showed that a specimen Gleason score 7 prostate cancer with a major grade component is significantly associated with a more advanced clinical stage, higher serum PSA, older age at the time of treatment and a higher proportion of African-American male patients. Overall, patients with 3 + 4 tumors experienced lower PSA recurrence compared to those with 4 + 3 prostate cancer. The 2- and 4-year recurrence rates for 3 + 4 patients were 11% and 39%, respectively, compared to 23% and 40% for 4 + 3 patients ($p < 0.0001$ in both cases overall). Analysis of patients with Gleason score 7 tumors and pathological organ-confined disease, taking into account preoperative PSA value, age, race and tumor volume, showed the major grade to be a significant predictor of survival ($p = 0.012$). In this cohort, patients with major grade 4 tumors experienced significantly higher biochemical recurrence compared to those with major grade 3 carcinoma ($p = 0.0021$) (Tables 3 and 4).

This analysis revealed that the primary grade pattern of Gleason score 7 adenocarcinoma correlated significantly with the clinical profile

Table 3 Correlation of major grade component with preoperative parameters

	Race		Age		Preoperative PSA		Clinical stage	
	African-American male	American-Caucasian male	< 55 years	≥ 55 years	≤ 10 ng/ml	> 10 ng/ml	T_{1c}	T_2
3 + 4 (n = 354)	141 (40%)	213 (60%)	78 (22%)	278 (78%)	270 (76%)	86 (24%)	113 (33%)	232 (67%)
4 + 3 (n = 178)	87 (49%)	91 (51%)	18 (10%)	160 (90%)	111 (62%)	67 (38%)	34 (19%)	143 (81%)
p Value*	0.047		0.001		0.001		0.001	

*χ^2 tests for general association; PSA, prostate-specific antigen

Table 4 Correlation of major grade component with pathological stage and tumor volume in radical prostatectomy specimens

	Pathological stage					Tumor volume			
	Organ confined	Positive surgical margin	Extra prostatic extension	Seminal vesicle invasion	Positive lymph node	0–2 cc	2–4 cc	4–10 cc	≥ 10 cc
3 + 4 (n = 354)	178 (50%)	95 (27%)	65 (18%)	17 (5%)	1 (< 1%)	87 (24%)	126 (35%)	114 (32%)	29 (8%)
4 + 3 (n = 178)	59 (33%)	31 (17%)	48 (27%)	30 (17%)	10 (6%)	31 (17%)	49 (28%)	77 (43%)	21 (11%)
p Value*	0.001					0.003			

* Mantel–Haenzsel χ^2 tests for non-zero association

of patients scheduled for radical prostatectomy following new diagnosis. Tumors with a major grade 4 component occurred in older patients who had more advanced clinical stage and serum PSA. With respect to pathological parameters in the radical prostatectomy specimen, tumors with a composition of major 4 with a minor 3 grade were of significantly more advanced pathological stage and larger tumor volume. This study suggests the importance of quantitating the proportion of less different-iated, higher-grade tumor components of prostate cancer, as they appear to correlate with other pathological parameters of aggressiveness and biochemical recurrence, particularly for the increasing subsets of patients with patho-logical organ-confined disease.

Equipped with a better understanding of the importance of accurate quantification of Gleason scores as well as the significant impact on prognosis by subgrouping of pathological Gleason scores < 7, 7 and > 7, we undertook another study to determine whether the biopsy Gleason score correlates with the prostatectomy Gleason score. Furthermore, we evaluated whether or not a biopsy Gleason score was as predictive of disease-free survival as a patho-logical Gleason score for each grade category < 7, 7 and > 7.

Accurate correlation was noted between biopsy and pathological Gleason scores in only 54.8%, 66.8% and 47.4% of Gleason scores < 7, 7 and > 7, respectively, with an overall accuracy of 58.3%. About 45.2% of biopsy Gleason scores < 7 were upgraded, while 52.6% of biopsy Gleason scores > 7 were downgraded. For biopsy Gleason 7 cancers, there was almost equal distribution of up- and downgrading. The biopsy Gleason score also correlated with overall disease-free survival ($p = 0.0005$). The difference in disease-free survival between biopsy Gleason scores < 7, 7 and > 7 were highly

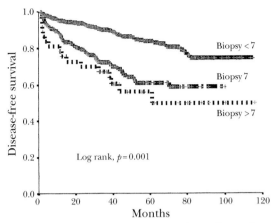

Figure 2 Kaplan–Meier curve for disease-free survival comparing biopsy Gleason score < 7, 7, > 7

significant ($p = 0.001$) (Figure 2). This was also true for the specimen Gleason scores < 7, 7 and > 7 ($p = 0.001$). When the overall disease-free survival was compared between biopsy Gleason and specimen Gleason scores of < 7, the specimen Gleason score had significant survival advantage over the biopsy Gleason score ($p = 0.001$). While the overall disease-free survival was similar between biopsy and specimen Gleason score 7 ($p = 0.12$), a significantly better disease-free survival was noted for biopsy Gleason score > 7 when compared to specimen Gleason score > 7 ($p = 0.02$) (Table 5; Figures 3–6).

Overall, exact agreement in grading between biopsy and prostatectomy specimens has ranged

Table 5 Correlation of biopsy and prostatectomy Gleason scores

| Biopsy Gleason score | Prostatectomy Gleason score | | | Total |
	< 7	7	> 7	
< 7	366 (54.8%)	273 (40.9%)	29 (4.3%)	668
7	43 (13.2%)	217 (66.8%)	65 (20.0%)	325
> 7	3 (7.9%)	17 (44.7%)	18 (47.4%)	38
Total	412	507	112	1031

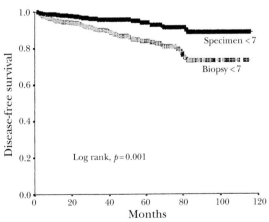

Figure 3 Kaplan–Meier curve for disease-free survival comparing specimen and biopsy Gleason score < 7

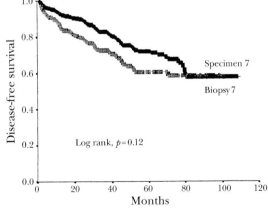

Figure 4 Kaplan–Meier curve for disease-free survival comparing specimen and biopsy Gleason score 7

from 31% to 81%[7,8]. There are several explanations for the discrepancy between the biopsy and pathological Gleason scores. First, prostate cancer is a multifocal disease with each separate tumor often having a different Gleason score. Traditionally, we have used the worst Gleason score in the biopsy specimen to determine the Gleason score for the entire biopsy specimen, but it may be more appropriate to use a combination of the Gleason scores that may better reflect the prostatectomy Gleason score pattern. In addition, many of the tumors now identified in the PSA era are relatively small and the biopsy material is scant. This results in a limited amount of tumor seen on core-needle biopsy. Frequently, there is inadequate tissue to provide a full Gleason score on the biopsy specimen and, instead, only one Gleason pattern is available. Steinberg and colleagues specifically identified four reasons for discrepancies between core-needle biopsy and radical prostatectomy grade[9]:

(1) Pathology error in the grading of the core-needle biopsy and radical prostatectomy specimen;

(2) A tumor with a pattern that straddles two grades in core-needle biopsy or prostatectomy specimens, in which, because of limited tissue, it is difficult to decide the best classification;

(3) Sampling error, in which the core-needle biopsy misses one of the grades present in the prostatectomy;

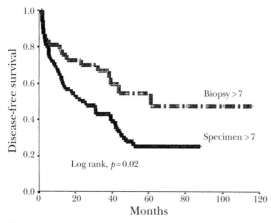

Figure 5 Kaplan–Meier curve for disease-free survival comparing specimen and biopsy Gleason score > 7

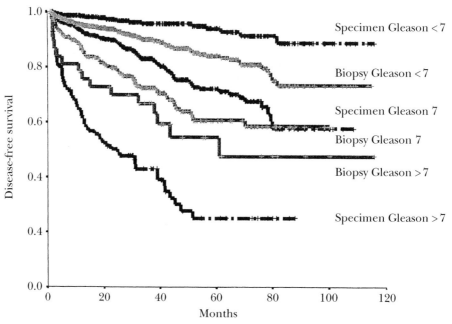

Figure 6 Kaplan–Meier curve for disease-free survival comparing specimen and biopsy Gleason score < 7, 7, and > 7

(4) Reverse sampling, in which the core needle samples a very minor grade component present in the prostatectomy that, because of its limited presence, is not incorporated in the radical prostatectomy score.

Interobserver and intra-observer variations also play an important role in histological grading. For the pattern of a tumor to be incorporated within the Gleason score, it should occupy at least 5% of the tumor. Less prevalent tumor patterns are usually commented on in a note, not in the Gleason score. Recently Pan and co-workers evaluated the impact of a tertiary (third most prevalent) pattern and determined that the tertiary high-grade components, especially for pathological Gleason scores 5–6 and 7, also have an adverse impact on biological behavior and are significant prognostically[10]. Perhaps, modifying the biopsy Gleason grading system to include the tertiary pattern may help to better reflect the overall disease-free survival.

With the widespread use of serum PSA tests and transrectal ultrasound, many more men are undergoing prostate biopsy today than in the past. Pathologists are being called to accurately diagnose limited cancer in core-needle biopsies and to accurately quantify and grade these cancers. Many preoperative and postoperative parameters have been thoroughly studied for their prognostic implications in guiding therapy for prostate cancer. As noted in our series, Kupelian and colleagues also demonstrated that the pathological Gleason score is a better predictor than the biopsy Gleason score in predicting disease-free survival[3]. However, the specimen Gleason score is not available preoperatively when discussing the treatment options with the patient. One is often left with the biopsy Gleason score to make a decision on whether to follow the patient expectantly, treat definitively or consider the cancer too advanced for curative therapy. Overall survival differences were compared between biopsy Gleason scores < 7, 7 and > 7 and pathological score to see whether patients could be better informed of their prognosis based on the biopsy Gleason score.

Our experience revealed that for Gleason score < 7 cancers, the specimen Gleason score had better overall disease-free survival compared to the biopsy Gleason score. This is probably due to the fact that almost half of all biopsy Gleason sum < 7 cancers are upgraded to Gleason 7 or > 7 in the final prostatectomy specimen. Inversely, for Gleason score > 7 cancer, the specimen Gleason score had a worse overall disease-free survival compared to the biopsy Gleason score. This is again probably due to downgrading of the biopsy Gleason score to Gleason score 7 or < 7 in half the patients. On the other hand, the biopsy Gleason score 7 mimics the overall disease-free survival achieved for the pathological Gleason score 7 since roughly half of the biopsy Gleason score 7 are either downgraded to < 7 or upgraded to > 7.

In conclusion, it appears that the biopsy Gleason score, although frequently not correlating strongly with the prostatectomy Gleason score, is an important prognostic factor and should be used in counselling patients. In addition, the percentage of Gleason pattern 3 or 4 may be an important prognostic factor in stratification of Gleason 7 cancers.

References

1. Lerner SE, Blute ML, Bergstralh EJ, *et al.* Analysis of risk factors of progression in patients with pathologically confined prostate cancer after radical retropubic prostatectomy. *J Urol* 1996; 156:137–43

2. Partin AW, Yoo J, Carter HB, *et al.* The use of prostate specific antigen, clinical stage and Gleason score to predict pathological stage in men with localized prostate cancer. *J Urol* 1993;150:110–14

3. Kupelian P, Katcher J, Levin H, *et al.* Correlation of clinical and pathologic factors with rising prostate-specific antigen profiles after radical prostatectomy alone for clinically localized prostate cancer. *Urology* 1996;48:249–60

4. Montie JE. Current prognostic factors for prostate carcinoma. *Cancer* 1996;78:341–4

5. Gleason D. Histologic grading of prostate cancer: a perspective. *Hum Pathol* 1992;23:273–9

6. Epstein JI, Pound CR, Partin AW, *et al.* Disease progression following radical prostatectomy in men with Gleason score 7 tumors. *J Urol* 1998; 160:97–101

7. Cookson MS, Fleshner NE, Soloway SM, *et al.* Correlation between Gleason score of needle biopsy and radical prostatectomy specimen: accuracy and clinical implications. *J Urol* 1997;157:559–62

8. Babaian RJ, Grunow WA. Reliability of Gleason grading system in comparing prostate biopsies with total prostatectomy specimens. *Urology* 1985;25:564–7

9. Steinberg D, Sauvageot J, Epstein JI. Correlation of prostate needle biopsy and radical prostatectomy: Gleason grade in academic and community settings. *Med Pathol* 1996;9:83A

10. Pan CC, Potter SR, Partin AW. The prognostic significance of tertiary Gleason patterns of higher grade in radical prostatectomy specimens: a proposal to modify the Gleason grading system. *Am J Surg Pathol* 2000;24:563–9

Laparoscopic radical prostatectomy: assessment after 350 procedures

13

B. Guillonneau and G. Vallancien

Introduction

The objectives of laparoscopic surgery are, not only, the reduction of perioperative morbidity compared to conventional surgery, but also, and may be more importantly, to allow a more precise operative procedure. Indeed, quality of surgery can be improved by a better visualization of the operative site due, on the one hand, to the optical magnification and, on the other hand, to the maneuverability of the laparoscope, providing hitherto unobtainable anatomical views. Hence, a laparoscopic approach for radical prostatectomy, which is responsible for significant operative morbidity and functional sequelae, could improve the postoperative course, and also, more particularly, could allow better preservation of periprostatic vascular, muscular and neurovascular structures.

Laparoscopic radical prostatectomy was first performed in 1991 by Schuessler and colleagues[1] and an initial series with nine cases was published in 1997[2]. However, the conclusions were not encouraging since the authors concluded that 'laparoscopy is not an efficacious surgical alternative to open prostatectomy for malignancy'.

Moving on from this initial disappointing outcome, using our experience in both retropubic radical prostatectomy and laparoscopic surgery, we initiated the development of laparoscopic radical prostatectomy at the Montsouris Institute in January 1998[3,4]. Since this date, all consecutive patients who were candidates for radical prostatectomy have been operated on, where there were no anesthetic contraindications, using a laparoscopic approach. Technical aspects of the procedure have obviously evolved, step by step, in the light of accumulated experience[5]. Each difficult point has been evaluated, modified and progressively improved to make a currently feasible, reproducible and subsequently teachable technique.

This chapter is the sum of our accumulated experience following the first 350 consecutive laparoscopic radical prostatectomies, performed between January 1998 and May 2000.

Specific contraindications

There is no specific anatomical contraindication to laparoscopic radical prostatectomy that can be foreseen in preoperative staging. There are, however, cases that make the operation more difficult. From the anatomical point of view, a small prostate volume (less than 20 g) generally makes dissection difficult, as in conventional surgery, since the anatomic limits of the gland can hardly be seen. On the other hand, mobilization of a large prostate (more than 80 g) is uncomfortable because of the weight of the gland and because its volume leads to poor visibility making lateral dissection difficult, particularly when the pelvis is deep and narrow. In addition, large glands often present with a prostatic median lobe that makes the preservation of the muscular fibers in the bladder neck impossible in practice.

Previous history of prostate surgery (cervicoprostatic monoincision, transurethral resection of the prostate or even transvesical prostatectomy) is not by itself a contraindication for the laparoscopic approach but it is, as in conventional surgery, a source of further difficulties.

Finally, neoadjuvant endocrine therapy is usually linked with surgical difficulties, being related to a small prostate volume and, perhaps, also to the modification of the periprostatic dissection planes.

Preoperative care

Antibiotic prophylaxis, using a single intravenous dose of a third-generation cephalosporin, is prescribed 2 h before the operation.

Antithrombotic prevention is an essential element of the perioperative care, especially since it involves three risk factors: cancer surgery, pelvic surgery and the laparoscopic procedure. The proposed protocol is a daily subcutaneous injection of low molecular weight heparin (3500 anti-Xa IU), the dose of which is adjusted according to the patient's risk. It must be started 3 h before the operation and be continued 15 days after. In addition, compression stockings should be worn by the patient while in hospital.

No skin (patients are no longer shaved) or digestive preparation is necessary, and admission on the day of the operation is proposed at a time convenient to the patient.

Preparation of the patient

The operation is performed under general anesthesic. The patient is placed in the dorsal supine position. Shoulder supports are not appropriate since there is a risk of postoperative pain caused by compression of the shoulders; a thoracic wrap using an elastic adhesive tape is more suitable and comfortable for the patient. Arms are placed along the body in such a way as to avoid the risk of brachial plexus elongation. Legs are placed in the flexion–abduction position on a foam support, and buttons at the end of the operating table to allow intraoperative rectal and urethral access.

After the usual skin preparations, the abdomen, from the costal margins to the perianal region, is disinfected and the patient is draped, each leg being draped individually. A Foley catheter is inserted and the bladder drained. The monitor is placed between the patient's legs, as close as possible to the surgeon's eye level. A right-handed surgeon stands on the patient's left with his assistant opposite. The scrub nurse stands on the surgeon's left with the instrument table.

After a radial inferior umbilical incision, a Verres needle is introduced and insufflation is started after the safety maneuvers, without exceeding a pressure of 12 mmHg. A 10-mm trocar is then inserted into the umbilicus for passage of the $0°$ laparoscope. Only then is the patient placed in the exaggerated Trendelenburg's position, so as to improve access to the pelvic region, by the spontaneous movement under gravity of the intestine and, in particular, the sigmoid colon. The operating table must then be lowered, or the surgeon positioned on a platform, so as to operate with his shoulders relaxed and comfortable.

Four other trocars are inserted: a 5-mm trocar into the left iliac fossa, a midline 5-mm trocar, half-way between the umbilicus and the pubis, a 5-mm trocar at the level of the umbilicus in the right pararectal fossa and, finally, a 10-mm trocar in the right iliac fossa at McBurney's point. (This latter trocar is for the introduction of the needles and the laparoscopic bag only.)

The operative technical steps

Transperitoneal pelvic lymphadenectomy is performed according to the usual technique[6]. Radical prostatectomy is performed according to a now standardized technique, in seven steps.

First step: posterior approach of the prostate

Freeing the seminal vesicles The first landmark is the vas deferens, found behind the peritoneum, at the inferior peritoneal reflection, posterior to the bladder. The sigmoid colon is held gently by the assistant, and the rectum retracted superiorly. The surgeon should then notice the appearance of two peritoneal arches. The superior arch represents the approximate location of the ureters and the trigone. The inferior arch, deep in the peritoneal reflection, is created by the meeting of the vasa in the midline.

The posterior vesical peritoneum must be incised transversely along the peritoneal arch. The vasa deferentia are separated, coagulated with bipolar forceps and then sectioned. One must be aware of the presence of the deferential artery that runs along the vas and must be carefully coagulated. Dissection of the vasa deferentia allows access to the seminal vesicles, which are dissected and left attached at their base. It is essential to cauterize the two vascular pedicles, one at the tip and the second at the base, to completely release the vesicles before the prostate dissection.

Opening the Denonvillier's fascia   Incision into the Denonvillier's fascia allows an easier and safer dissection later in the operation, taking the rectum away from the prostatic pedicles. To make the exposure easier, the assistant should move the vasa deferentia upwards to place the Denonvillier's fascia on tension. Sagittal striations will be visible under the magnification of the laparoscope. The Denonvillier's fascia is incised horizontally along the reflection line between the prostatic base and the posterior surface of the seminal vesicles. As soon as a shallow incision is made, prerectal fat is seen and provides a safe plane of dissection to the posterior surface of the rectum. The prostate is released from the anterior surface of the rectum in the midline, as far as possible towards the apex. The posterior surface of the prostate is gradually dissected after inserting a Hegar intrarectal bougie to improve, if needed, tactile perception of the anterior rectal wall.

Second step: anterior approach of the prostate

Entering the Retzius space   The bladder is filled with approximately 120 cc of saline, to help to identify the contours and to pull it posteriorly. The anterior parietal peritoneum is incised from one umbilical ligament to the other. It is unnecessary to divide the medial umbilical ligaments. By staying close to the medial aspect of the medial umbilical ligaments and heading laterally and caudally from here, the pubic ramii are encountered. This dissection allows clear identification of the urachus which can be

sectioned last, thus minimizing the risk of injuring the bladder. It is essential to free the bladder well from its anterior and lateral attachments in order to permit a tension-free vesicourethral anastomosis at the end of the operation. After the bladder is freed anteriorly and laterally, it is then emptied with a syringe; since the patient is in an exaggerated Trendelenburg's position, spontaneous emptying is never complete.

Exposure of the endopelvic fascia   The fat over the fascia covering the prostate must be swept cephalad and laterally in order to expose clearly the intrapelvic fascia and the puboprostatic ligaments. The superficial dorsal vein is easily identified; it must be coagulated with bipolar current and then sectioned.

The endopelvic fascia is identified lateral to the prostate, and incised along the line of reflection, allowing a lateral approach to the levator ani muscles. Towards the puboprostatic ligaments, one small venous complex is often found laterally which must be coagulated and transected to allow the freeing of the prostate from the lateral pelvic muscles.

Incision of the puboprostatic ligaments is carried out to facilitate the dissection and exposure of the dorsal venous complex, and later on of the urethra. This section is carried out using curved scissors, as close as possible to the pubic bone.

Ligating the dorsal venous complex   Santorini's plexus is clearly visible anteriorly and laterally to the urethra. It is ligated with a 2–0 resorbable suture passed with a number 36 needle underneath the venous plexus from one side to the other. For a right-handed surgeon, the needle must be passed via the right 10-mm port, from the right side of the plexus to the left side with the back hand; the needle should be angled so that the curve of the needle follows the curve of the symphysis. Depending on the breadth of the plexus, a second separate suture can be placed to make the ligation safer. In any case, the complex must not be sectioned at this step, so as to avoid excess bleeding.

A backbleeding stitch, ligating the pre-prostatic venous drainage, can be made, since it is helpful during the subsequent section of the venous complex.

Third step: bladder neck dissection

This is a difficult step since there are no clear anatomical landmarks. To identify the bladder neck area, the anterior prevesical fat is retracted superiorly, causing a faint outline of the prostatovesical plane. Gentle tractions on the Foley catheter can be also useful in helping the surgeon identify this zone. The preprostatic fascia is then incised transversely at its junction with the bladder, and the bladder muscular fibers are encountered and followed as far as an avascular plane of dissection between the bladder and the prostate. This plane is dissected with a sharp and blunt dissection. It is often necessary to control minor vessels with the bipolar forceps. The urethra, entering into the prostate, can be and must be perfectly identified before incising its anterior wall to expose the Foley catheter. The catheter balloon is then deflated and the tip of the catheter pulled up and into the abdomen to expose the lateral and posterior walls which are incised with the scissors. The Foley catheter is removed, and the assistant holds the posterior neck of the prostate with forceps, while the surgeon exposes the posterior face of the bladder neck, holding the posterior bladder mucosal incision. Since the bladder neck is thus preserved, the ureteral orifices are distant from the bladder incision and no search is made for them.

As one proceeds to incise the posterior junction between the prostate and the bladder, it is important to direct the dissection in a straight line posteriorly, following the posterior bladder wall. This dissection does not present the urologist with a distinct and clear plane. It is often useful to enlarge the dissection laterally in order to avoid an imprecise dissection into a well. The major risk is the development of a 'natural' plane which may be easily entered, but which corresponds to the adenomectomy plane.

With a meticulous dissection in a straight line posterior to the posterior bladder neck, one can access the previously dissected retrovesical space, after transversely incising a final fascia, the 'anterior layer' of the Denonvillier's fascia. The vasa deferentia and the seminal vesicles are brought into the operating field by the assistant, thus exposing on both sides the prostatic pedicles since they have already been completely dissected medially and laterally.

Fourth step: lateral dissection of the prostate

Incising the prostatic pedicles In the antegrade laparoscopic operation, the pedicles are laid virtually bare before they are incised. To best expose them, the assistant grasps the vasa and the seminal vesicles through the space of dissection between the prostate and the posterior bladder neck, and pulls them up to expose the pedicle to be incised. Owing to the magnification, the pedicle's vessels are well vizualized and they must be systematically coagulated with a bipolar current. Because of the traction on the seminal vesicles, the vessels appear to rise vertically which facilitates their exposure but is a distortion of their natural orientation. It is important to remember that the neurovascular bundles are also attracted. Thus, it is then essential for the surgeon to reorient himself periodically during the dissection of the pedicles to keep in mind the location of the posterolateral neurovascular bundles, and to avoid a definitive injury to these bundles by a close dissection to the prostate. The incision of the pedicle must be continued until an entrance is made into a fat plane in which the posterolateral neurovascular bundle runs.

Preserving the neurovascular bundles After transection of the pedicles, the surgeon will find a flimsy tube of fat, nerves and vessels that runs along the posterolateral surface of the prostate, from the base to its entrance into the pelvic muscular floor. To best preserve the bundles, it is necessary to make a lateral incision of a thin visceral fascia that laterally covers the peribundle fat, and medially to extend the incision of the Denonvillier's fascia that reflects along the prostatorectal contact zone. These two fascial incisions make the fat tube surrounding the bundles thinner thus exposing the bundle more clearly and perforating the capsular arteries which rise vertically into the prostate. These small arteries must be coagulated with thin bipolar forceps to diminish the risk of thermal injury. There are more arteries towards the back near the prostatic pedicle, than in the foreground near the apex, where the bundles must be dissected off the prostate with a blunt and sharp dissection. At the apex, the neurovascular bundles diverge from the prostate and the urethra, but must be followed until they enter into the pelvic floor in order to avoid the risk of later injury. Hemorrhage around the bundles is always minor, and for the sake of neurovascular integrity, should be ignored.

Fifth step: apical dissection of the prostate

At this moment, the prostate is attached only by three structures which will be individually sectioned downwards: the Santorini's complex, the urethra and the rectourethralis muscle.

Sectioning the dorsal venous complex Because the dorsal vein has been ligated and the pedicles have been incised, there will be little bleeding when the dorsal complex is incised, but it can be useful to complete the hemostasis using bipolar coagulation. The incision is tangential to the prostate in order to avoid capsular incision at this place. Gradually, the dorsal vein complex is retracted anteriorly to reach an avascular plane of dissection situated between the venous complex and the urethra. This plane must be developed to perfectly expose the anterior urethral wall.

Incising the urethra Laterally, the urethra must be separated from the fibrotic structures, and it is often possible to dissect the posterior wall to simplify the next step.

A metal sound with an 'S' shape (Beniqué's catheter) is introduced to help identify the urethra by improving the tactile perception of its limits, and to make the incision easier.

The urethral wall is then incised with a retractable cold knife to obtain a sharp incision. The urethral bougie is pushed through the anterior urethrotomy and into the pelvis to expose the lateral and posterior urethral walls. The back wall of the urethra is now similarly incised with the laparoscopic knife or scissors.

Sectioning the rectourethralis After complete section of the urethra, the rectourethralis appears rather attenuated with this approach and represents the final attachments of the prostate. In order to avoid injury to the neurovascular bundles, it is necessary to section the rectourethralis laterally locating precisely the bundle on the side where the surgeon sections the rectourethralis. This division of the rectourethralis close to the prostate completely frees the specimen which is temporarily placed inside an endoscopic bag, in a paracolic gutter.

Sixth step: urethrovesical anastomosis

It is not necessary to evert the bladder mucosa nor is it necessary to narrow the bladder neck since its preservation has been correctly performed. The number of stitches depends on the size of the bladder neck. The objective is to obtain a watertight anastomosis and, in order to reach this goal, currently we prefer to perform the anastomosis with 12 stitches.

Throughout this part of the procedure, the surgeon works with two needleholders. The anastomosis is made with interrupted stitches of a 3–0 resorbable suture with a number 26 needle. All ties are thrown intracorporally and, therefore, a 6-inch length is sufficient.

The first three sutures are place posteriorly at 5, 6 and 7 o'clock, going inside-out on the urethra and outside-in on the bladder neck. Therefore, these stitches are tied intra-luminally. The metal sound (Beniqué's catheter with a depressed tip) helps guide the needle into the urethra and places the sutures, which glide into the lumen as the sound is retracted.

Six other sutures are symmetrically placed at 4 and 8, then 3 and 9, then 2 and 10 o'clock and tied outside the lumen. As a rule, for a right-handed surgeon, the right-sided stitches go outside-in on the bladder (right hand, forehand) and inside-out on the urethra (left hand, backhand); the left-sided stitches go outside-in on the bladder neck (left hand, forehand) and inside-out on the urethra (right hand, backhand). Three final anterior stitches are placed at 1, 11 and 12 o'clock, but not immediately tied. As a rule, the stitches go outside-in on the urethra (right hand, forehand) and inside-out on the bladder neck (right hand, forehand or left hand, forehand depending on the placement). The Foley catheter is inserted under visual control and its correct position is checked. Then the two anterior sutures can be safely tied without any risk of piercing the catheter. The balloon is inflated with 10 ml and the bladder is filled with 120 cc of saline to check the watertightness of the anastomosis.

Seventh step: completing the operation

The abdominal pressure is lowered to 5 mmHg, to check for venous bleeding. The peritoneal incisions are left open and a suction drain is passed to the pelvis through the left-sided 5-mm port. The 5-mm trocars are removed and the orifices are once more checked to eliminate parietal vascular injury. The lower 10-mm trocar is removed and the specimen inside its sac is extracted through an enlargement of 4–5 cm of this small McBurney's incision, depending on the size of the specimen. Lastly, the incisions are conventionally closed and dressed.

Operative variants

Placement of the trocars

The trocars can be placed according to the habits of the surgeon. Often, they are placed 'like a fan' round the umbilicus, with two 5-mm trocars in the left iliac fossa and one 5-mm and one 10-mm trocar in the right iliac fossa. In any case, a 10-mm trocar must be used for the passage of the needle and the insertion of the extraction bag for the operative specimen.

Instruments and technical points   The use of different instruments is technically possible. In particular, endoscopic staplers can be used for the section and the hemostasis of the prostatic pedicles. Apart from the cost, the major disadvantage is the non-sparing of the neurovascular bundles that are attracted into the line of section. The use of harmonic scissors is conceivable in order to decrease the heat diffusion at the level of the capsular arteries, and to protect the neurovascular bundles from thermal injury. No data are presently available to confirm or dispute this theory of bipolar coagulation. In this spirit, metal clips are unnecessary and crude.

Urethrovesical anastomosis can be carried out correctly with a running suture, but in our experience the procedure is longer and less comfortable than when using the interrupted suture, and we have now abandoned the running suture.

The extra-peritoneal approach   The subperitoneal approach has been described[7] and is technically feasible but it appears, with experience, that the key to the operation lies in the first approach to the deferentiovesical complex which can only be performed via the transperitoneal route. No series has reported this extraperitoneal approach. Rassweiler and co-workers[8] reported recently an approach that is close to this latter method[8], since the radical prostatectomy is performed through a transperitoneal route but without the initial dissection of the vesicular complex which is dissected last, as in a conventional retropubic prostatectomy.

The use of robotics   In our Institute, the laparoscope is manipulated by means of a voice-controlled robot (Computer Motion, Goleta, CA, USA). The use of this robotic arm allows the surgeon to control rapidly and safely the optic mobilization, improving the operative ergonomy. All is commanded by the voice of the surgeon so everything depends on his visualization of the operative site. This allows the release of one of the assistant's hands so that he can fully assist the surgeon by using both his hands. Finally, the robotic arm ensures excellent stability of the image which avoids the stress and tiredness of the surgeon when he has to control permanently any involuntary movement of his assistant.

Postoperative care

Analgesics The usual analgesic protocol for the first 24 h consists of: paracetamol, 6 g/24 h, tiemonium, 40 mg/24 h, and noramidopyrine, 8 g/24 h, but often no parenteral analgesia is requested by the patient since pain is scored as 2 or less by the Visual Analog Scale in 60% of patients on the second postoperative day. Major analgesics are necessary only rarely, and post-operative complications should be suspected in such cases.

Nutrition Feeding is usually resumed 12 h after the operation; parenteral fluids are generally stopped between 12 and 24 h after the operation.

Antithrombotic care This is of major importance given the increased risk after a pelvic cancer operation and a laparoscopic approach in which the venous return is diminished, in spite of the exaggerated Trendelenburg's position. Pre- and postoperative prevention is based on antithrombotic prophylaxis started before the operation (low molecular weight heparin) and continued for a fortnight after the operation, use of compression stockings while in hospital and early mobilization of the patient on the first day after the operation. This essential preventive element is possible because of the absence of postoperative pain which allows early autonomous mobility.

Bladder catheter removal Depending on the quality of the anastomosis the urethral catheter is removed from the second postoperative day, at present without any radiological control. As a rule, if there has been preservation of the bladder neck and if the anastomosis was leak-proof during the operation, the bladder catheter can be removed as early as the second day after the operation. If there is doubt about the quality of the anastomosis or if preservation of the bladder neck has not been possible, the urethral catheter is removed after the fifth day following the operation. Obviously, the Foley catheter must not be removed if there is drainage of urine through the suction drain (after the first postoperative hours).

In our first 50 patients, the mean time before removal of the bladder catheter postoperatively was 7.8 days, which was based on previous experience. However, we progressively reduced the duration, as the quality of anastomosis improved, to 7 days on average for the next 50 patients, and to 4.2 days for the last 150 patients. This short catheterization time perfectly reflects the quality of the anastomosis achieved by the laparoscopic procedure.

Hospital stay The mean postoperative stay was 5.2 days in the last group of 140 patients. In France, patients do not like to go home with a catheter and, hence, they defer their departure until the catheter has been removed. Given that most patients do not require analgesia post-operatively or specific care, in many cases, they can be discharged in even less time than in other health-care systems.

Technical feasibility

Surgical conversion

Surgical conversion to a conventional retro-pubic approach can be indicated in cases of intraoperative complications such as technical difficulties. The intraoperative complications are mainly due to hemorrhage of Santorini's venous plexus. It is necessary in this case to try to perform the hemostasis by clamping the plexus, and to put in a new ligature.

From our experience, the use of bipolar coagulation or the application of a clip is a transient and unsatisfactory solution. If the hemostasis seems impossible and if the decision to convert is taken, it is always possible to compress the plexus with a clamp or by the insertion of a nut through the 10-mm trocar while the laparotomy is performed.

Technical difficulties lie in dissection planes which may be difficult to visualize. An extra capsular tumor (pT3) may generate adhesions which are difficult to dissect, particularly on the posterior surface of the prostate when it is difficult to locate the posterior dissection plane safely. This also occurs in patients for whom neoadjuvant endocrine therapy has been prescribed. The prostate is small in these cases with no definite limits and dissection planes are often difficult to find.

Another cause of operative difficulties may be a history of prostatic surgery (transurethral resection of the prostate or transvesical prostatectomy). This makes dissection of the vasa deferentia very difficult, and the preservation of the bladder neck impossible.

Finally, it is important to stress the technical difficulty of achieving a correct and watertight urethrovesical anastomosis. When the urethrovesical anastomosis cannot be achieved correctly, a mini laparotomy must be carried out in order to perform the anastomosis in the conventional way, and advantage of the incision should be taken to extract the operative specimen.

In any case, it is necessary to warn the patient beforehand that there is always a risk of surgical conversion. It would be useless to attempt hazardous procedures which would, in no way, benefit the patient. Even if the conversion rate decreases with experience and now tends towards zero, there will always be difficult cases for which conventional surgery will be more efficient. One must keep in mind that the surgical benefit is for the patient and that the key word is safety; in cases of conversion to a conventional retropubic approach, there must be no hesitation.

Basically, in our first 40 cases, the conversion rate was 10%, in the following 40 cases, the rate decreased to 7.5%, and in the last 270 cases, there have been no conversions (0%).

Operative time

Laparoscopic prostatectomy is a long and difficult operation which necessitates a good technical knowledge of laparoscopic surgery and of the prostate anatomy. The surgeon will have to cope with stress fatigue in dealing with the different operative difficulties. At the end of the operation, the anastomosis is a very important surgical act. It is always difficult and determines the quality of the postoperative results. For this reason, it is necessary to perform this step of the operation in good conditions, physically and technically. The specific operating time for the bilateral lymph node dissection is about 30 min (range 20–50 min). With experience, the operating time of the whole procedure gradually decreases but it still remains a little longer than the time required for conventional surgery.

Obviously, the experience of the surgeon is essential. The mean operative time of the whole series was 232 min (range 115–360 min), but this time has decreased regularly as we have become more experienced. In our study, the mean operative time for the 50 first cases was 278 min, 240 min for the following 50 patients, and, for the last 140 patients, mean operative time was 195 min (range 115–240 min) which is more or less comparable to the operative time for the retropubic procedure.

Specific complications

There were no postoperative deaths in our series, and the morbidity of laparoscopic radical prostatectomy appeared very low in our experience, taking into account the technical difficulty of the procedure, in the absence of reference studies.

Hemorrhage

The dorsal venous complex   The vascular injury is visually an injury to Santorini's venous plexus. It is essential to bear in mind that a laparoscopic procedure cannot be continued in the case of bleeding as hemorrhaging interferes considerably with visibility and makes the operation uncertain and dangerous. It is safe to revert to conventional surgery if a hemostasis of good quality cannot be obtained. This complication occurred, initially, when an accurate technique of the ligation of the dorsal venous complex was not achieved regularly. At present, control of the venous complex is always perfect if carried out according to the technique we have described above.

The epigastric injury Another specific vascular risk is injury to the epigastric artery, due to the port insertion. On completion of the procedure, it is essential to examine carefully the point of entry of each secondary sheats into the abdomen. Even with this important precaution, the risk of secondary bleeding still exists. We report the cases of three patients (0.8%) in whom the diagnosis of epigastic artery injury was missed, and for whom a blood transfusion was necessary secondary to the hemorrhagic parietal syndrome. In addition, open control of the epigastric injury was vital for the first patient.

Overall, at present the transfusion rate is 5.4%, with a regular reduction as more experience is gained. The transfusion rate in the first 50 patients in our series was 15%, and then 6% in the next 50 patients. Finally, among the last 250 patients, the rate was only 2.8%. The indications were two patients with an epigastic artery injury (see above), two patients treated with intravenous heparin for an aortic cardiac valve and three patients for whom no explanation for postoperative bleeding was found. This reduction in transfusion rates is clearly parallel to the reduction of bleeding, which is, on average, 370 ml for the whole series, and 280 ml on average, in the last group of 140 patients. There are several explanations for this reduction. The pressure of the pneumo-peritoneum (12 mmHg or less) certainly contributes to the occlusion of small veins, but the other element concerns the technique itself. Since a laparoscopic procedure cannot be continued in a case of insufficient visibility, one of the objectives is to ensure excellent visibility of the operative site, and that requires systematic coagulation of all small vessels which are generally neglected in an open procedure. Finally, the quality of vision is improved by the magnification of the image and the various possible orientations of the laparoscope, which enable visualization of vascular structures not accessible by conventional surgery, due to the anatomy of the pelvis and the surgeon's limitations.

Digestive complications

Rectal injury Rectal injury may occur during two different steps of the procedure: first, when the Denonvillier's fascia is not incised at the base of the vesicles but too far on the posterior side; and, second, during the dissection of the lateral aspects of the prostate towards the apex when the Denonvillier's fascia is near the rectum and the dissection space becomes narrow. When new to the procedure and in cases of peroperative difficulties, the use of an intrarectal bougie, manipulated as required by the nurse, may facilitate the detection of the plane of Denonvillier's fascia and allow better detection of the limits of the rectal wall, by movement of the rectum, and by the tactile sensation produced by the bougie.

In our series, rectal injury occurred four times (1.14%), and, in all cases, at the end of the procedure during the section of the recto-urethralis because the posterior dissection was not completed. In all cases, the injury was immediately recognized and precisely sutured laparoscopically, without colostomy. The operative site was disinfected and antibiotic therapy prescribed. Oral feeding was delayed (after the 3rd day) and, in all cases, the immediate postoperative course was uneventful, but the bladder catheter was removed on the 8th postoperative day to diminish the risk of rectourethral fistula.

Colonic perforation One case occurred due to an instrumental injury. The wound was peroperatively recognized and sutured with an uneventful postoperative course.

Peritonitis One patient presented postoperative peritonitis secondary to an ileal injury, for which the etiology is still not clear (electric burn or trocar perforation).

Urological complications

Bladder injury Bladder injury occurs at the approach to the space of Retzius. The bladder extends up towards the umbilicus and the urachus must be sectioned as high as possible. A bladder injury is easily identified (the aspect of the vesicular mucosa; gas in the urine bag). It is necessary to perform extramucous sutures of the bladder and to leave the bladder catheter in place for 5 days.

Ureter injury We experienced three ureteric injuries (0.8%). In one case, the peritoneal incision was made too high and the ureter was mistaken for the vas deferens. The ureter was accurately sutured over a ureteral stent, and the postoperative course was uneventful.

The intravenous pyelography showed no dilatation after stent removal at day 8. This complication is exceptional but this case proves that there is a risk of ureteral injury if the landmarks are not considered carefully. The best way to avoid this complication is to follow the vas as far as the ampulla and the seminal vesicle, so that the vas is clearly identified as the vas deferens.

In two other cases, the injury was secondary to a peritoneal incision performed in order to mobilize the bladder. Initially, the two peritoneal incisions were joined, but the risk of ureteric injury taught us that this approach is not useful.

Urinary fistula Drainage of urine is the result of a leaking anastomosis. Transient aspiration at less than 24 h of a few milliliters of urine by the suction drain is frequent and usually has no secondary effects. If the aspiration of urine by the drain continues, it can be associated with some biological signs of the uroperitoneum (increase of creatinemia, metabolic acidosis, decrease of diuresis). It is then necessary to correct the acid–base balance generated by the reabsorption of urine, to restrict hydration, and to leave the peri-anastomotic suction in place. When there is a decrease in diuresis and an increase in serum creatinine, diuretics must not be prescribed, as they would only increase intraperitoneal diuresis and maintain the vicious circle. In any case, the bladder catheter should be left in place for sometime. It is possible to remove it when the fistula is drained, after radiological visualization of the lower urinary tract.

Performing a new anastomosis because of a persisting fistula was necessary in one patient. The indication was a persistent fistula beyond the first week. This secondary anastomosis was successfully performed laparoscopically on the 9th postoperative day. The peroperative observation was not certain, and the hypothesis that an eversion of the ureteral meatus out of the anastomotic lumen occurred cannot be excluded.

Thrombophlebitic complications

The association of pelvic surgery and laparoscopic surgery increases the thromboembolic risk, and, therefore, it is essential to use antithrombotic prophylaxis begun just before the operation, and continued for a fortnight after the operation.

Use of compression stockings by the patient while in hospital, and the patient getting up by himself on the first day after the operation also help.

To date, two patients have presented with phlebitis (0.57%). In each case, it was a secondary complication to a previous surgical complication, epigastric injury in one case, and peritonitis in the other case. Except for these two cases, no patient has presented with postoperative primary phlebitis.

Miscellaneous complications

Obturator nerve injury One lymphadenectomy was complicated by partial obturator nerve paralysis, probably secondary to an electric lesion. This paralysis resolved spontaneously without sequelae in less than 6 months.

Other We did not observe any neurological lesions due to stretching or compression of the peripheral nerves.

Oncological results

Oncological efficacy criteria are pathological examination of the operative specimen and biological non-progression.

The indication for radical prostatectomy in our study was based on a diagnosis of clinically localized prostate cancer ($\leq T_{2b}$ stage). The mean prostate-specific antigen (PSA) level was 10.9 ± 7 ng/ml (range 2.0–34.5). The mean number of positive sextant biopsies was 2.36 ± 1.29 (range 1–6), and the mean Gleason score was 5.8 ± 1 (range 2–8).

Preoperative staging included seminal vesicle biopsies whenever one or two sextant prostatic biopsies were positive at the base, according to our protocol[9] and radical prostatectomy was contraindicated in the case of positive seminal vesicle biopsies. Bone scintigraphy was requested when the PSA level was greater than 15 ng/ml. Laparoscopic pelvic lymphadenectomy was performed during the same operation in cases of clinical stage T_{2b} cancer, serum PSA level > 10 ng/ml, and predominant Gleason grade 4 on prostatic biopsies.

Lymphadenectomy

Lymphadenectomy was performed in 76 patients (22%). Frozen-section histological examination was negative in all cases and the final staging was pN_0 in these 76 patients, and N_x in the other 274 patients.

Prostate specimen

To date, pathological data are available for the first 330 specimens. Mean specimen weight was 56 ± 19.6 g (range 20–153 g). Definitive histological examination revealed prostatic intraepithelial neoplasia in two patients (0.6%), pT_{2a} in 24% of cases, pT_{2b} in 277 patients (59%), pT_{3a} in 31 patients (9.4%) and pT_{3b} in 22 patients (7%).

Positive surgical margins were found in 15.75% of all operative specimens. By pathological stage, three pT_{2a} specimens (3.8%), 29 pT_{2b} specimens (14.9%), 11 pT_{3a} specimens (35.5%) and ten pT_{3b} specimens (49%) were found to have positive surgical margins.

It is possible that most of these positive margins were surgically induced, because, in the first group of 100 pT_2 tumor patients, the number of specimens with positive margins was 15, but only ten in the next 120 patients. It seems from the literature that their prognosis is identical to that of totally organ-confined tumors[10], but long follow-up is needed for a proper judgement.

Biochemical progression

With regard to data on biochemical progression, to date, the follow-up has been too short to produce definitive conclusions (average follow-up 4.8 months (range 1–18)). However, at present, the biochemical results appear identical to those expected from our experience gained after the retropubic approach: among the group of 76 patients with a pT_{1-2} stage, with at least 12 postoperative months (range 12–24; average 14), the rate of patients with a PSA level below 0–1 ng/ml is 87%.

Parietal seeding

The question of an additional oncological risk related to the laparoscopic route is still controversial. The great majority of tumors operated in our series were intracapsular organ-confined tumors, which are, therefore, not exposed to the pneumoperitoneum, and which can be considered to have little or no risk of dissemination. Only one report of cutaneous metastases after lymphadenectomy for prostate cancer has been published in the literature[11]. This case concerned a highly undifferentiated tumor which was dissected with no particular technical precautions. The risk of cutaneous tumor seeding is, therefore, probably very low in view of the number of lymphadenectomies performed for prostate cancer throughout the world.

Functional results

No scoring scale is available to assess the functional value of radical prostatectomy and the surgeon's subjectivity is known to play an important role in interpretation of functional criteria. Sending to each patient a self-administered questionnaire to be completed at home seemed to us the best way to proceed[12].

Our available results are sketchy, since the mean follow-up is too short, and definitive assessment is of little relevance at present. Moreover, the continuous improvement of the technique does not allow us to draw conclusions from the experience of our first patients, who are the only ones to have had a sufficiently long follow-up.

Miction

To date, one of our patients has presented with a stricture of the anastomosis justifying an endoscopic procedure.

In order to evaluate continence as objectively as possible, we have prospectively sent the self-administered questionnaire validated by the International Continence Society to all our patients. Among the 194 patients with at least 6 months' follow-up, 190 patients answered (97.5%). The analysis of the self-administered questionnaire revealed that 143 patients are perfectly continent (without any pad, day or night), giving a 6-month continence rate of 75.3%. Forty-seven patients still wear pads at 6 months.

At 12 months, 109 patients received their questionnaire and 106 answered (97.2%). The analysis of the self-administered questionnaire revealed that 92 patients are perfectly continent (without any pad, day or night), giving a 12-month continence rate of 87%. Among the 14 patients still wearing pads, four suffered from severe incontinence for more than 12 months after the operation, and an artificial sphincter implantation was considered but, so far, these patients have not been implanted. Publications often report higher continence rates, but they correspond to subjective results obtained by clinical interview and not by self-administered questionnaire, which affects the results[12,13]. In our experience of retropubic surgery, using the same self-administered questionnaire and the same criteria, we found a continence rate of 73% at 12 months[14]. Under these conditions, the continence rate of 75% obtained at 6 months and 87% at 12 months after laparoscopic prostatectomy is very encouraging, especially as it relates to our first patients. The recovery period also appears to be short, less than 1 month in 50% of patients.

Sexual potency

Owing to the technical difficulties that we had to resolve, we were unable to systematically preserve neurovascular bundles at the beginning of our series, i.e. in the first 100 patients. Preservation of neurovascular pedicles was only regularly performed for the later patients. At present, with an extremely short follow-up of less than 3 months, in a highly selected group of 40 patients, the spontaneous postoperative erection rate is 45%. Among these patients, three are able to experience intercourse, without the assistance of oral or intracavernous medication. Since preservation of sexual potency is a critical point, it is hoped that this rate will improve with time and that the quality of erections will allow patients to resume a satisfactory sex life.

Conclusions

Radical prostatectomy can be routinely and safely performed by transperitoneal laparoscopy by a urological team experienced in laparoscopy and in radical prostatectomy. The operative and postoperative morbidity are very low. Postoperative pain is minimal, allowing a reduction in the length of the hospital stay. Oncological results appear satisfactory after a short follow-up. Improvement in the quality of intraoperative visibility by magnification of the image allows a more precise procedure. This subjective improvement in the quality of dissection will allow a reduction in the usual functional sequelae of conventional radical prostatectomy, such as incontinence and impotence. This will need to be confirmed by a larger series of operations with a longer follow-up.

Laparoscopic radical prostatectomy is now performed routinely and is proposed as the first-line surgical treatment for localized prostatic cancer in our department.

References

1. Schuessler W, Kavoussi LR, Clayman R, *et al.* Laparoscopic radical prostatectomy: initial case report. *J Urol* 1992;4:246A
2. Schuessler W, Schulam P, Clayman R, *et al.* Laparoscopic radical prostatectomy: initial short-term experience. *Urology* 1997;50:854–7
3. Guillonneau B, Cathelineau X, Barret E, *et al.* Prostatectomie radicale cœlioscopique. Première évaluation après 28 interventions. *Presse Med* 1998;27:1570–4
4. Guillonneau B, Vallancien G. Laparoscopic radical prostatectomy: initial experience and preliminary assessment after 65 operations. *Prostate* 1999;39:71–5
5. Guillonneau B, Valancien G. Laparoscopic radical prostatectomy: the Montsouris experience. *J Urol* 2000;163:418–22
6. Griffith D, Schuessler W, Nickell K, *et al.* Laparoscopic pelvic lymphadenectomy for prostatic adenocarcinoma. *Urol Clin North Am* 1992;19:407–15
7. Raboy A, Ferzli G, Albert P. Initial experience with extraperitoneal endoscopic radical retropubic prostatectomy. *Urology* 1997;50:849–53
8. Rassweiler J, Seemon O, Abdel-Salam Y, *et al.* Laparoscopic radical prostatectomy; the Heilbron technique. *J Endourol* 1999;13(Suppl 1): A46
9. Guillonneau B, Debras B, Veillon B, *et al.* Indications for preoperative seminal vesicle biopsies in staging of clinically localized prostatic cancer. *Eur Urol* 1997;32:160–5
10. Ohori M, Wheeler TM, Kattan MW, *et al.* Prognostic significance of positive surgical margins in radical prostatectomy specimens. *J Urol* 1995;154:1818–26
11. Bangma C, Chadia W, Schröder F. Cutaneous metastasis following laparoscopic pelvic lymphadenectomy for prostatic carcinoma. *J Urol* 1995;153:1635–6
12. Bates TS, Wright MPJ, Gillatt DA. Prevalence and impact of incontinence and impotence following total prostatectomy assessed anonymously by the ICS-Male questionnaire. *Eur Urol* 1998;33:165–9
13. Öjdeby G, Clarzon A, Brekkan E, *et al.* Urinary incontinence and sexual impotence after radical prostatectomy. *Scand J Urol Nephrol* 1996;30: 473–7
14. Guillonneau B, Cathelineau X, Cour F, *et al.* Up-date of the morbidity of radical prostatectomy. Retrospective analysis of 100 consecutive operations for the period 1996–1997 (French). *Prog Urol* 1999;9:662–7

Section IV

Management of localized prostate cancer and preventive approaches

Watchful waiting or early endocrine treatment in 'low-risk' prostate cancer

14

P. J. Van Cangh, B. Tombal and J. L. Gala

The past 15 years have witnessed a profound change in the prostate cancer population. The widespread use of prostate-specific antigen (PSA) has induced a dramatic increase in the prevalence of low tumor burden prostate cancers: patients are now diagnosed with prostate cancer much earlier and failure of radical therapy is also detected at a very early stage. An ever-increasing cohort of asymptomatic patients now present to urologists with minimal disease and prolonged expected survival[1]. In addition, significant advances in medical care have allowed correction of previously lethal co-morbidities, thereby increasing the likelihood of longer survival.

The question of when to initiate endocrine therapy therefore becomes more pressing, as endocrine therapy is not curative and side-effects of treatment, especially of long duration, are considerable[2]. In low-risk low-volume prostate cancer it has now become urgent to ascertain whether or not the potential benefits of immediate endocrine treatment positively balance its inconveniences[3].

The arguments

Until now, in our view, no study has convincingly demonstrated a definitive advantage to giving androgen suppression early in low-risk low-volume prostate cancer[3]. Through the years, supporters and opponents of early or delayed treatment have argued over the optimal solution.

Arguments in favor of early endocrine therapy include the following:

(1) Experimental animal models indicate that androgen withdrawal is more effective when started early in the development of a tumor[4–6].

(2) The precise relationship between the intensity of the response to androgen withdrawal and the extent of the metastatic disease is unclear. However, several studies have suggested that a favorable response is more likely to occur in smaller than in bigger tumors and that the number and location of bone metastases have a strong impact on prognosis. Several studies conducted by the National Cancer Institute (NCI), the European Organization for Research and Treatment of Cancer (EORTC), and others have shown that patients with less than five metastases limited to the axial skeleton and with good performance status will derive the most benefit from treatment[7,8]. However, this was not shown to lead to advantage in survival.

(3) The need for ancillary procedures (i.e. transurethral prostatic resection (TURP), JJ stents) and the emergence of life-threatening complications (i.e. pathological fractures, spinal cord compression and paraplegia) are less likely to occur when patients are treated early[9].

(4) Progression of prostate cancer is not truly asymptomatic since most patients will suffer from malaise, fatigue and a sense of unhealthiness. In addition, some patients will die without having the opportunity of receiving treatment[9,10].

Arguments against early administration of endocrine therapy include the reasons for recommending delayed treatment, as well as the necessity for strict long-term follow-up with the inherent risk of undertreating those patients delaying or lost to follow-up.

Arguments in favor of delaying treatment include the following:

(1) Since endocrine therapy is only palliative, and asymptomatic patients have no symptoms to palliate, delaying treatment avoids androgen ablation and its poorly tolerated side-effects[11]. When symptomatic progression occurs – and it will inevitably if the patient lives long enough – effective treatment is still available.

(2) Observation means watchful waiting and not neglect – rapid progression and complications can be detected early by PSA-based follow-up and modern imaging technology; treatment can, therefore, be started early enough to prevent catastrophic complications[12]. Sequential observation allows the determination of the velocity of rising PSA levels (usually reported as doubling time or PSAdt). PSAdt has been demonstrated to be one of the most important parameters in the evaluation of the patient with progressing disease[13,14]. In addition, several new parameters are under investigation such as the level of urinary PSA, the ratio of free/total PSA in the urine, the results of anastomotic biopsy samples, and the detection of circulating prostate cells by PSA reverse transcriptase–polymerase chain reaction (RT–PCR) after surgery[15].

(3) Well-differentiated prostate cancer progresses slowly and many such patients will die of other causes, with cancer rather than from cancer.

(4) Cost is reduced.

Against delaying endocrine therapy stand all the arguments for early treatment, including patient anxiety when confronted with the advice of now neglecting a rising PSA level, which had earlier been the compelling argument to accept aggressive local treatment.

The rising problem of early or low-volume prostate cancer

The combined influence of three factors involving PSA – *de facto* PSA screening, earlier diagnosis of failure by rising PSA after radical therapy and earlier diagnosis of advanced disease – has shifted the prostate cancer population towards a larger proportion with low-volume disease. In the most recent studies, a majority (up to 78%) of patients presents at an earlier stage of the disease ($T_{1-2}N_0M_0$) and the incidence of N_+/M_+ patients is consequently reduced[16,17].

PSA screening

Interim analysis of the ongoing European Randomized Study of Screening for Prostate Cancer reports a contemporary incidence of N_+ and M_+ disease as low as 2% and a shift towards lower-grade tumors (Gleason score < 7 in 90% of patients)[17]. By contrast, a retrospective analysis of data collected between 1989 and 1994 in a neighboring area, reported up to 24% of N_+/M_+ patients[1]. Similarly, in most recent studies, the incidence of N_+ patients has dramatically decreased from 20–40% in the late 1980s to less than 5%[18].

PSA failure

At present, approximately two-thirds of men diagnosed with prostate cancer will be offered radical therapy, and 40% of those – representing one-quarter of today's prostate cancer patients – will relapse, usually with a rising PSA. Progression of prostate cancer is, therefore, diagnosed much earlier following regular PSA testing in this rapidly growing cohort of patients with truly low-volume disease for which a long survival might be expected. This is well illustrated in a landmark longitudinal study of patients treated at the Brady Urological Institute in whom PSA failure occurred after radical prostatectomy for localized disease ($\leq T_2$): the median actuarial time to clinical metastases was 8 years, and the median actuarial time for progression from metastasis to death was an additional 5 years[13].

Faced with the problem of PSA failure, the urologist must decide whether the cause of failure is local, distant, or both distant and local[19]. In case of local recurrence only, there is a possibility of cure by additional treatment to the primary site. In practice, two complementary approaches exist: either to estimate the probabilities of recurrence based on statistical risk factors, or to try to obtain a positive identification of recurrent disease by imaging studies and by biopsy.

The risk factors of recurrence have been well studied and several models and nomograms have been constructed based on major but individual center experiences. A popular model comes from the Johns Hopkins Hospital in Baltimore (the Partin tables) based on pathological data of the radical prostatectomy specimen[20]. By combining serum PSA, Gleason sum and status of surgical margins (positive or negative), three risk groups have been identified. Both the Baylor University experience (Scardino nomogram) and the CAPSURE database have been analyzed and produced the same type of model. Other authors[21] have produced prognostic factors from preoperative data, essentially based on initial serum PSA level, preoperative prostate biopsy and clinical stage. The importance of tumor grade has been repeatedly emphasized[22-24]. Similar models have been constructed for radiotherapy-treated patients. Such models are helpful, as they not only identify poor-risk patients who require immediate therapy, but also good-risk patients who might safely benefit from observation. Positive identification of recurrent disease is a challenging task in this situation of small tumor burden. Bone scans and computerized tomography (CT) scans are of little help, except when serum PSA levels and/or PSA doubling time are high (> 20 ng/ml or > 20 ng/ml/year, respectively). Immunoscintigraphy (Prostascint

scan) offers the prospect of specifically detecting the site of recurrence. Ideally, when the scan is positive only in the prostatic fossa, results of adjuvant local therapy should be optimal; in reality, the study only has a positive predictive value of 50% and a negative predictive value of 17%. Systematic biopsy of the prostatic fossa is debatable, especially when digital rectal examination (DRE) is normal, as sampling errors are common; adjuvant radiation therapy is indeed known to decrease PSA levels in > 50% of negative biopsies. The significance of post-radiation biopsy is a hotly debated topic, and not addressed in this review.

New definition of advanced disease

The third reason for the growing importance of the timing of androgen ablation is the radical change in the definition of advanced prostate cancer. Classically, advanced disease consisted of patients with clinically apparent extra-prostatic disease, and nodal (N_+) or distant (M_+) metastases. At present, cases of microscopic extracapsular disease (pT_3), those with a high risk of failure (Gleason grade 4–5, Gleason score 8–10, high initial PSA level (> 20 ng/ml), elevated acid phosphatase), as well as those with biochemical failure only (rising PSA) or even molecular failure (positive RT–PCR) are also included in this category. Patients are therefore considered to have advanced disease at a much earlier stage of evolution and with a substantially lower tumor burden; they have a much longer life expectancy and if therapy is initiated early, a much longer duration of treatment must be expected. Side-effects (especially long-term) as well as cost, become significant determinants; before initiating a long-term palliative treatment, that will sooner or later be met with resistance, especially in an asymptomatic patient, the potential benefits must be thoughtfully weighed against the potentially negative impact on quality of life and general health (longer survival must compensate for the side-effects of androgen ablation)[3,11,14].

Natural history of low-risk low-volume disease

Several Swedish studies have demonstrated the prolonged survival of selected patients with clinically localized prostate cancer[25,26]. In a study of early-stage initially untreated prostate cancer patients based on the population of the Swedish county of Orebro, Johansson and colleagues found that the corrected 15-year survival rate was similar in 223 patients with deferred treatment (81%; 95% confidence interval (CI) 72–89%) and in 77 who received initial treatment (81%; 95% CI 67–95%)[25].

The data from the Connecticut tumor registry carefully analyzed by Albertsen and co-workers clearly demonstrated the importance of age, co-morbidities and tumor histology: men with a low Gleason score (2–4) faced only a 4–7% risk of dying from prostate cancer within 15 years of diagnosis; those patients conservatively treated incurred no loss of life expectancy compared to the general population[27].

A large compilation study showed that grade 1 prostate cancer patients have an excellent 10-year survival rate[22]. Similarly, Lu Yao and Yao analyzed the data from 59 876 patients demonstrating again the prolonged survival of patients with well-differentiated prostate cancer[28].

A false interpretation of the impact of PSA elevation after radical therapy and, especially, after radical prostatectomy, induces a compulsive concern about PSA, and pushes physicians towards the automatic administration of hormonal therapy with the sole advantage of relieving the patient's (and their own) anxiety, even though the main objective of treating biochemical failure is to prevent metastasis and death from prostate cancer[12,14]. Since progression to symptomatic M_+ disease is unpredictable, advocating hormonal manipulation in every patient with biochemical failure is clearly excessive[29,30].

Data presently exist to facilitate the decision of the timing of hormonal therapy. The series of 1997 radical prostatectomy performed at the Johns Hopkins Hospital, in which patients received no additional treatment until symptoms or metastases occurred, offers a unique opportunity to analyze the predictive factors of poor outcome[13]. First, these data demonstrate that all men with detectable metastatic disease who died (33% of those with a rising PSA level), did so due to progression of prostate cancer, after escaping adequate endocrine treatment. This stresses the need to identify those patients at risk of developing detectable disease and to enrol them in therapeutic protocols. Second, the authors identify three significant ($p < 0.001$) prognostic factors: the Gleason score of the primary tumor (5–7 versus 8–10), the time to biochemical progression (≤ 2 years versus > 2 years) and PSA doubling time (< 10 months versus ≥ 10 months). The initial Gleason score together with the PSA level, age and pathological stage, are the most powerful predictors of outcome. Hopefully we should soon be able to elaborate accurate predictive algorithms and decide who is at risk, who should be treated and which therapy should be used (androgen suppressive or non-hormonal). In addition, such algorithms would help to reassure patients with a high probability of a favorable outcome, for whom watchful waiting is the most appropriate approach.

Early endocrine treatment – expected benefits

What will it do for me?

Historically, prior to the introduction of PSA, pivotal studies have addressed the issue of the timing of hormonal therapy[10]. Although of considerable interest in the past, they offer little help to today's patients presenting earlier with a much lower tumor burden. Several modern (in the post-PSA era) clinical trials have reconsidered this issue; conclusions are at best contradictory, some demonstrating an overall survival advantage for early androgen deprivation, and many others showing no or minimal advantage.

In a prospective, randomized study conducted by the Eastern Cooperative Oncology Group (ECOG), 98 patients with low-stage prostate cancer and a negative metastatic work-up were found to have positive nodes at the time of radical prostatectomy[31]. They were randomized to immediate castration ($n = 46$) or delayed endocrine treatment at the time of progression ($n = 52$). After a median follow-up of 7.1 years, the patients who had received immediate endocrine therapy had a significantly improved outcome compared to those who had been observed and had received delayed therapy: cancer deaths were 4.3% compared to 31%, respectively ($p < 0.001$). These data, if corroborated by additional research, are applicable to this population with early disseminated cancer, but cannot be generalized to patients with earlier disease, such as PSA failure after radical therapy. Of note, the cancer-specific survival rate in the delayed group was surprisingly poorer (62%) compared to some other contemporary series (around 80% in the Mayo Clinic series[32]), indicating a possible imbalance in risk factors. Moreover, the timing of hormonal therapy in the observation group was not clearly defined, raising the possibility of a deleterious delay in some patients. Reported at the same time, a non-randomized study from Rotterdam University of a similar size ($n = 91$) reached opposite conclusions[33]. In this study, in contrast to the previous one, delayed endocrine therapy of M_0N_+ patients provided a significant survival advantage over immediate treatment: 21% versus 49% cancer mortality, respectively ($p < 0.04$). There is, however, an imbalance of prognostic factors in favor of the 'delayed-treatment' group. These preliminary results will need longer follow-up for a more definitive answer.

A randomized study on N_+ patients has been conducted by the EORTC (30846) comparing immediate versus delayed endocrine treatment (goserilin + cyproterone acetate) in $pN_{1-3}–M_0$ prostate cancer. Hopefully, final results will soon be available and provide more definitive arguments for counselling patients. An interim analysis revealed a highly significant difference in time to progression, but no difference in cancer-related or overall survival[34].

The South Sweden Prostate Cancer Study Group enrolled 285 previously untreated localized prostate cancer patients in a randomized study aiming to determine if early endocrine treatment (parenteral and/or oral estrogens) prolongs the interval to metastasis and/or cancer-related or overall survival[35]. There was a significant difference ($p = 0.03$) among the groups in disease-free survival and in the probability of dying of prostatic cancer with the highest risk in the surveillance group, but there was no difference in overall survival. Similarly to the classical Veterans Administration studies, the increased cardiovascular mortality from estrogens may have obscured a therapeutic benefit.

The Medical Research Council (MRC) conducted a randomized study to compare the effects of endocrine therapy on the course of advanced prostate cancer when started at diagnosis or deferred until clinical progression[9]. Symptomatic clinical progression was delayed in the immediate group, and severe complications from disease progression were significantly less frequent. Differences in mortality were not statistically significant in patients with M_1 and M_x disease, whereas in M_0 patients a statistically significant difference was observed ($2p = 0.02$ for overall survival, and $2p < 0.001$ for disease-specific survival). Final conclusions have, however, been challenged due to the fact that 29 of the 54 men who died of prostate cancer in the delayed group never received endocrine therapy. Similar criticisms were raised against the Veterans Administration Co-operative Urological Research Group-2 studies in which 17% of the 278 asymptomatic patients on deferred treatment died of prostate cancer without being given the possible benefit of endocrine treatment[36]. In addition, since the MRC trial was conducted before the routine use of PSA and only an annual follow-up was required, it might be argued that closer PSA monitoring and a more regular follow-up would have allowed an earlier diagnosis of disease progression and avoided catastrophic complications. Moreover, with a longer follow-up and more maturity (818/934 have died), the overall survival benefit in M_0 is no longer significant, suggesting an adverse effect of prolonged hormone treatment in increasing mortality

Table 1 Early versus delayed endocrine therapy

Study	Stage	Number of patients	Follow-up (years)	Treatment	Overall survival	Notes
MRC-PCWPIG, 1997[9]	locally advanced M_0 asymptomatic M_+	938	—	early vs. delayed endocrine therapy	(+) early in M_0, but ...$\Rightarrow$ (no advantage in M_+)	(−) study with longer follow-up update 2000 (Kirk[37])
EORTC 22863, 1997[39], 1999[40]	T_{2b}–T_4	401	5	1 month neoadjuvant endocrine therapy (CPA) + radiation therapy + 3 years adjuvant LHRH analog	(+) early 79 vs. 62%	prolonged effect of endocrine therapy?
ECOG, 1999[31]	T_{1-2} N_+	98	7.2	post-radical prostatectomy	(+) 85 vs. 65%	small volume cancer (80% had non-detectable PSA)
EORTC 30846 interim analysis[34]	N_+ M_0	—	> 6	no radical prostatectomy, early vs. delayed endocrine therapy	(−)	
EORTC 30891	asymptomatic M_0	—	—	no radical treatment, early vs. delayed endocrine therapy	(−)	
RTOG 85–31[41] RTOG 85–31 update[43]	T_{3-4}	945	4.5 5.6	radiation therapy + endocrine therapy started at end of radiation therapy	(−) (+) in subgroup Gleason 8–10, $p = 0.036$	only after 9 years
Umea[38]	T_{1-4} M_0 pN_{0-3}	91	9.3	pelvic lymph node dissection, early vs. delayed castration 1 month before radiation therapy	(+) only for N_+ (not for N_-) 61 vs. 38%; $p = 0.02$	
Goteborg-SSPCSG[35]	M_0	—	—	early vs. delayed estrogen	(−)	> mortality for estrogens

CPA, cyproterone acetate; LHRH, luteinizing hormone releasing hormone; PSA, prostate-specific antigen; MRC, Medical Research Council; PCWPIG, Prostate Cancer Working Party Investigators Group; EORTC, European Organization for Research and Treatment of Cancer; ECOG, European Cooperative Oncology Group; RTOG, Radiation Therapy Oncology Group; SSPCSG, South Sweden Prostate Cancer Study Group; (+), positive study for early endocrine therapy

from other causes[37]. Here, also, the study addressed advanced disease, and to apply its conclusions to earlier disease stages would require additional studies.

Another EORTC study (30891) compared early versus delayed castration (surgical or medical) in previously untreated patients with non-metastatic asymptomatic prostate cancer, not suitable for local curative treatment. No difference in survival has been detected so far, but final results of this are not yet available since, to date, an insufficient number of patients have died.

The effect of immediate androgen suppression in conjunction with external beam radiation therapy (EBRT) versus EBRT alone and delayed treatment at relapse, has been evaluated by several radiotherapy teams.

Investigators from Umea County in Sweden recruited 91 patients with clinically localized cancer who underwent surgical lymph node staging and were thereafter randomized to receive definitive EBRT with immediate or delayed orchidectomy. After a median follow-up of 9.3 years, overall survival was statistically better in the immediate arm (61 vs. 38%; $p = 0.02$), but only for node-positive patients, demonstrating again the importance of selection factors[38].

The EORTC conducted a randomized study (22863) in prostate cancer patients treated with radiation therapy and receiving either immediate luteinizing hormone releasing hormone (LHRH) analog administered for 3 years or delayed hormonal treatment at the time of relapse[39]. With a mean follow-up of 5 years, disease-free and overall survival were significantly better in the early treatment group (75 vs. 40% and 78 vs. 62%; $p = 001$, respectively)[40]. Unfortunately, no pelvic lymph node dissection was performed, contrary to the Umea study, and a control arm of endocrine treatment alone is missing; such a study, however, is in progress (RTOG 97–02).

Randomized phase III studies were conducted by the RTOG in order to evaluate the role of hormonal management adjuvant to radiotherapy in high-risk patients (T_2N_+, T_3 and also pT_3 and/or positive seminal vesicle after radical prostatectomy) (RTOG 85–31)[41] and in patients with bulky tumors (RTOG 86–10). In a subset analysis of post-prostatectomy patients, early treatment improved progression-free survival and biochemical recurrence in particular, but with a median follow-up of 4.5 years no difference was noted in distant failure and overall survival[42]. An update of RTOG 85–31 at 5.6 years, reported similar overall survival in general, but an improved survival in a selected subgroup of patients with Gleason score 8–10 cancers[43]. These radiotherapy data suggest a synergistic action of combined therapies, whereas studies of neoadjuvant endocrine therapy in radical prostatectomy series have demonstrated a reduction in the rate of positive surgical margins, but, so far, no benefit in time to progression or survival.

The analysis of these studies suggests that the beneficial impact of early androgen ablation is stronger in patients with aggressive and (relatively) extensive disease (Table 1). In patients with less bulky disease, the survival advantage is less clear. In our view, there are no conclusive arguments to recommend systematic early androgen deprivation in the contemporary 'low-risk' prostate cancer patient diagnosed by PSA screening or biological failure after radical treatment of curative intention[3].

Androgen deprivation – side-effects

What will it do to me?

For many years, oral estrogens have been the sole alternative to surgical castration. Although relatively cheap and effective, they present significant side-effects: besides gynecomastia and decreasing libido and sexual potency, they may lead to fluid retention, congestive heart failure, deep venous thrombosis, pulmonary embolism, myocardial infarction and strokes. LHRH analogs were rapidly shown to provide a reliable means of suppressing testosterone to be equal in effectiveness and side-effects to bilateral orchidectomy[44]. Owing to their intrinsic mechanism of action, however, they have been administered with an antiandrogen during the first weeks of treatment in order to prevent a tumor flare-up by agonistic androgenic stimulation. In an attempt to preserve sexual function and libido, antiandrogens have been developed to inhibit directly the intracellular action of dihydrotestosterone (DHT) on prostatic cells by interfering with receptor steroid binding or nuclear translocation of the androgen receptor. By interrupting a normal feedback mechanism, antiandrogens slightly raise LH and testosterone levels and this is thought to permit the preservation of libido and potency in a significant proportion of patients. Legitimate concerns have been raised as to whether peripheral blockade alone provides sufficient androgen withdrawal. Recently, however, it has been suggested that antiandrogens could offer a valuable option in patients with low disease burden by providing a comparable efficiency while improving quality of life[45]. A recent analysis of two multicenter, randomized trials suggests that the non-steroidal antiandrogen bicalutamide is as effective as castration in M_0 patients with significant improvement in sexual interest and physical capacity[46]. The steroidal antiandrogen, cyproterone acetate, is as effective as estrogen therapy and has a better side-effect profile. Compared with flutamide as monotherapy for good-risk metastatic prostate cancer patients (EORTC study 30892), preliminary results show less toxicity for cyproterone acetate (gynecomastia, diarrhea, nausea and liver function deterioration) with no significant difference in sexual potency[2]. Greater concern has been raised against potential toxicity related to prolonged androgen suppression. Sustained exposure to endocrine treatment may cause anemia resulting in fatigue, pale appearance of the patients and impaired cardiac function[47]. Osteoporosis and osteoporotic fractures are other time-dependent side-effects of castration especially in elderly men with disseminated prostate carcinoma. Several studies have demonstrated that the incidence of osteoporosis increases significantly in castrated men after 2–4 years of hormonal suppression and leads to a cumulative incidence of osteoporotic fractures as high as 50% at 10 years[48].

The impact of androgen deprivation on quality of life has recently attracted well-deserved attention. In an important 'preference' trial of different strategies of androgen deprivation in asymptomatic patients the question was raised again as to whether early androgen deprivation for prostate cancer does more harm than good: the majority of men who chose androgen deprivation therapy reported significantly more fatigue, additional emotional distress and worse general health compared to men who did not receive androgen suppression[11].

Clearly if androgen deprivation is required for prolonged periods, better treatment modalities should be investigated, with fewer side-effects and a less negative impact on quality of life and general health. Ongoing trials on antiandrogen monotherapy[45,46], 'step-up' therapy[2] and intermittent androgen suppression[49] address this important issue.

Conclusions: when to start endocrine therapy in low-risk prostate cancer – early or late?

This apparently simple question has no straightforward answer because of the unpredictability of the two main variables: the evolution of a particular tumor cannot be reliably anticipated and the precise survival of a particular prostate cancer patient is unknown. It comes, therefore, as no surprise that the answer is at best controversial. There are, however, useful data that can help the urologist and his patient to make an informed choice. Patients with well-differentiated tumors, low initial PSA level and slow PSA doubling time clearly do not need immediate therapy, local or general. Patients with severe co-morbidities that limit foreseeable survival also can be observed expectantly. By contrast, patients with high-grade cancers, high initial PSA levels and rapidly progressing disease should be treated immediately. For the intermediate cohort of patients, strict watchful waiting is an option with initiation of therapy at early signs of progression. As demonstrated by the catastrophic complications such as spinal cord compression and ureteral obstruction occurring in the delayed arm of the MRC study[9], treatment should not be started too late. Unfortunately, no strict clinical or biological criteria exist to trigger a change in therapeutic attitude. Early treatment offers advantages in time to progression and disease-specific survival, but there is no convincing evidence that it provides a clinically significant survival advantage counterbalancing its well known side-effects, especially in low-risk low-volume disease. The timing of hormonal therapy in low-risk prostate cancer remains a matter of controversy as there are no solid data produced by randomized studies addressing this precise question.

References

1. Rietbergen JB, Hoedemaeker RF, Kruger AE, et al. The changing pattern of prostate cancer at the time of diagnosis: characteristics of screen detected prostate cancer in a population based screening study. *J Urol* 1999;161:1192–8

2. Schröder FH. Endocrine treatment of prostate cancer – recent developments and the future. I. Maximal androgen blockade, early vs. delayed endocrine treatment and side-effects. *Br J Urol Int* 1999;83:161–70

3. Van Cangh PJ, Gala JL, Tombal B. Immediate versus delayed androgen deprivation for prostate cancer. *Prostate* 2000;45(Suppl 10):19–25

4. Bruchovsky N, Rennie PS, Coldman AJ, et al. Effects of androgen withdrawal on the stem cell composition of the Shionogi carcinoma. *Cancer Res* 1990;50:2275–82

5. Isaacs JT. The timing of androgen ablation therapy and/or chemotherapy in the treatment of prostatic cancer. *Prostate* 1984;5:1–17

6. Henry JM, Isaacs JT. Relationship between tumor size and the curability of metastatic prostatic cancer by surgery alone or in combination with adjuvant chemotherapy. *J Urol* 1988; 139:1119–23

7. Denis L, Smith PH, De Moura JL, et al. Orchidectomy vs. Zoladex plus flutamide in patients with metastatic prostate cancer. The EORTC GU Group. *Eur Urol* 1990;18:34–40

8. Crawford ED, Eisenberger MA, McLeod DG, et al. A controlled trial of leuprolide with and without flutamide in prostatic carcinoma. *N Engl J Med* 1989;321:419–24

9. The Medical Research Council Prostate Cancer Working Party Investigators Group. Immediate versus deferred treatment for advanced prostatic cancer: initial results of the Medical Research Council Trial. *Br J Urol* 1997;79:235–46

10. Byar DP. Proceedings of the Veterans Administration Cooperative Urological Research Group's studies of cancer of the prostate. *Cancer* 1973;32:1126–30

11. Herr H, O'Sullivan M. Quality of life of asymptomatic men with nonmetastatic prostate cancer on androgen deprivation therapy. *J Urol* 2000;163:1743–6

12. Jhaveri FM, Zippe CD, Klein EA, et al. Biochemical failure does not predict overall survival after radical prostatectomy for localized prostate cancer: 10-year results. *Urology* 1999; 54:884–90

13. Pound CR, Partin AW, Eisenberger MA, et al. Natural history of progression after PSA elevation following radical prostatectomy. *J Am Med Assoc* 1999;281:1591–7

14. Scher HI. Management of prostate cancer after prostatectomy. Treating the patient, not the PSA. *J Am Med Assoc* 1999;281:1642–5

15. Gala JL, Heusterspreute M, Hanon F, et al. Expression of prostate-specific antigen and prostate-specific membrane antigen in blood cells: implications for the detection of hematogenous prostate cells and standardization. *Clin Chem* 1998;44:472–81

16. Haese A, Huland E, Graefen M, et al. Supersensitive PSA-analysis after radical prostatectomy: a powerful tool to reduce the time gap between surgery and evidence of biochemical failure. *Anticancer Res* 1999;19: 2641–4

17. Schröder FH, Kranse R, Rietbergen J, et al. The European Randomized Study of Screening for Prostate Cancer (ERSPC): an update. Members of the ERSPC, Section Rotterdam. *Eur Urol* 1999;35:539–43

18. Ghavamian R, Bergstralh EJ, Blute ML, et al. Radical retropubic prostatectomy plus orchiectomy versus orchiectomy alone for pTxN+ prostate cancer: a matched comparison. *J Urol* 1999;161:1223–7

19. Jhaveri FM, Klein EA. How to explore the patient with a rising PSA after radical prostatectomy: defining local versus systemic failure. *Semin Urol Oncol* 1999;17:130–4

20. Partin AW, Yoo J, Carter HB, et al. The use of PSA, clinical stage, and Gleason score to predict pathological stage in men with localized prostate cancer. *J Urol* 1993;150:110–18

21. Kattan MW, Wheeler TM, Scardino PT. Postoperative nomogram for disease recurrence after radical prostatectomy for prostate cancer. *J Clin Oncol* 1999;17:1499–507

22. Chodak GW, Thisted RA, Gerber GS, et al. Results of conservative management of clinically localized prostate cancer. *N Engl J Med* 1994;330: 242–8

23. Stamey TA, Yemoto CM, McNeal JE, et al. Prostate cancer is highly predictable: prognostic equation based on all morphological variables in radical prostatectomy specimen. *J Urol* 2000;163: 1155–60

24. Graefen M, Noldus J, Pichlmeier U, et al. Early PSA relapse after radical prostatectomy: prediction on the basis of preoperative and postoperatuve tumor characteristics. *Eur Urol* 1999;36:21–30

25. Johansson JE, Holmberg L, Johansson S, et al. Fifteen-year survival in prostate cancer. A

prospective population-based study in Sweden. *J Am Med Assoc* 1997;277:467–71

26. Adolfsson J, Steineck G, Hedlund PO. Deferred treatment of locally advanced nonmetastatic prostate cancer: a long term follow-up. *J Urol* 1999;161:505–8

27. Albertsen PC, Hanley JA, Gleason DF, *et al.* Competing risk analysis of men aged 55 to 74 years at diagnosis managed conservatively for clinically localized prostate cancer. *J Am Med Assoc* 1998;280:975–80

28. Lu Yao GL, Yao SL. Population-based study of long-term survival in patients with clinically localised prostate cancer. *Lancet* 1997;349:906–10

29. Boccon-Gibod L. Introduction: rising PSA after radical prostatectomy: a burning issue. *Semin Urol Oncol* 1999;17:125–6

30. Bhayani SB, Andriole GL. Hormonal manipulation for rising PSA after radical prostatectomy. *Semin Urol Oncol* 1999;17:148–53

31. Messing EM, Manola J, Sarosdy M, *et al.* Immediate hormonal therapy compared with observation after radical prostatectomy and pelvic lymphadenectomy in men with node-positive prostate cancer. *N Engl J Med* 1999; 341:1781–8

32. Zincke H, Bergstralh EJ, Larson-Keller JJ, *et al.* Stage D1 prostate cancer treated by radical prostatectomy and adjuvant hormonal treatment. Evidence for favorable survival in patients with DNA diploid tumors. *Cancer* 1992;70:311–23

33. Wijburg C, Boeken Kruger AE, van der Cruijsse I, *et al.* Immediate or delayed endocrine treatment for lymph node metastasized prostate cancer, is there a best choice? *J Urol* 1999;161:1149A

34. Van den Ouden D, Tribukait B, Blom J, *et al.* and the EORTC GU Group. DNA ploidy of core biopsies and metastatic lymph nodes of prostate cancer patients: impact on time to progression. *J Urol* 1993;150:400–6

35. Lundgren R, Nordle O, Josefsson K. Immediate estrogen or estramustine phosphate therapy versus deferred endocrine treatment in non-metastatic prostate cancer: a randomized multicenter study with 15 years of follow-up. The South Sweden Prostate Cancer Study Group. *J Urol* 1995;153:1580–6

36. Handley R, Carr TW, Travis D, *et al.* Deferred treatment for prostate cancer. *Br J Urol* 1988;62:249–53

37. Kirk D and the MRCPC Working Party Group. Immediate vs. deferred hormone treatment in advanced prostate cancer: review of data after longer period of follow-up. *Br J Urol Int* 2000; 86(Suppl 3):220, A-MP6.1.07

38. Granfors T, Modig H, Damber JE, *et al.* Combined orchiectomy and external radio-therapy versus radiotherapy alone for non-metastatic prostate cancer with or without pelvic lymph node involvement: a prospective randomized study. *J Urol* 1998;159:2030–4

39. Bolla M, Gonzalez D, Warde P, *et al.* Improved survival in patients with locally advanced prostate cancer treated with radiotherapy and goserilin. *N Engl J Med* 1997;337:295–300

40. Bolla M, Colette L, Gonzalez D, *et al.* Long term results of immediate adjuvant hormonal therapy with goserilin in patients with locally advanced prostate cancer treated with radiotherapy. *Eur J Cancer* 1999;35(Suppl 4):abstr 266

41. Pilepich MV, Caplan R, Byhardt RW, *et al.* Phase III trial of androgen suppression using goserilin in unfavorable prognosis carcinoma of the prostate treated with definitive radiotherapy: report of RTOG Group Protocol 85–31. *J Clin Oncol* 1997;15:1013

42. Corn BW, Winter K, Pilepich MV. Does androgen suppression enhance the efficacy of postoperative irradiation? A secondary analysis of RTOG 85–31. *Urology* 1999;54:495–502

43. Lawton C, Winter K, Murray K, *et al.* Updated results of the Phase-II RTOG trial 85–31 evaluating the potential benefit of androgen deprivation following standard radiation therapy for unfavorable prognosis carcinoma of the prostate. *Proc ASCO* 1999;18:93–8

44. Prostate Cancer Trialists' Collaborative Group. Maximum androgen blockade in advanced prostate cancer: an overview of the randomized trials. *Lancet* 2000;355:1491–8

45. Schröder FH. Antiandrogens as monotherapy for prostate cancer. *Eur Urol* 1998;34(Suppl 3):12–17

46. Iversen P, Tyrrell CJ, Anderson JB, *et al.* Comparison of 'Casodex' (Bicalutalide) 150 mg monotherapy with castration in previously untreated non-metastatic prostate cancer: mature survival results. *J Urol* 2000;163:159,A-704

47. Strum SB, McDermed JE, Scholz MC, *et al.* Anaemia associated with androgen deprivation in patients with prostate cancer receiving combined hormone blockade. *Br J Urol* 1997; 79:933–41

48. Daniell HW, Dunn SR, Ferguson DW, *et al.* Progressive osteoporosis during androgen deprivation therapy for prostate cancer. *J Urol* 2000;163:181–6

49. Van Cangh PJ, Tombal B, Gala JL. Intermittent endocrine treatment. *W J Urol* 2000;18:183–9

Biochemical outcome after radical prostatectomy, external beam radiation therapy or interstitial radiation therapy for clinically localized prostate cancer

15

A. V. D'Amico, R. Whittington, S. B. Malkowicz, D. Schultz, K. Blank,
J. E. Tomaszewski, A. A. Renshaw, I. Kaplan, C. J. Beard and A. Wein

Introduction

Recommendations for treatment of clinically localized adenocarcinoma of the prostate should be made using the results of evidence-based medicine. To date, there are no completed prospective randomized trials comparing definitive local treatment options for this disease. Retrospective comparisons[1,2] stratified by the known prognostic factors and using actuarial analyses have been published comparing radical prostatectomy to external beam radiation therapy. However, a direct comparison of the results of ultrasound-guided interstitial prostate radiation therapy to radical prostatectomy or radiation therapy stratified by the pretreatment prognostic factors has not been reported previously.

Use of pretreatment prostate-specific antigen (PSA) measurements[3], the biopsy Gleason score[4] and the American Joint Commission on Cancer Staging (AJCC) T-stage system[5] in predicting post-radiation[6–10] and postoperative[11–16] PSA failure-free survival (biochemical no-evidence of disease, bNED) has been published previously by several investigators. Therefore, in order to accurately compare the bNED outcome amongst each of the local treatment modalities, it is important to control for the values of these known prognostic factors.

The purpose of this study is to provide bNED outcome data stratified by pretreatment PSA level, biopsy Gleason score and AJCC T-stage

in men treated with radical prostatectomy, radiation therapy or interstitial prostate radiation therapy, with or without the addition of neoadjuvant androgen deprivation for clinically localized prostate cancer.

Methods

Patient population

Between January 1989 and October 1997, 1872 men with clinically localized prostate cancer underwent definitive local therapy. Local therapy received was radical prostatectomy ($n = 888$) or implant ± neoadjuvant androgen deprivation therapy ($n = 218$) at the Hospital of the University of Pennsylvania, or conformal radiation therapy ($n = 766$) at the Joint Center for Radiation Therapy.

Staging

In all cases, staging evaluation included a history and physical examination including a digital rectal examination (DRE), serum PSA measurement, computed tomography (CT) of the pelvis or an endorectal and pelvic coil magnetic resonance imaging (MRI) scan of the prostate and pelvis, bone scan and a transrectal ultrasound-guided (TRUS) needle biopsy of the prostate with Gleason score histological

147

grading[4]. A sextant biopsy was performed using an 18-gauge Tru-Cut needle (Travenol Laboratories, Deerfield, Illinois, USA) via a transrectal approach. The clinical stage was obtained from the DRE findings using the current 1992 AJCC staging system[5]. Radiological and biopsy information were not used to determine clinical stage. The PSA was obtained on an ambulatory basis prior to radiological studies and biopsy. All PSA measurements[3] were made using the Hybritech, Tosoh or Abbot assays.

Treatment

A referee genitourinary pathologist reviewed the diagnostic biopsy specimens for all patients undergoing surgery or implant treatment at the Hospital of the University of Pennsylvania (J.E.T.) and external beam radiation therapy at the Joint Center for Radiation Therapy (A.A.R.). Surgical treatment consisted of a radical retropubic prostatectomy and bilateral pelvic lymph node sampling.

All patients managed with definitive external beam radiation therapy were treated using ≥ 10 MV photons and a conformal shaped 4-field technique. Those patients with AJCC clinical stage $T_{1,2a}$ disease and who also had PSA levels < 10 ng/ml and a biopsy Gleason sum of 2–6 were given treatment to the prostate only, with a 1.5-cm margin. The median prescription dose was 66 Gy (66–70 Gy) and was delivered using 2-Gy fractions. All other patients with clinically localized disease received a median prescription dose of 45 Gy (45–50.4 Gy) in 1.8-Gy fractions to the prostate and seminal vesicles plus a 1.5-cm margin. This was followed by treatment to the prostate alone using a shrinking field technique with a 1.5-cm margin to a median prescription dose of 22 Gy (18–22 Gy) in 1.8–2.0 Gy fractions. A 95% normalization was used routinely.

Interstitial prostate radiation was performed using palladium 103 seeds, a perineal template-guided, peripheral loading technique and a Bruel and Kjaer ultrasound unit. The minimum peripheral dose to the prostatic capsule was 115 Gy. A transrectal ultrasound probe was used to image the prostate at 5-mm intervals pre-operatively to ascertain the optimal number and location of seeds needed to deliver the minimum peripheral dose to the entire prostate gland volume. Individual seed strength ranged from 1.58 to 1.64 mCi and the total amount of mCi implanted ranged from 35.3 to 194.3 mCi. Post-implant dosimetry was performed routinely on all patients based on films obtained at 4 weeks after the implant. For the first 143 patients, orthogonal films were used while, for the remaining 75 patients, computerized tomography was used. Of the 218 patients who received implant therapy, 152 (70%) received neoadjuvant androgen deprivation for a median of 3 months (2–10 months). Hormonal therapy consisted of a luteinizing hormone releasing hormone (LHRH) agonist which was preceded by the use of a non-steroidal anti-androgen for 7–10 days. Most patients (96/116, 83%) received 3 months of neoadjuvant androgen deprivation therapy. The remaining patients underwent varying lengths of treatment: two (1.33%), 15 (10%), 14 (9%), 20 (13%), one (1%), two (1.33%) and two (1.33%) received 2, 4, 5, 6, 7, 9 and 10 months of neoadjuvant androgen deprivation therapy, respectively.

Follow-up

The median follow-up of the 888 surgically managed patients at the Hospital of the University of Pennsylvania was 38 months (8–100 months). The median follow-up for the 766 and 218 radiation-managed patients at the Joint Center for Radiation Therapy and the Hospital of the University of Pennsylvania was 38 months (8–75 months) and 41 months (3–72 months), respectively. The patients were seen 1 month postoperatively or after the end of radiation therapy, then at 3-month intervals for 2 years, every 6 months for 5 years, and annually thereafter. At each follow-up, a serum PSA measurement was obtained prior to performing the DRE. All pretreatment PSA values were obtained within 1 month of the date of surgery or start of radiation. No patient was lost to follow-up and all patients were alive at the time of this analysis.

Statistical analyses

In order that the results of the Cox regression multivariate analyses were applicable in the clinical setting for an individual patient, three risk groups were defined. These risk groups were established from a review of the literature[6-19] and are based on the known prognostic factors: PSA level, biopsy Gleason score and the 1992 AJCC T-stage findings. Patients with AJCC clinical T-stage $T_{1c,2a}$, and a PSA level ≤ 10 ng/ml and a biopsy Gleason score ≤ 6 have been identified to be at low risk ($< 25\%$ at 5 years) for post-therapy PSA failure. Conversely, patients with AJCC stage T_{2c} disease and a PSA level > 20 ng/ml or a biopsy Gleason score ≥ 8 have a high risk ($> 50\%$ at 5 years) of post-therapy PSA failure. The remaining patients with PSA levels > 10 and ≤ 20 ng/ml or a biopsy Gleason score 7 or AJCC clinical stage T_{2b} have been found to have an intermediate risk (25–50% at 5 years) of post-therapy PSA failure. Patients with AJCC clinical stage $T_{1a,1b}$ were not managed using interstitial radiation therapy because of the significant rate of urinary incontinence noted[17] using this approach in patients with a history of a transurethral resection of the prostate. Therefore, patients with AJCC clinical stage $T_{1a,1b}$ disease managed with radical prostatectomy or radiation therapy were excluded from the study in order to ensure statistically valid comparisons.

A Cox regression multivariate analysis[20] was used to compare bNED outcome among the therapies within each risk group. For each analysis, the assumptions of the Cox model were tested and satisfied. Coefficients from the Cox regression model were used to calculate the overall relative risk of PSA failure for patients managed with radiation therapy or implant ± neoadjuvant androgen suppression, as compared to patients managed with radical prostatectomy. For the purposes of the multivariate analysis, the type of therapy was treated as a categorical variable indicating radical

prostatectomy at the Hospital of the University of Pennsylvania, radiation therapy, implant or implant plus neoadjuvant androgen deprivation. Radical prostatectomy at the Hospital of the University of Pennsylvania was defined as the baseline group for the purposes of the multivariate analyses.

PSA failure was defined according to the American Society of Therapeutic Radiation and Oncology (ASTRO) 1996 consensus statement[21] for all study patients. The definition required that a patient should have three consecutive rising PSA values, each obtained at least 3 months apart, before PSA failure was scored. The time of PSA failure was defined as the midpoint between the time of the PSA nadir value and the time of the first rising PSA value. Time zero was defined as the date of diagnosis for all study patients.

Pairwise comparisons were made using the log rank test. In the case where n comparisons were made, the level of significance, in order to be called statistically significant, was lowered from the convention of 0.05 to $0.05/n$ as per the Bonferroni methodology[22]. For the purpose of illustration, estimates of bNED outcome were calculated using the actuarial method of Kaplan and Meier[23] and graphically displayed. In the low-, intermediate- and high-risk patient groups, the sample size and the number of events in this study were sufficient to detect a 12%, 17% and 15% difference in bNED survival, respectively, with 80% power at a 0.05 level of significance. This was calculated for a baseline bNED survival of 85%, 60% and 30% at 5 years in the low-, intermediate- and high-risk patients, respectively.

Results

Risk group analysis

The clinical pretreatment characteristics of the 1872 patients used in the time-to-PSA-failure analyses are listed in Table 1 and are stratified by the type of treatment. Table 2 lists the clinical characteristics of the study patients within each risk group. The pairwise p values from the comparative analyses of the proportion of

Table 1 Clinical pretreatment characteristics of the 1872 patients used in the time-to-PSA-failure analyses are shown stratified by the type of treatment

Clinical factor	RP at U_{PENN} (n = 888)		RT at JCRT (n = 766)		Implant (n = 66)		Implant + H (n = 152)	
	n	%	n	%	n	%	n	%
PSA (ng/ml)								
> 0–4	85	10	77	10	5	8	16	10.5
4.1–10	510	57	329	43	37	56	111	73
10.1–20	210	24	198	26	16	24	24	16
> 20	83*	9	162[†]	21	8**	12	1[††]	0.5
Gleason score								
2–4	164	19	109	14	6	9	10	7
5–6	517	58	376	49	47	71	110	72
7	133	15	192	25	10	15	29	19
8–10	74	8	89	12	3	5	3	2
AJCC T-stage								
T_{1c}	256	29	222	29	15	23	57	37.5
T_{2a}	388	44	246	32	35	53	68	45
T_{2b}	93	10	141	18	5	7	7	4.5
T_{2c}	151	17	157	21	11	17	20	13

U_{PENN}, Hospital of the University of Pennsylvania; JCRT, Joint Center for Radiation Therapy; AJCC, American Joint Commission on Cancer Staging; H, neoadjuvant hormonal therapy; *PSA range: 20.3–243 ng/ml; median: 29.8 ng/ml; [†]PSA range: 20.1–561 ng/ml; median: 32.6 ng/ml; **PSA range: 20.4–96.7 ng/ml; median: 26 ng/ml; [††]PSA range: 26.9 ng/ml; median: 26.9 ng/ml

patients having a specific pretreatment clinical characteristic between the treatment groups are shown in Table 3. After adjustment for the multiple comparisons[22], no significant differences were noted in low-risk and intermediate-risk patients. High-risk patients managed with implant plus neoadjuvant androgen deprivation had an increased proportion of patients with PSA levels < 10 ng/ml and a decreased proportion of patients with PSA levels > 20 ng/ml compared to patients managed with radical prostatectomy ($p = 0.003$) or radiation therapy ($p = 0.0002$). Both of these differences could bias the comparisons of bNED survival in favor of the implant plus neoadjuvant androgen suppression patient cohort. The use of multiple comparisons between treatment modalities ($n = 6$) required that the level of statistical significance as per the Bonferroni methodology[22] be redefined as < 0.05/6 or < 0.0083.

Time-to-PSA-failure analyses

Table 4 lists the p values from the Cox regression multivariate analyses evaluating the effect of the treatment type on time to post-therapy PSA failure stratified by risk group. The relative risks of PSA failure with a 95% confidence interval are also shown. No significant difference ($p \geq 0.25$) in outcome was noted in low-risk patients ($T_{1c,2a}$, PSA level ≤ 10 ng/ml and Gleason score ≤ 6) across all treatment modalities. The 95% confidence intervals for the relative risk of PSA failure relative to radical prostatectomy for all patients included 1.0 values. High-risk patients (T_{2c} or PSA level > 20 ng/ml or Gleason score ≥ 8), however, treated using a radical prostatectomy or radiation therapy did significantly better ($p \leq 0.012$) then those managed with implant therapy with or without neoadjuvant androgen deprivation. Specifically, high-risk patients managed with implant therapy had at least a 2.2-fold increased

Table 2 Detailed description of the clinical pretreatment characteristics of the 1872 patients used in the time-to-PSA-failure analyses stratified by risk group and the type of treatment

Risk group	RP at U_{PENN}		RT at JCRT		Implant		Implant + H	
	n	%	n	%	n	%	n	%
Low risk								
Total n	402	100	225	100	32	100	91	100
PSA > 0–4 ng/ml	68	17	42	19	4	13	12	13
PSA 4.1–10 ng/ml	334	83	183	81	28	87	79	87
Gleason Score 2–4	104	26	53	24	4	12	7	8
Gleason Score 5–6	298	74	172	76	28	88	84	92
AJCC T_{1c}, T_{2a}	402	100	225	100	32	100	91	100
Intermediate risk								
Total n	247	100	232	100	15	100	38	100
PSA > 0–4 ng/ml	9	4	23	10	1	7	1	3
PSA 4.1–10 ng/ml	100	40	82	35	4	27	19	50
PSA 10.1–20 ng/ml	138	56	127	55	10	66	18	47
Gleason Score 2–4	31	13	31	13	3	20	3	8
Gleason Score 5–6	126	51	91	39	6	40	12	32
Gleason Score 7	90	36	110	48	6	40	23	60
AJCC T_{1c}, T_{2a}	179	72	138	59	12	80	31	82
AJCC T_{2b}	68	28	94	41	3	20	7	18
High risk								
Total n	239	100	309	100	19	100	23	100
PSA > 0–4 ng/ml	8	3	12	4	0	0	3	13
PSA 4.1–10 ng/ml	76	32	64	21	5	26	13	57
PSA 10.1–20 ng/ml	72	30	71	23	6	32	6	26
PSA > 20 ng/ml	83	35	162	52	8	42	1	4
Gleason score 2–4	29	12	25	8	0	0	0	0
Gleason score 5–6	93	39	113	36	12	63	14	61
Gleason score 7	43	18	82	27	4	21	6	26
Gleason score 8–10	74	31	89	29	3	16	3	13
AJCC T_{1c}, T_{2a}	63	26	105	34	6	31	3	13
AJCC T_{2b}	25	11	47	15	2	11	0	0
AJCC T_{2c}	151	63	157	51	11	58	20	87

U_{PENN}, Hospital of the University of Pennsylvania; JCRT, Joint Center for Radiation Therapy; AJCC, American Joint Commission on Cancer Staging; H, neoadjuvant hormonal therapy

risk of PSA failure compared to those treated with radical prostatectomy, even if neoadjuvant androgen deprivation therapy was used. Intermediate-risk patients (T_{2b} or Gleason score 7 or PSA levels > 10 and ≤ 20 ng/ml) did significantly worse ($p ≤ 0.003$) if managed by implant alone, but fared equivalently ($p = 0.18$) to those patients managed with radical prostatectomy if androgen deprivation was also administered. Intermediate-risk patients managed with implant therapy alone had a 3.1-fold increased risk of PSA failure compared to those patients managed with radical prostatectomy. These results remained

unchanged when patients were stratified using the traditional groups of biopsy Gleason score. Specifically, patients with biopsy Gleason scores 2–6 had no statistical difference in their estimates of PSA failure-free survival across all the treatment modalities evaluated in this study. However, patients with biopsy Gleason scores 8–10 who were managed with implant ± neoadjuvant androgen deprivation therapy had a lower PSA failure-free survival that approached statistical significance ($p ≤ 0.07$) when compared to those patients managed with radical prostatectomy or radiation therapy. Patients with biopsy Gleason score 7 disease did not have statistically different PSA failure-free survival when managed with radical prostatectomy, radiation therapy or implant + neoadjuvant androgen deprivation

Table 3 Pairwise p values comparing the proportion of patients with the given pretreatment clinical characteristic shown in Table 2 across treatment modalities. Because of the multiple comparisons, the level of significance as per Bonferroni methodology[22] was defined as < 0.05/6 or < 0.0083

Risk group	PSA	Gleason score	Clinical stage
Low risk			
RP vs. RT	0.580	0.521	1.00
RP vs. implant	0.579	0.092	1.00
RP vs. implant + H	0.384	0.009	1.00
RT vs. implant	0.389	0.159	1.00
RT vs. implant + H	0.241	0.011	1.00
Implant vs. implant + H	0.921	0.801	1.00
Intermediate risk			
RP vs. RT	0.193	0.267	0.009
RP vs. implant	0.477	0.563	0.575
RP vs. implant + H	0.604	0.018	0.235
RT vs. implant	0.688	0.771	0.115
RT vs. implant + H	0.125	0.299	0.009
Implant vs. implant + H	0.276	0.343	1.00
High risk			
RP vs. RT	0.0003*	0.090	0.014
RP vs. implant	0.78	0.975	0.936
RP vs. implant + H	0.003*	0.036	0.051
RT vs. implant	0.55	0.095	0.851
RT vs. implant + H	0.0002*	0.69	0.009
Implant vs. implant + H	0.006*	1.00	0.058

*Significant values; RP, radical prostatectomy; H, neoadjuvant hormonal therapy; RT, external beam radiation therapy

therapy ($p \geq 0.59$). However, these patients did statistically worse ($p \leq 0.003$) if managed by implant alone.

For the purpose of illustration, estimates of bNED outcome with pairwise p values evaluating the comparisons between treatment types were calculated using the actuarial method of Kaplan and Meier[23] and are graphically displayed by risk group in Figures 1–3.

Comment

Several studies from the urological[12–16] and oncological[6–11,17–19] literature confirm that the combination of the AJCC clinical T-stage system, pretreatment PSA levels and biopsy Gleason score can predict the pathological organ confinement rate, biochemical failure rate and subsequent metastatic rates in patients managed with definitive local therapy for clinically localized prostate cancer. Therefore, when attempting to compare bNED outcome across different treatment modalities, it is important to control for the values of these three prognostic factors. Using the results of the published literature[6–19], the risks of postradiation and postoperative PSA failure were classified into three groups based on the pretreatment prognostic factors.

Using a multivariate time-to-PSA-failure analysis to compare bNED outcome after radical prostatectomy, radiation therapy or implant with or without neoadjuvant androgen deprivation therapy for patients stratified by the defined pretreatment risk groups, several

Table 4 p Values from the Cox regression analyses evaluating the ability of a treatment modality to predict the time to post-therapy PSA failure stratified by risk group. The relative risk (RR) is defined as the proportional increase in PSA failure expected with a given treatment modality when compared to radical prostatectomy (RP). This value is shown with a 95% confidence interval (CI)

Treatment	Low risk		Intermediate risk		High risk	
	p	RR (95% CI)	p	RR (95% CI)	p	RR (95% CI)
RP at U$_{PENN}$	—		—		—	
RT at JCRT	0.79	1.1 (0.5–2.7)	0.26	0.8 (0.5–1.2)	0.26	0.9 (0.7–1.1)
Implant	0.91	1.1 (0.3–3.6)	0.006	3.1 (1.5–6.1)	0.0002	3.0 (1.8–5.0)
Implant + hormones	0.21	0.5 (0.1–1.9)	0.22	1.6 (0.8–3.3)	0.02	2.2 (1.2–4.0)

RT, radiation therapy; U$_{PENN}$, Hospital of the University of Pennsylvania (baseline group); JCRT, Joint Center for Radiation Therapy

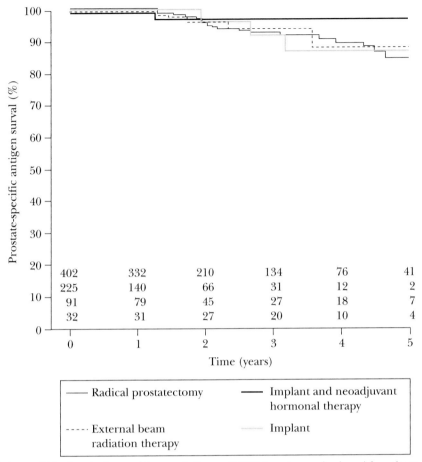

Figure 1 Estimated biochemical no-evidence of disease (bNED) outcome for low-risk patients stratified by treatment modality. All pairwise p values are > 0.25. Adapted from *J Am Med Assoc* 1998;280:969

observations were noted. First, the group of patients defined to be at low risk for post-therapy PSA failure were estimated to derive equal benefit from treatment with radical prostatectomy, radiation therapy or implant (Figure 1) at 5 years. Moreover, the addition of neoadjuvant androgen deprivation to implant therapy in low-risk patients provided no further benefit in the estimated 5-year bNED outcome. Second, patients at high risk for post-therapy PSA failure did significantly worse with implant therapy despite the addition of neoadjuvant hormonal deprivation when compared to patients treated with radical prostatectomy or radiation therapy (Figure 3). It is important to note that a statistically significant increase in favorable prognostic factors was present in the high-risk patients managed with implant plus neoadjuvant androgen suppression (i.e. PSA levels < 10 ng/ml) compared to patients managed with radical prostatectomy or radiation therapy (Tables 2 and 3). Despite this potential bias in favor of the patients managed with implant + neoadjuvant androgen suppression, the bNED outcome of these patients was still inferior to those patients managed with radical prostatectomy or radiation therapy. Finally, patients in the intermediate category for post-therapy PSA failure did significantly worse when managed with implant alone as compared to patients managed with radical prostatectomy, radiation therapy or implant plus neoadjuvant

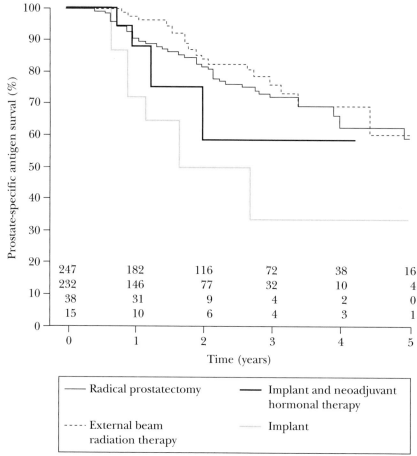

Figure 2 Estimated biochemical no-evidence of disease (bNED) outcome for intermediate-risk patients. Pairwise p values: radical prostatectomy vs. radiation therapy, 0.26; radical prostatectomy vs. implant + androgen ablation, 0.18; radical prostatectomy vs. implant, 0.003; radiation therapy vs. implant+androgen ablation, 0.009; radiation therapy vs. implant, 0.0002; implant+androgen ablation vs. implant, 0.14. Adapted from *J Am Med Assoc* 1998;280:969

androgen deprivation (Figure 2). While a statistical difference may exist for intermediate-risk patients managed with implant plus neoadjuvant androgen deprivation therapy versus radical prostatectomy or radiation, this study was not adequately powered to detect this difference.

Further follow-up is needed to ascertain if these results are maintained. In particular, low-risk patients can sustain late PSA failures (i.e. beyond 5 years). Moreover, men with low-grade or low-risk disease have a relatively low rate of PSA progression requiring numbers of patients much larger than presented in this study in order to prove a statistical difference.

Therefore, while small differences may exist, they are unlikely to reach statistical significance. In addition, the intermediate-risk patients managed with a median of 3 months of neoadjuvant androgen deprivation and implant therapy may be experiencing a hormone-induced delay in PSA failure and not a true therapeutic gain. With only nine patients at risk after 2 years in the implant plus androgen deprivation group compared to 116 and 77 in the radical prostatectomy and radiation therapy managed groups, respectively, it is too soon to make conclusions regarding the relative efficacy of these three treatments. Therefore, because of the small number of patients and relatively short

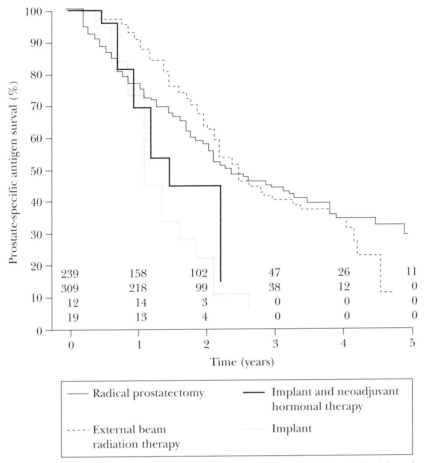

Figure 3 Estimated biochemical no-evidence of disease (bNED) outcome for high-risk patients. Pairwise p values: radical prostatectomy vs. radiation therapy, 0.25; radical prostatectomy vs. implant+androgen ablation, 0.012; radical prostatectomy vs. implant, 0.0005; radiation therapy vs. implant+androgen ablation, 0.0007; radiation therapy vs. implant, < 0.0001; implant + androgen ablation vs. implant, 0.41. Adapted from *J Am Med Assoc* 1998;280:969

follow-up, particularly in the patients receiving neoadjuvant androgen deprivation, the results must be viewed as preliminary and need to be subjected to longer follow-up. However, these early data suggest that in high-risk patients, who are in greater need of treatment and who have the most to lose by ineffective therapy, implant therapy with or without the addition of a median of 3 months of neoadjuvant androgen deprivation was less effective than radical prostatectomy or radiation therapy at maintaining bNED survival. When examining the PSA failure-free survival using the traditional groupings of the biopsy Gleason score, the same results were

found as those noted when the data were analyzed according to the risk groups, lending further support to the findings of this study.

Several issues remain that are not addressed by the data in this study. First, the comparison of PSA outcome for expectant management versus treatment is lacking. This comparison would be particularly relevant in the low-risk patients where 5 year PSA progression rates numerically approximate to the 10-year clinical progression rates noted from expectant management series[24,25]. Second, the PSA outcomes of the now widely practiced combination therapies of external beam radiation therapy plus implant with or without neoadjuvant androgen deprivation therapy need to be prospectively compared to the PSA outcomes achieved after radical prostatectomy, radiation therapy or implant. These comparisons would be particularly relevant in the high-risk and intermediate-risk groups where implant therapy alone may be insufficient. A final unanswered question remains. That is, whether the use of palladium-103 (^{103}Pd), as opposed to the conventional iodine-125 (^{125}I), affected the PSA outcome data reported in this study. The physical characteristics of these two radionuclides differ in that the half-life and mean photon energy are 60 days, 27 keV and 17 days, 21 keV for^{125}I and ^{103}Pd, respectively. These differences result in an initial dose rate of 0.0772 Gy/h and 0.197 Gy/h for ^{125}I and ^{103}Pd,

respectively. It is, therefore, conceivable that the higher dose rate of palladium could have affected the results. Further investigations of these issues are needed.

Nevertheless, considering the widespread increase in the use of interstitial radiation therapy, these data serve to heighten awareness to the possibility that this form of prostate cancer therapy may only be clinically efficacious in a select subgroup of patients and possibly inadequate in others. While no definitive conclusions can be reached using non-randomized retrospective data, these analyses can provide the basis on which to design prospective randomized clinical trials that could definitively compare bNED, cause-specific and overall survival outcomes amongst treatment modalities.

References

1. Kupelian P, Katcher J, Levin HS, et al. Stage T1–2 prostate cancer: a multivariate analysis of factors affecting biochemical and clinical failures after radical prostatectomy. Int J Radiat Oncol Biol Phys 1997;37:1043–52
2. D'Amico AV, Whittington R, Kaplan I, et al. Equivalent biochemical failure free survival after external beam radiation therapy or radical prostatectomy in patients with a pretreatment prostate specific antigen of > 4–20 ng/ml. Int J Radiat Oncol Biol Phys 1997;37:1053–8
3. Oesterling JE, Jacobsen SJ, Klee GG, et al. Free, complexed and total serum prostate specific antigen: the establishment of appropriate reference ranges for their concentrations and ratios. J Urol 1995;154:1090–5
4. Gleason DF and the Veterans Administration Cooperative Urological Research Group. Histologic grading and staging of prostatic carcinoma. In Tannenbaum M, ed. Urologic Pathology. Philadelphia, PA: Lea & Febiger, 1977:171–87
5. Beahrs OH, Henson DE, Hutter RVP. American Joint Committee on Cancer, Manual for Staging Cancer, 4th edn. Philadelphia, PA: JP Lippincott, 1992
6. Zagars GK, Pollack A, Kavadi VS, et al. Prostate specific antigen and radiation therapy for

clinically localized prostate cancer. Int J Radiat Oncol Biol Phys 1995;32:293–306
7. Pisansky TM, Kahn MJ, Rasp GM, et al. A multiple prognostic index predictive of disease outcome after irradiation for clinically localized prostate cancer. Cancer 1997;79:337–44
8. Lee WR, Hanks GE, Schultheiss TE, et al. Localized prostate cancer treated by external beam radiotherapy alone: serum prostate specific antigen driven outcome analysis. J Clin Oncol 1995;13:464–9
9. Pisansky TM, Cha SS, Earle JD, et al. Prostate specific antigen as a pretherapy prognostic factor in patients treated with radiation therapy for clinically localized prostate cancer. J Clin Oncol 1993;11:2158–66
10. Zietman AL, Coen JJ, Shipley WU, et al. Radical radiation therapy in the management of prostatic adenocarcinoma: the initial prostate specific antigen value as a predictor of treatment outcome. J Urol 1994;151:640–5
11. Hanks GE, Lee WR, Schultheiss TE. Clinical and biochemical evidence of control of prostate cancer at 5 years after external beam radiation. J Urol 1995;154:456–9
12. Partin AW, Piantadosi S, Sanda MG, et al. Selection of men at high risk for disease recurrence for experimental adjuvant therapy

following radical prostatectomy. *Urology* 1995;45: 831–8

13. Lerner SE, Blute ML, Bergstralh EJ, *et al.* Analysis of risk factors for progression in patients with pathologically organ confined prostate cancers after radical retropubic prostatectomy. *J Urol* 1996;156:137–43

14. Zietman AL, Edelstein RA, Coen JJ, *et al.* Radical prostatectomy for adenocarcinoma of the prostate. The influence of preoperative and pathologic findings on biochemical disease-free outcome. *Urology* 1994;43:828–33

15. D'Amico AV, Whittington R, Malkowicz SB, *et al.* PSA failure despite pathologically organ confined and margin negative disease: the basis for an adjuvant therapy trial. *J Clin Oncol* 1997; 15:1465–9

16. D'Amico AV, Whittington R, Malkowicz SB, *et al.* Outcome based staging for clinically localized adenocarcinoma of the prostate. *J Urol* 1997; 158:1422–6

17. Ragde H, Blasko JC, Grimm PD, *et al.* Interstitial iodine-125 radiation without adjuvant therapy in the treatment of clinically localized prostate carcinoma. *Cancer* 1997;80:442–53

18. Blasko JC, Wallner K, Grimm PD, *et al.* Prostate specific antigen based disease control following ultrasound guided I 125 implantation for stage T1/T2 prostatic carcinoma. *J Urol* 1995; 154:1096–9

19. Wallner K, Roy J, Harrison L. Tumor control and morbidity following transperineal Iodine 125 implantation for stage T1/T2 prostatic carcinoma. *J Clin Oncol* 1996;14:449–53

20. Cox DR. Regression models and life tables. *J Roy Stat Soc* B 1972;34:187–9

21. Cox JD for the American Society for Therapeutic Radiology and Oncology Consensus Panel. Consensus statement: guidelines for PSA following radiation therapy. *Int J Radiat Oncol Biol Phys* 1997;37:1035–41

22. Neter J, Wasserman W, Kutner M, eds. Simultaneous inferences and other topics in regression analysis-1. *Applied Linear Regression Models,* 1st edn. Homewood, Illinois: Richard D. Irwin, Inc., 1983:150–3

23. Kaplan EL, Meier P. Non-parametric estimation from incomplete observations. *J Am Stat Assoc* 1958;53:457–500

24. Chodak GW, Thisted RA, Gerber GS, *et al.* Results of conservative management of clinically localized prostate cancer. *N Engl J Med* 1994; 330:242–8

25. Adolfsson J, Steineck G, Hedlund PO. Deferred treatment of clinically localized prostate cancer: actual 10-year and projected 15-year follow-up of the Karolinska series. *Urology* 1997;50:722–6

Table 1 Age-adjusted mortality rates (per 100 000 population) in some European countries and the USA for the periods 1990–1993[7] and 1994–1997[4]

Country	1990–1993	1994–1997
Norway	22.1	23.2
Sweden	21.1	21.4
Denmark	19.5	19.9
Netherlands	18.4	19.4
Finland	18.3	17.6
USA	17.5	15.9

since the 1950s[8–12], whereas in Sweden a slight decline was observed between 1975 and 1981[13].

Long-term monitoring of the mortality rate provides detailed information on trends through the years. The recent decline observed in the age-adjusted prostate cancer death rate for US men was preceded by a continuous increase, going back as far as 1930[7]. This turn in mortality rate may have been influenced by several factors, such as changes in competing causes of death, improvements in treatment practices and shifts in the current medical procedure for prostate cancer treatment[14,15]. Decreased exposure to risk factors and increased prevention strategies such as modifications in nutritional factors and chemoprevention can also reduce mortality[16,17]. On the other hand, the mortality rate for prostate cancer can be both negatively and positively affected by the accuracy of diagnosing and recording the disease on death certificates as the underlying cause of death[18–21]. Moreover, the increasing male life expectancy[22] could possibly enhance the likelihood of dying from prostate cancer[23,24].

A very important factor (if not the most essential one) is the putative control of prostate cancer by early detection, since the advanced stage of the disease has a poor prognosis and is, practically, not curable. In the past two decades, PSA screening has gained much popularity as a screening instrument above digital rectal examination (DRE) and transrectal ultrasonography (TRUS). This increased interest in early detection of prostate cancer is assumed to be partially responsible for the recent downturn

in the mortality rate in the USA. However, to evaluate the effectiveness of screening on reduction in mortality, it is necessary to combine mortality data with the specific data from screened and unscreened individuals.

Proof due to screening?

The best method to determine the effectiveness of screening in reducing mortality is a randomized controlled trial. In this study design, invited men are randomly assigned to either the screen group that is offered screening or to the control group which (ideally) would not receive any screening. However, a randomized controlled trial is costly, requires a large number of participants and a long follow-up period, and they are prone to lack of compliance in the screened group and contamination in the control group, in some countries more than others. To date, results of one randomized controlled trial on prostate cancer screening have been reported, the Quebec Prospective Randomized trial, conducted between November 1988 and December 1996[25]. Briefly, this study included 46 193 eligible men from the metropolitan area of Quebec, of which 30 956 were invited for screening with PSA and DRE (DRE only on the first visit). The remaining 15 237 uninvited men served as an unscreened group and were followed according to standard medical health care. Only 23.1% of the invited men from the screening arm actually attended screening (7155 men out of 30 956), whereas in the control group, 6.5% underwent screening. Despite this high rate of non-compliance in the screened group and contamination in the control group, the authors claimed that this first prospective randomized controlled trial showed a 69% decrease in death from prostate cancer[25]. However, this figure has been disputed in particular, because of the method of analysis applied by the authors[26,27]. This decrease in mortality was based on an analysis in which screening data of the invited and screened men and those screened in the control group were combined and compared with the data of invited and uninvited men who never underwent screening. By adopting this method, it is likely that the 'healthy-volunteer effect' would be introduced into the results. This means that the two groups are no longer comparable, which is an essential feature of a randomized controlled trial, because the screened men become a self-selected group, most likely health conscious and aware of the disease and its symptoms. In addition, the length of observation of prostate cancer mortality strongly differed for the screened and unscreened men, approximately 3 and 7 years, respectively[26,27]. This meant that a man diagnosed with prostate cancer before his date of first screening opportunity would be allocated to the 'unscreened' group, a procedure that artificially emphasizes a non-existent benefit of screening. Analysis of a randomized controlled trial is always between the initial randomized (comparable) screening and control arms. The same data then show no effect of screening in this very small-scale Quebec randomized trial. Out of a total of 46 193 eligible men, 97 deaths from prostate cancer occurred among the 30 956 invited men and 45 deaths from prostate cancer occurred among the 15 237 not-invited men accounting for a risk ratio of 1.06, $(97/30\ 956)/(45/15\ 237)^{26}$.

In the absence of randomized controlled trial proof, case–control studies could possibly provide some evidence on the effectiveness of a screening program[28]. The exposure to screening in both cases and control subjects is measured retrospectively[29,30]. This study design is less costly and not lengthy compared to a randomized controlled trial and does not require a large number of subjects, but it is susceptible to bias[28,29]. Again, it is likely that the underlying risk for the disease differs between screened and unscreened men. Differentiation between a screening and a diagnostic test for prostate cancer can also be a limitation for this design[31]. The case–control studies reported to date on the mortality of prostate cancer and screening have yielded ambiguous results, and the screening modality applied was DRE. Friedman and colleagues[32] and Richert-Boe and colleagues[33] found no beneficial effect of DRE screening on the reduction of the prostate

cancer mortality rate in their population selected from the medical-care program of large health-maintenance organizations. In contrast, Jacobsen and co-workers[30] showed that DRE screening was much less common in the cases who died of prostate cancer, compared to the matched-control group, representing a 50–70% reduction if this result proves to be causal. In their recent paper, Connor and co-workers[34] showed that the criteria for selecting matched controls to cases, the choice of the timescale of screening and the method used to measure exposure to screening in case–control studies can considerably affect the results due to introduced bias.

Important information on screening can also be gathered by other observational designs such as cohort studies, where a group of individuals is followed-up over a period of time, and trend analyses, which are based on examination of (aggregated) data of populations across time. On the issue of prostate cancer mortality reduction and early detection by screening, trend analyses are more frequently reported than cohort studies. In Tyrol, Austria, a mass screening project was begun in 1993 with PSA testing as the initial test and DRE and TRUS for further examination[35]. Preliminary results of this study showed a difference of 42% in prostate cancer mortality when comparing regional mortality data from the Tyrol region[36], bearing in mind that this figure arose from the comparison of 96 prostate cancer deaths in 1993 with 65 cases in 1996. Although this outcome strongly contributes to the progress of the early detection of prostate cancer, the study was not randomized and comprised self-selected participants who may have been more health conscious and perhaps different in their characteristics relating to the development of prostate cancer.

Expected reduction of mortality rate in screening studies can also be analyzed by computer simulation using the actual screening performances of the population under study, as recently shown in the Dutch nation-wide breast cancer screening program[37]. By applying this analysis method, it was found that a *statistically significant* decline in the breast cancer mortality rates attributable to screening could be expected from 1997 onward, approximately 8 years after the program started nationwide. In simulation programs essential randomized controlled trial data are necessary to make predictions.

Different time-trend analyses have been reported in an attempt to explain the 6.3% decrease in prostate cancer mortality between 1991 and 1995 in the USA[38] in light of the widespread implementation of PSA screening[15,18,39–42]. These time-trend analyses, which are particularly based on the Surveillance, Epidemiology and End Results (SEER) registry data, have as yet not made it possible to make definite inferences on the benefit of screening. After thorough evaluation of the prostate cancer incidence-based mortality 0–5 years rates, Merrill and Stephenson[42] considered that the observed decline in the mortality rates after the peak in 1992 can be attributed primarily to patients whose diagnosis was made within the PSA era. Dennis and Resnick[41] reported an analysis of trends in the incidence and mortality of prostate cancer in which the mortality of prostate cancer was examined based on the 2-year mortality rate from prostate cancer or metastases by year of diagnosis. A decrease in the 2-year mortality rate, after a stable rate in the period 1973–1989 and an upswing between 1990 and 1991, was observed and the authors implied that this finding supports the effectiveness of screening for prostate cancer. These authors all assume a very early effect of screening on the prostate cancer mortality rate. On the other hand, Feuer and colleagues[18] concluded that the increase and subsequent decrease in mortality is to some extent influenced by misclassification of the underlying cause of death. After analyzing the prostate cancer mortality trends by computer simulation, Etzioni and co-workers[39] also indicated that screening can only partially explain the observed trends, taking the lead time of the disease into account. With screening, the disease is detected earlier than it would have been diagnosed in cases of manifestation of the symptoms. Hence, a decline in mortality rate of the disease due to

these screening practices could (only) be seen after this lead time, which is on average estimated to be 5.5 years for prostate cancer[43]. The observed drop in the mortality rate of prostate cancer occurred in the very same time period as the dramatic increase in screening by PSA testing. There is also a concern about translating survival rate improvements into evidence for the effectiveness of screening; these rates might rather reflect lead-time bias than true increases in survival, since early detection increases the time between diagnosis and death regardless of the effects of treatment.

Nonetheless, many feel that reasonable proof has been achieved for cervical cancer screening with analysis of time trends in mortality. Läärä and associates[44] reported the evaluation of mortality from cervical cancer between 1953 and 1982 in the Scandinavian countries where organized cervical cancer screening programs using PAP smears have been introduced, but no randomized controlled trial has ever been conducted for the evaluation of the effectiveness of such screening. The comparisons between the countries were carried out based on the analysis of the age-specific mortality rate in the respective age groups in different (specific) time periods. This study demonstrated large reductions in the cervical cancer mortality rate in the time periods that screening with the PAP test was implemented, the reductions being more obvious in the target age groups. Then again, the number that in fact received or did not receive screening remains unknown. This uncontrolled character of the study design makes trend analyses not quite suitable for providing strong evidence for the effectiveness of screening, especially at the present time considering the changes in risk factors and competing causes of death and, very importantly, the improvements in cancer treatment. The latter is currently an issue of debate in the breast cancer screening program in England and Wales, i.e. whether the reduction in breast cancer mortality can be attributed to screening or to improvements in treatment[45]. Similarly, in The Netherlands, the breast cancer mortality rate following the introduction of screening has been showing a downward trend, implying that changes in treatment practices should also be considered in the analysis of the Dutch program[37].

No proof, but is it likely? ERSPC and PLCO trials

To date, no conclusive evidence has been presented on the benefit of prostate cancer screening in the reduction of the prostate cancer mortality rate. However, it is very likely that this outcome would ultimately be achieved, seeing the considerable shift in the stage of the disease. The various studies analyzing the US trends in prostate cancer incidence and mortality show a changing trend in the stage at which disease is detected towards detection of more localized organ-confined tumors, whereas the incidence of distant-stage disease is decreasing. These observations are supported by studies in which men were actually screened using PSA, DRE or TRUS as screening tools; the majority of the cancers detected in such studies are at early stages. In the multicenter project on prostate detection of the American Cancer Society, started in 1987 with PSA testing, and DRE and TRUS examination, 92% of the cancers detected were the early-stage A_1–B_2 tumors[46]. Similarly, Catalona and colleagues[47] demonstrated that in both initial and serial screening (6–37 months after initial screening) based on PSA testing, 99% of tumors detected were localized. In the part of the Tyrol screening project, where PSA measurements were done in blood samples of asymptomatic blood donors, pathological staging of the detected cancers showed that five out of six men aged 40–49 years (83%) and 50 out of 58 men aged 50–65 years (86%) had non-palpable to organ-confined disease (A_1–B_2). Therefore, the trends in stages of the prostate cancer detected by screening are optimistic, since curative treatment is possible for patients with localized, organ-confined stage disease, while advanced disease at the time of diagnosis is not curable. Moreover, the progress in treatment of these early-stage tumors with surgery and radiotherapy is promising for the patients' survival.

There is no doubt that PSA testing in particular has in part affected the 'incidence' of prostate cancer. It is tempting to assume that screening combined with treatment of the localized, potentially curable prostate cancers would eventually result in a reduction of mortality. However, this has not yet been convincingly proven, as noted earlier; the evidence until now has been circumstantial and deduced from population-based data, data obtained from uncontrolled studies. The strongest evidence for the effectiveness of screening on the reduction in prostate cancer mortality can only be obtained by conducting randomized controlled trials. Two large-scale, randomized studies were started in 1994 in Europe and the USA, the European Randomized Study of Screening for Prostate Cancer (ERSPC trial) and the Prostate, Lung, Colorectal and Ovarian Cancer Screening Trial (PLCO trial), respectively. The characteristics of these trials (Table 2) have been extensively documented before[48] and the most recent results are pending publication. The initial and serial screenings are based on PSA testing, while DRE and TRUS are used for further examinations. Both the PSA cut-off levels and the screen interval differ among the various centers which, in addition to the USA, at present, include Belgium, Finland, Italy, The Netherlands, France, Spain, Sweden and Switzerland. Currently, more than 80% of the target population in all the centers combined have been enrolled (de Koning and colleagues 2000, submitted for publication) and, based on present data, the statistical power of the study has been re-evaluated.

It is still too soon to make any inference or prediction on the benefit of screening in reducing prostate cancer mortality. As PSA testing is gaining more popularity, the extent of contamination within the control arm of the trial should be closely monitored. A rather restrictive attitude towards PSA testing of healthy men now will ensure that the ongoing trials are not jeopardized, and may eventually give the important public health, clinical and individual answers. Some patience now may save lives in the end.

Table 2 Characteristics of the study design in the countries participating in the European Randomized Study of Screening for Prostate Cancer (ERSPC) trial and the Prostate, Lung, Colorectal and Ovarian Cancer Screening (PLCO) trial

	ERSPC trial						PLCO trial
	Belgium	Finland	Italy	Spain	Sweden	The Netherlands	USA (10 sites)
Age at entry (years)	55–74	55/59/63/67	55–70	50–70	51–66	55–74	55–74
Screening interval (years)	4	4	4	4	2	4	1
Type of trial	volunteer	randomized population	randomized population	volunteer	randomized population	volunteer	volunteer
Randomization	after consent	before consent	before consent	after consent	before consent	after consent	after consent
Period of initial recruitment	1992–99	1996–99	1996–99	1996–99	1995–96	1994–99	1993–2001
Identification of source population	population registry	population registry	population registry	population registry	population registry	population registry	mail, mass media
Exclusion criteria							
Pre-existent prostate cancer	yes	yes	yes	yes	yes	yes	yes
Prior PSA	no	no	no	no	no	no	> 1 last 3 years
Target sample size							
Intervention group	8750	22 500	7000	5000	9973	20 000	37 000
Control group	8750	45 000	7000	5000	9973	20 000	37 000
*Screening tests/biopsy**							
PSA (ng/ml)	4.0	4.0 PSA driven 3.0–3.9/F/T	4.0 PSA driven 2.5–3.9	4.1	3.0	4.0/3.0	4.0
DRE	all	no	PSA driven	no	no	all/1.0/no	all
TRUS	all	no	PSA driven	no	no	all/1.0/no	no
Source of follow-up information							
Incidence	active	cancer registry	cancer registry	active	cancer registry	cancer registry	active (annual study update)
Mortality	population registry	population registry	population registry	active	population registry	population registry	active
Death certificate	all	all	all	all	all	all, death review	all
Endpoints							
Death from prostate cancer	yes	yes	yes	yes	yes	yes	yes
Quality of life	possibly	yes	yes	possibly	yes	yes	planning
Cost-effectiveness	possibly	yes	yes	possibly	yes	yes	planning
Biorepository	serum, prostate tissue	serum	no	no	serum, prostate tissue	serum, buffy coat	serum, cells, tissue, buffy, red blood cells
Pilot study	conducted	conducted	conducted	conducted	conducted	conducted	conducted

PSA, prostate-specific antigen; DRE, digital rectal examination; TRUS, transrectal ultrasonography
*The cut-off level for PSA/criteria for application of other screening tests

References

1. Jensen OM, Esteve J, Moller H, *et al.* Cancer in the European Community and its member states. *Eur J Cancer* 1990;26:1167–256
2. Parkin DM, Whelan SL, Ferlay J, *et al.* eds. *Cancer Incidence in Five Continents.* Vol. VII. Lyon: International Agency for Research on Cancer, 1997
3. Black RJ, Bray F, Ferlay J, *et al.* Cancer incidence and mortality in the European Union: cancer registry data and estimates of national incidence for 1990. *Eur J Cancer* 1997;33:1075–107
4. Greenlee RT, Murray T, Bolden S, *et al.* Cancer statistics, 2000. *CA Cancer J Clin* 2000;50:7–33
5. Potosky AL, Miller BA, Albertsen PC, *et al.* The role of increasing detection in the rising incidence of prostate cancer. *J Am Med Assoc* 1995;273:548–52
6. National Cancer Institute. *SEER Cancer Statistics 1973–1996.* Bethesda, MD: National Cancer Institute, 2000
7. Parker SL, Tong T, Bolden S, *et al.* Cancer statistics, 1996. *CA Cancer J Clin* 1996;46:5–27
8. Harvei S, Tretli S, Langmark F. Cancer of the prostate in Norway 1957–1991 – a descriptive study. *Eur J Cancer* 1996;32A:111–17
9. Brasso K, Friis S, Kjaer SK, *et al.* Prostate cancer in Denmark: a 50-year population-based study. *Urology* 1998;51:590–4
10. Post PN, Straatman H, Kiemeney LA, *et al.* Increased risk of fatal prostate cancer may explain the rise in mortality in The Netherlands. *Int J Epidemiol* 1999;28:403–8
11. Post PN, Kil PJ, Crommelin MA, *et al.* Trends in incidence and mortality rates for prostate cancer before and after prostate-specific antigen introduction. A registry-based study in southeastern Netherlands, 1971–1995. *Eur J Cancer* 1998;34: 705–9
12. Van der Gulden JW, Kiemeney LA, Verbeek AL, *et al.* Mortality trend from prostate cancer in The Netherlands (1950–1989). *Prostate* 1994;24: 33–8
13. Gronberg H. *Prostate Cancer. Epidemiological Studies.* Umea: Umea University, Department of Oncology and Urology & Andrology, 1995:124
14. Mettlin CJ, Murphy GP, Rosenthal DS, *et al.* The National Cancer Data Base report on prostate carcinoma after the peak in incidence rates in the U.S. The American College of Surgeons Commission on Cancer and the American Cancer Society. *Cancer* 1998;83:1679–84
15. Hankey BF, Feuer EJ, Clegg LX, *et al.* Cancer surveillance series: interpreting trends in prostate cancer. 1. Evidence of the effects of screening in recent prostate cancer incidence, mortality, and survival rates. *J Natl Cancer Inst* 1999;91:1017–24
16. Thompson IM, Coltman CA Jr, Crowley J. Chemoprevention of prostate cancer: the Prostate Cancer Prevention Trial. *Prostate* 1997; 33:217–21
17. Brawley OW, Parnes H. Prostate cancer prevention trials in the USA. *Eur J Cancer* 2000;36:1312–15
18. Feuer EJ, Merrill RM, Hankey BF. Cancer surveillance series: interpreting trends in prostate cancer. 2. Cause of death misclassification and the recent rise and fall in prostate cancer mortality. *J Natl Cancer Inst* 1999;91:1025–32
19. Newschaffer CJ, Otani K, McDonald MK, *et al.* Causes of death in elderly prostate cancer patients and in a comparison nonprostate cancer cohort. *J Natl Cancer Inst* 2000;92:613–21
20. Hsing AW, Tsao L, Devesa SS. International trends and patterns of prostate cancer incidence and mortality. *Int J Cancer* 2000;85:60–7
21. Albertsen PC, Walters S, Hanley JA. A comparison of cause of death determination in men previously diagnosed with prostate cancer who died in 1985 or 1995. *J Urol* 2000;163:519–23
22. Nusselder WJ, Mackenbach JP. Lack of improvement of life expectancy at advanced ages in The Netherlands. *Int J Epidemiol* 2000;29:140–8
23. Neal DE, Donovan JL. Screening for prostate cancer. *Ann Oncol* 1998;9:1289–92
24. Neal DE, Leung HY, Powell PH, *et al.* Unanswered questions in screening for prostate cancer. *Eur J Cancer* 2000;36:1316–21
25. Labrie F, Candas B, Dupont A, *et al.* Screening decreases prostate cancer death: first analysis of the 1988 Quebec prospective randomized controlled trial. *Prostate* 1999;38:83–91
26. Boer R, Schröder FH. Quebec randomized controlled trial on prostate cancer screening shows no evidence for mortality reduction. *Prostate* 1999;40:130–4
27. Alexander FE, Prescott RJ. Reply to Labrie *et al.* Results of the mortality analysis of the Quebec Randomized/controlled trial (RCT). *Prostate* 1999;40:135–7
28. Denis L, Mettlin C, Carter HB, *et al.* Early detection and screening. In Murphy G, Khoury S, Partin A, *et al*, eds. *Prostate Cancer.* 2nd edn. Plymouth: Health Publisher Ltd., 2000:221–33
29. Cronin KA, Weed DL, Connor RJ, *et al.* Case–control studies of cancer screening: theory and practice. *J Natl Cancer Inst* 1998;90:498–504

30. Jacobsen SJ, Bergstralh EJ, Katusic SK, *et al.* Screening digital rectal examination and prostate cancer mortality: a population-based case–control study. *Urology* 1998;52:173–9

31. Barry MJ. PSA screening for prostate cancer: the current controversy – a viewpoint. Patient Outcomes Research Team for Prostatic Diseases. *Ann Oncol* 1998;9:1279–82

32. Friedman GD, Hiatt RA, Quesenberry CP Jr, *et al.* Case–control study of screening for prostatic cancer by digital rectal examinations. *Lancet* 1991;337:1526–9

33. Richert-Boe KE, Humphrey LL, Glass AG, *et al.* Screening digital rectal examination and prostate cancer mortality: a case–control study. *J Med Screen* 1998;5:99–103

34. Connor RJ, Boer R, Prorok PC, *et al.* Investigation of design and bias issues in case–control studies of cancer screening using microsimulation. *Am J Epidemiol* 2000;151:991–8

35. Hominger W, Reissigl A, Rogatsch H, *et al.* Prostate cancer screening in the Tyrol, Austria. Experience and results. *Eur J Cancer* 2000;36:1322–35

36. Magee J. Drop in PCa deaths attributed to PSA screening. *Urology Times* 2000, June (www.findarticles.com)

37. Van den Akker-van Marle E, de Koning H, Boer R, *et al.* Reduction in breast cancer mortality due to the introduction of mass screening in The Netherlands: comparison with the United Kingdom. *J Med Screen* 1999;6:30–4

38. Office of Cancer Communications. *Cancer Death Rate Declined for the First Time Ever in the 1990s.* Bethesda, MD: National Cancer Institute, 1996

39. Etzioni R, Legler JM, Feuer EJ, *et al.* Cancer surveillance series: interpreting trends in prostate cancer. III. Quantifying the link between population prostate-specific antigen testing and recent declines in prostate cancer mortality. *J Natl Cancer Inst* 1999;91:1033–9

40. Brawley OW. Prostate carcinoma incidence and patient mortality: the effects of screening and early detection. *Cancer* 1997;80:1857–63

41. Dennis LK, Resnick MI. Analysis of recent trends in prostate cancer incidence and mortality. *Prostate* 2000;42:247–52

42. Merrill RM, Stephenson RA. Trends in mortality rates in patients with prostate cancer during the era of prostate specific antigen screening. *J Urol* 2000;163:503–10

43. Gann PH, Hennekens CH, Stampfer MJ. A prospective evaluation of plasma prostate-specific antigen for detection of prostatic cancer. *J Am Med Assoc* 1995;273:289–94

44. Läärä E, Day NE, Hakama M. Trends in mortality from cervical cancer in the Nordic countries: association with organised screening programmes. *Lancet* 1987;1:1247–9

45. Blanks RG, Moss SM, McGahan CE, *et al.* Effect of NHS breast screening programme on mortality from breast cancer in England and Wales, 1990–8: comparison of observed with predicted mortality. *Br Med J* 2000;321:665–9

46. Mettlin C, Murphy GP, Babaian RJ, *et al.* The results of a five-year early prostate cancer detection intervention. Investigators of the American Cancer Society National Prostate Cancer Detection Project. *Cancer* 1996;77:150–9

47. Catalona WJ, Smith DS, Ratliff TL, *et al.* Detection of organ-confined prostate cancer is increased through prostate-specific antigen-based screening. *J Am Med Assoc* 1993;270:948–54

48. Auvinen A, Rietbergen JB, Denis LJ, *et al.* Prospective evaluation plan for randomised trials of prostate cancer screening. The International Prostate Cancer Screening Trial Evaluation Group. *J Med Screen* 1996;3:97–104

Chemo-endocrine prevention: recent achievements and potential

17

F. H. Schröder

Background

The incidence and mortality of human prostate cancer show very strong variations between different parts of the world. The highest incidence is seen in Northern European countries and in the United States. World-wide, the risk of acquiring prostate cancer and of dying of this disease is highest in African-American men. These large differences in reported prostate cancer mortality, which are in the range of 10–15-fold in favor of most Asian countries as opposed to what is called the Western world, have remained unexplained so far[1]. Racial background, endocrine factors and environmental factors including diet have been considered and have been the subject of research in the past and at present. As will be shown in this chapter, racial predisposition may explain a small part of these differences but is unlikely to be a major factor. It is of great interest that, with respect to breast cancer, similar differences in incidence and mortality are encountered in comparing the same regions. Adlercreutz[2] has proposed and elaborated the concept of Eastern and Western diet. His group has also shown for the first time that dietary and endocrine factors may be linked[3]. De Jong and colleagues[4] have shown, in a prospective study comparing in an age-matched fashion the endocrine status of Japanese men in the region of Kyoto to Dutch men living in the area of Rotterdam, that plasma androgen levels are significantly lower in Japanese men. Observed differences with respect to 5α-reductase levels in groups of men with high and low incidences of prostate cancer may also be due to dietary habits, but could also have a racial background[5].

In spite of intensive research conducted by means of retrospective studies, cohort studies and case–control protocols, a conclusive explanation for the important regional differences in the incidence of clinical prostate cancer and prostate cancer mortality has so far not been found. Recent reviews of potential risk factors and the related evidence are available[6]. This chapter will concentrate on potential approaches to chemo-endocrine prevention, evidence coming from prospective randomized studies with respect to potential mechanisms, the issue of endpoints of future studies and, finally, the results of a recent double-blind, randomized, cross-over, tertiary prevention study conducted at the author's institution.

Rationale for prevention studies

Next to the large regional differences in prostate cancer incidence and mortality, information is available from recent literature with respect to possible precursor lesions and the steps in the morphogenesis of prostate cancer, which may be influenced by environmental factors. Furthermore, regional differences in lesions relating to initiation and progression of prostate cancer can be and have been identified by autopsy studies. Migrant studies of men moving from low incidence to high incidence areas provide support for the 'environmental hypothesis'.

Precursor lesions

High-grade prostatic intraepithelial neoplasia (HGPIN) has been intensively investigated with respect to its possible role as a precursor lesion of prostate cancer. Here, we discuss a few facts that are directly related to prevention studies. In autopsy studies using step-sectioning of prostates which are not harboring prostate cancer, HGPIN has been found in 9–43% of cases[7]. In the same concise and complete review, it is shown that HGPIN shows a strong age dependence. Caucasian men in their third, fourth, fifth and sixth decades in the Wayne State autopsy series harbored 0%, 2%, 5% and 12% of HGPIN, respectively. The prevalence in African-Americans was at least two times as high. Two autopsy series from Japan, which is one of the regions with an at least historically low incidence of clinical prostate cancer, show prevalence rates of HGPIN that are comparable to US and European autopsy data. In clinical settings, on average about one-half of HGPIN cases are associated with invasive carcinoma. Clearly, the frequency of HGPIN exceeds the prevalence of cancer by about two-fold. These data are in sharp contrast to the prevalence of HGPIN in biopsy specimens. These figures vary from 0.8 to 15%; the prevalence is dependent on the choice of populations and is low in a population-based screening study[7,8]. It is higher in institutional case-finding studies of men who present with the wish to be screened or because of symptoms[9].

The high autopsy prevalence of HGPIN, which exceeds the presence of biopsy detectable clinical cancer in the same population by at least ten-fold, satisfies the requirement that precursor lesions should be more frequent than the related cancer. In considering prostate cancer prevention, it is of great relevance to identify the step in the morphogenesis of this tumor that represents the watershed between *initiation* and *progression*. Prior to the extensive research effort that has established PIN as a possible precursor lesion of prostate cancer[10], it has been shown that the frequency of small latent carcinomas in autopsy series is also exceedingly frequent, age-related and independent of the presence of large invasive cancers[11]. These findings were confirmed in prostate specimens removed with radical cystoprostatectomy carried out for bladder cancer[12]. Typically, these tumors are well-

differentiated, multifocal and have a volume of between 0.02 and 0.2 ml. For these small cancers, it has also been shown that their prevalence in autopsy specimens is independent of the large geographical variations of the incidence of clinical prostate cancer[13,14]. These data, because of the high and similar frequency of PIN and latent focal carcinoma, and by the fact that they are equally frequent in areas of high and low incidence of clinical prostate cancer, allow the identification of these lesions as being related to the process of *initiation*, whatever the mechanism may be. It becomes, therefore, highly likely that the mechanism of progression to clinically manifest disease originating from PIN and latent focal cancer is governed by those environmental factors that differ geographically. Obviously, environmental factors may not be the only risk factors that lead to clinically manifest disease.

A recent publication on the very large Scandinavian twin study[15] shows that, with regard to all cancers under study, about 85% are related to environmental factors. Surprisingly, for prostate cancer, in comparing the prevalence in identical twins to the sporadic cancers occurring in non-identical twins, 45% of all cancers can be explained by an identical genetic background, meaning that we have to assume that environmental risk factors may be determinants in 45% of men with prostate cancer. This is not in line with the present estimate based on segregation analyses, which explains about 9% of all prostate cancers as being potentially determined by inheritance.

Epidemiological evidence of risk factors

To date, epidemiological evidence for the presence of risk factors is not conclusive. Vitamins E, D and A, endocrine factors, such as the low estrogenic activity of isoflavanoids and other components of soy, as well as the exposure to heavy metals and to selenium, animal fats and the consumption of vegetables have been identified as being either protective or related to an increased risk[6,16]. A review of dietary factors is given by Schuurman and colleagues[17].

Endocrine factors are probably of impor- tance. Anecdotal evidence reveals that early castrates do not develop prostate cancer. On the other side of the spectrum, bodybuilders using large dosages of androgenic steroids have been described as developing very aggressive prostate cancer at a very early age. Some of the effects of diet, according to what is known about mechanisms, may in fact be related to a lowering of androgen production and plasma androgen levels[4]. Interfering with 5α-reductase activity, the use of Finasteride® in patients with minimal residual disease, evidenced by a rising prostate-specific antigen (PSA) level after radical prostatectomy, has been shown to delay PSA progression by 8 months in a blinded treat- ment period of 12 months[18]. Relevant questions relating to this and similar observations are whether PSA changes relate to tumor mass in a given situation of interference and whether clinical observations with minimal disease may translate into a preventive effect if such regimens are applied to men at risk without known prostate cancer.

Migrant studies

Strong support for the concept of promotion of progression of prostate cancer from a precursor or latent/focal stage to the clinically manifest disease is provided by migrant studies and comparative autopsy studies between areas of high and low clinical prevalence[13,19]. Next to confirmation of the very similar prevalence of latent focal disease in regions of high and low clinical incidence of prostate cancer, these studies show that migration from Japan to Hawaii or to the mainland of the United States leads to an increase in clinical incidence of prostate cancer. This increase occurs in the first generation but is enhanced during the second and subsequent generations[20]. While the possibility of registration errors is an explan- ation for some of these findings, it is very unlikely that the autopsy data are not reliable. The migrant studies confirm the concept that environmental factors promote the biological progression of prostate cancer from the latent/ focal state and possibly from HGPIN to the

clinically relevant and potentially lethal form of this disease.

Case selection and endpoints

The most simple and most logical approach to studies of chemo- or endocrine preventive agents and regimens is the prospective, random- ized, double-blind, placebo-controlled clinical trial. Conceptionally, identifying risk groups by age and using prostatic cancer incidence in the two arms as the endpoint seems to be the most logical approach. However, this approach is loaded with difficulties. These are related to the potential long duration of such trials, the issue of compliance with prescribed treatment over very long periods, the interference with the endpoint by PSA-based screening, the contam- ination by the utilization of other potentially protective regimens and others. Also, the definition of 'incidence' is very problematic if one considers that the lead time produced by screening may amount to 6–10 years. Further- more, a trial of this type will have to recruit between 20 000 and 30 000 men in the age groups at risk and utilize follow-up periods of 10 years or longer. The follow-up period can be shortened by using biopsy evidence as an endpoint parameter. This necessitates requiring all participants to have a biopsy taken after a given period of time. A modification of this approach was utilized in the randomized, placebo-controlled study of Finasteride, which is conducted by the National Cancer Institute of the USA in conjunction with the Southwest Oncology Group (SWOG). This trial has completed recruitment of about 18 000 men; the follow-up period is 7 years and is concluded by a biopsy of the prostate. The outcome is pending[21]. Obviously, there is a great need to identify risk factors and endpoints that allow a decrease in the sample size and duration of preventive trials. Such end- points will have to have a well-documented significant relation to outcome parameters, especially prostate cancer mortality and overall survival. In other words, it will be necessary to establish surrogacy of such markers, a difficult task.

HGPIN has a precursor lesion, and T_{1a} focal carcinoma identified at transurethral resection or open prostatectomy may represent proper entry criteria related to a higher risk of developing prostate cancer within a shorter period of time than characterization of study participants by age only. However, even with repeated biopsy or with a repeated transurethral resection, co-existing manifest prostate cancer cannot be excluded with certainty. Also, while the risk of the subsequent development of prostate cancer associated to A1 lesions is reasonably well-understood and is probably in the range of 15–20%[22] over an average period of 8 years, the time course with respect to the development of clinical cancer after the biopsy diagnosis of presumably isolated HGPIN is unknown at this time. Another complicating factor lies in the low rate of biopsy-detectable isolated PIN, which is dependent on the population and ranges from 0.7 to 15%[7]. Other potential precursor lesions, such as atrophy or a typical adenomatous hyperplasia (AAH), are even less developed and are not suitable at this time for the use of risk factors that would allow the streamlining of prevention trials. These problems are in sharp contrast to the need to screen a very large number of substances if one wishes to establish their effectiveness in prostate cancer prevention. A procedure that allows for screening of risk factors with a reasonably large throughput capacity is urgently needed, especially with respect to potentially protective agents. The search for surrogate markers should have a top research priority. By definition, a surrogate marker should correlate significantly with an improvement of survival or prostate cancer mortality in a randomized study, showing an advantage for a given treatment regimen. This definition is exceedingly difficult to fulfil. Revealing a significant correlation of the presence or absence of a given risk factor with prostate cancer mortality in a non-randomized situation may approach the definition value of 'surrogacy'[23].

It would be of great importance to know whether a PSA response obtained in men with minimal residual disease has surrogate value. This can be evaluated in long-term studies using prostate cancer mortality and overall survival as the endpoint. Still, such studies will have to be of long duration, considering the slow biological progression rate of this disease[24]. Subsequently, it will be necessary to establish whether PSA response in minimal residual disease will translate into an advantage in terms of prevention if the same principle is applied to populations at risk. In a situation where the enormous cost and effort to be put into formal prevention studies limit their feasibility to the extremes, compromise algorithms, such as the one presented in Table 1, should be seriously considered. Figure 1 gives a schematic representation of the use of PSA in a placebo-controlled, randomized prevention study. The prolongation of the PSA doubling time obviously translates into an advantage in PSA progression. The clock seems to be turned back

Table 1 Algorithm for screening potentially protective agents and risk factors

Setting	Parameters	Next steps
(1) *In vitro* and animal studies (PC lines, xenotransplants, transgenic animals)*	tumor mass PSA, apoptosis	proceed to study 2 with positive or negative study
(2) Patients with minimal or maximal, residual PC and rising PSA*	PSA (slope, doubling time (DT))	if studies 1 + 2 are +/+, proceed to study 3; if −/+, consider study 3; if +/− or −/−, discard the risk factor from further analysis
(3) Risk factor-based human prevention study	PC on biopsy or clinical, PSA slope/DT, apoptosis, other markers	if positive, introduce, combine with other factors

*Studies 1 and 2 can be carried out simultaneously

by this procedure. Animal studies can confirm whether a PSA response to a given regimen will correspond to a reduction in tumor mass[25]. The algorithm in Table 1 should provide the possibility of discarding positive or negative risk factors from expensive and time-consuming prevention studies that are based on risk factors, such as HGPIN.

Results of randomized studies

A number of randomized prevention studies are ongoing or have recently been completed. The latter have led to important information that will be utilized in future studies. The Scandinavian twin study[15] sets the target: 55% of all prostate cancers are likely to be related to non-hereditary environmental factors. Their identification and practical application could produce significant progress by leading to a profound decrease in the risk of clinical prostate cancer and the related mortality. A recent review is given in references 21 and 26.

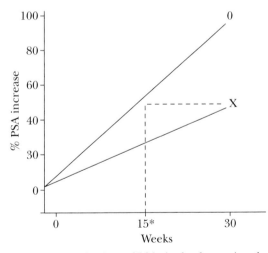

Figure 1 Gain in time of PSA rise by decreasing the doubling time of PSA rise from 60 to 30 weeks (hypothetical sketch assuming a linear PSA rise. The assumption of linearity leads to a wrong projection. Because the rise is exponential, the decrease in doubling time from 60 weeks (placebo) to 29.5 weeks (verum) translates into a gain of 8 weeks time with a 6-week verum period. 0, placebo, X = verum)

Completed randomized studies

Clark and colleagues[27,28] reported on a randomized, placebo-controlled, double-blind study of 200 mg selenium per day to study the incidence of basal cell or squamous cell carcinoma of the skin. A brief summary of the trial and its outcome is given in Table 2. The trial resulted in a significant reduction to 0.37 of the relative risk of developing prostate cancer in the selenium group. The value of this information is limited by the fact that prostate cancer was not the primary endpoint of the study and the study was not powered for prevention of prostate cancer. Still, selenium may, on the basis of this study and the remaining epidemiological evidence, be considered as one of the main protective factors identified so far. Evidence on the protective value of vitamin E at a dosage of 50 mg per day in combination with betacarotene (20 mg per day) was obtained in a similar way[29]. The placebo-controlled, randomized study using this regimen was set up to study the effect on lung cancer. Other cancers were included. The only positive result related to prostate cancer. In the cohort of men who received 50 mg of α-tocopherol, the incidence and mortality of prostate cancer increased by 32% and 41%, with a median follow-up of 6.1 years. Again, the data resulting from this trial are summarized in Table 3. The only randomized prevention study based on minimal residual disease with a rise of PSA was recently reported by Schröder and colleagues[30]. In this placebo-controlled, randomized, cross-over trial, PSA slope was used as the only endpoint. A run-in period was followed by a 6-week active period applying placebo versus control, by a 2-week wash-out

Table 2 Selenium – controlled prevention trial[27,28]

Randomized, placebo-controlled, double-blind study of 200 μg selenium/day in 1312 male (±75%) and female (±25%) patients with basal cells or squamous carcinoma of the skin

Follow-up, 6.5 years (median)

Among endpoints: prostate cancer incidence

Results: Se 13, placebo 35 cases, RR Se 0.37 (6464 man-years). No effect on skin cancers

Table 3 Vitamin E – controlled prevention trial[29]

Open, randomized study of 29 133 male smokers treated with α-tocopherol (50 mg/day) or β-carotene (20 mg/day) versus placebo (age 50–69 years)

Endpoints: incidence and mortality of lung and other cancers

Follow-up: 5 years, median 6.1 years

Results: α-tocopherol ($n = 14\,560$): 32% decrease (95% CI, −47 to −12%) in PC incidence, 41% decrease (95% CI, −4 to −59%) in PC mortality (246 cancers, 62 deaths)

β-carotene increased incidence and mortality by 23% and 15%

period and then by a 6-week cross-over period, which was again followed by a run-out or reference period. The self-developed supplement contained a soy extract, a green tea extract, phytosterols, carotenoids, selenium and vitamin E. The supplement was applied daily in addition to a regular diet. Betacarotene, lycopene, luteine, vitamin E, diadzeine and genisteine were determined in the blood at regular intervals and served, among others, as compliance markers. Endocrine parameters studied in serum included testosterone, 5α-dihydro-testosterone, sex hormone binding globulin, free androgen index and luteinizing hormone. A total of 37 patients were recruited. In comparing placebo and verum periods for all men who had completed the study without missing data ($n = 19$), a comparison of the 2 Log PSA slopes in the verum and the placebo periods revealed differences in doubling times amounting to 29.5 and 60 weeks for the verum and placebo treatments ($p < 0.05$, one-sided). A definitive manuscript is in preparation. This study will be followed by a number of similar protocols, which will also be associated with animal studies. The goal will be to identify the active compounds, producing longer-term data and studying the effectiveness in hormone-unresponsive PSA progression.

Ongoing randomized trials

The Finasteride study has already been briefly described above. Other randomized studies undertaken by the early detection and prevention branch of the NCI/USA include a study of selenium (SELECT study) and of the anti-androgen flutamide. Details can be found in reference 21.

Conclusions

The very large, existing, epidemiological differences between areas of high and low incidence and mortality of prostate cancer are so far incompletely explained. Major leads are identifiable from the epidemiological literature; very few are confirmed in a randomized setting. These latter include selenium 200 mg per day, vitamin E 50 mg per day, and, in a study of minimal residual disease by means of PSA slope, a dietary supplement containing a soy extract, green tea extract, phytosterols, carotenoids, selenium and vitamin E.

The methodological difficulties in conducting proper prevention studies in the field of prostate cancer are pointed out. These relate to the identification of proper risk factors and endpoints, which will allow cutting down the size, the duration and the cost of future studies. An algorithm is proposed. Essential questions relate to the surrogacy of alternative endpoints, to the value of PSA, to the feasibility of the use of precursor lesions, and to the validity of data resulting from studies in minimal residual disease in relation to prevention. If the large observed geographical differences in prostate cancer incidence and mortality could be utilized in effective preventive regimens, this would probably produce the largest progress in the field of prostate cancer achieved to date. The development of short cuts to utilize alternative designs and step-up schemes in the development of preventive regimens should represent a top research priority.

References

1. Whelan SL, Parkin DM, Masuyer E. *Patterns of Cancer in Five Continents*. Lyon: IARC Scientific Publications No. 102; 1990

2. Adlercreutz H. Western diet and Western diseases: some hormonal and biochemical mechanisms and associations. *Scand J Clin Lab Invest Suppl* 1990;201:3–23

3. Hamalainen E, Adlercreutz H, Puska P, Pietinen P. Diet and serum sex hormones in healthy men. *J Steroid Biochem* 1984;20:459–64

4. de Jong FH, Oishi K, Hayes RB, *et al.* Peripheral hormone levels in controls and patients with prostatic cancer or benign prostatic hyperplasia: results from the Dutch–Japanese case–control study. *Cancer Res* 1991;51:3445–50

5. Ross RK, Bernstein L, Lobo RA, *et al.* 5-alpha-reductase activity and risk of prostate cancer among Japanese and US white and black males. *Lancet* 1992;339:887–9

6. Kolonel LN. Nutrition and prostate cancer. *Cancer Causes Control* 1996;7:83–94

7. Sakr WA, Billis A, Ekman P, Wilt T, Bostwick DG. Epidemiology of high-grade prostatic intra-epithelial neoplasia. *Scand J Nephrol Suppl* 2000; 205:11–18

8. Hoedemaeker RF, Kranse R, Rietbergen JB, Kruger AE, Schroder FH, van der Kwast TH. Evaluation of prostate needle biopsies in a population-based screening study: the impact of borderline lesions. *Cancer* 1999;85:145–52

9. Schröder FH, van der Cruijsen-Koeter I, de Koning HJ, Vis AN, Hoedemaeker RF, Kranse R. Prostate cancer detection at low prostate specific antigen. *J Urol* 2000;163:806–12

10. McNeal JE, Bostwick DG. Intraductal dysplasia: a premalignant lesion of the prostate. *Hum Pathol* 1986;17:64–71

11. Franks LM. Latent carcinoma of the prostate. *J Path Bact* 1954;68:603–16

12. Ohori M, Dunn JK, Scardino PT. Is prostate-specific antigen density more useful than prostate-specific antigen levels in the diagnosis of prostate cancer? *Urology* 1995;46:666–71

13. Breslow N, Chan CW, Dhom G, *et al.* Latent carcinoma of prostate at autopsy in seven areas. The International Agency for Research on Cancer, Lyons, France. *Int J Cancer* 1977;20: 680–8

14. Yamabe H, ten Kate FJW, Gallee MPW, *et al.* Stage A prostatic cancer: a comparative study in Japan and The Netherlands. *World J Urol* 1986; 4:136–40

15. Lichtenstein P, Holm NV, Verkasalo PK, *et al.* Environmental and heritable factors in the causation of cancer. *N Engl J Med* 2000;343: 78–85.

16. Oishi K, Okada K, Yoshida O, *et al.* A case–control study of prostatic cancer with reference to dietary habits. *Prostate* 1988;12:179–90

17. Schuurman AG, van den Brandt PA, Goldbohm RA. Prospective epidemiological studies on dietary risk factors for prostate cancer: a review. In *Diet and Other Risk Factors for Prostate Cancer*. Thesis, A.G. Schuurman. Maastricht: University of Maastricht, 1999: 9–29

18. Andriole G, Lieber M, Smith J, *et al.* Treatment with finasteride following radical prostatectomy for prostate cancer. *Urology* 1995;45:491–7

19. Haenszel W, Kurihara M. Studies of Japanese migrants. I. Mortality from cancer and other diseases among Japanese in the United States. *J Natl Cancer Inst* 1968;40:43–68

20. Akazaki K, Stemmerman GN. Comparative study of latent carcinoma of the prostate among Japanese in Japan and Hawaii. *J Natl Cancer Inst* 1973;50:1137–44

21. Thompson IA, Coltman CA. Chemoprevention of cancer of the prostate. In Resnick MI, Thompson IM, eds. *Advanced Therapy of Prostate Disease*. London: BC Decker Inc., 2000: 428–45

22. Epstein JI, Paull G, Eggleston JC, Walsh PC. Prognosis of untreated stage A1 prostatic carcinoma: a study of 94 cases with extended followup. *J Urol* 1986;136:837–9

23. Schröder FH, Kranse R, Barbet N, Hop WC, Kandra A, Lassus M. Prostate-specific antigen: a surrogate endpoint for screening new agents against prostate cancer? *Prostate* 2000;42:107–15

24. Pound CR, Partin AW, Eisenberger MA, Chan DW, Pearson JD, Walsh PC. Natural history of progression after PSA elevation following radical prostatectomy. *J Am Med Assoc* 1999;282:1591

25. Thalmann GN, Sikes RA, Chang S-M, Johnston DA, von Eschenbach AC, Chung LWK. Suramin-induced decrease in prostate-specific antigen expression with no effect on tumor growth in the LNCaP model of human prostate cancer. *J Natl Cancer Inst* 1996;88:794–801

26. Schulman CC, Zlotta AR, Denis L, Sakr WA. Prevention of prostate cancer. *Scand J Urol Nephrol Suppl* 2000;205:50–61

27. Clark LC, Combs JGF, Turnbull BW, *et al.* Nutritional Prevention of Cancer Study Group. Effects of selenium supplementation for cancer prevention in patients with carcinoma of the skin. A randomized controlled trial. *J Am Med Assoc* 1996;276:1957–63

28. Clark LC, Dalkin B, Krongrad A, *et al.* Decreased incidence of prostate cancer with selenium supplementation: results of a double-blind cancer prevention trial. *Br J Urol* 1998;81:730–4

29. Heinonen OP, Albanes D, Virtamo J, *et al.* Prostate cancer and supplementation with alpha-tocopherol and beta-carotene: incidence and mortality in a controlled trial. *J Natl Cancer Inst* 1998;90:440–6

30. Schröder FH, Kranse R, Dijk MA, *et al.* Tertiary prevention of prostate cancer by dietary intervention: results of a randomised, double blind, placebo controlled, cross-over study. *Eur Urol* 2000;37(Suppl 2):24, Abstr 96

Section V

Prostate cancer: endocrine treatment

The molecular mechanisms of hormone resistance in prostate cancer

18

F. C. Hamdy

'We found the patient complaining of excruciating pains in various parts of the body, which could be compared to nothing except the pains under which persons afflicted with carcinoma occasionally labour. He could void no urine without the assistance of a catheter. The prostate gland, examined by the rectum was found to be much enlarged and of a stony hardness. I continued to visit him in consultation for nearly a year, at the end of which time he suddenly lost the use of the muscles of his lower limbs and died a fortnight afterwards.'

Sir Benjamin Brodie, 1842

Introduction

Prostate cancer is the second most common malignancy in males in the Western world, with over 35 000 men dying from the disease every year in Europe alone[1]. Patients with advanced disease can present in a variety of ways, including bladder outflow obstruction, irritative bladder symptoms secondary to trigonal involvement and hematuria. Metastatic disease may present with skeletal pain, or with general systemic manifestations, including weight loss, weakness and anorexia. With locally advanced disease, prostate cancer may manifest itself as renal failure secondary to bilateral ureteric orifice involvement. The clinical picture tends to be dominated by the problem of bone metastases, which occur in 85% of patients. They represent the most important cause of morbidity, with pain requiring substantial analgesia, and resulting complications including pathological fractures and spinal compression.

In 1940, Charles Huggins discovered the beneficial effects of androgen deprivation in patients with metastatic prostate cancer[2]. Since then, hormonal manipulation has remained the mainstay of treatment in advanced stages of the disease. It is still expected that approximately 85% of all patients with advanced prostate cancer will respond to androgen blockade. Patients will show both subjective and objective responses, manifested by considerable and rapid symptomatic improvement, particularly in metastatic skeletal pain, together with local and distant regression of the disease. This is complemented by normalization of serum tumor markers. Relapse, however, is common at a mean interval of 2 years following initiation of treatment. The disease is then hormone resistant and prognosis becomes extremely poor. Methods of hormonal manipulation include bilateral orchidectomy, estrogen preparations which are rarely prescribed nowadays, in view of the serious cardiovascular side-effects encountered with the recognized 3 mg daily dose, which is required in order to achieve castrate levels. The use of the smaller dose of 1 mg daily remains controversial, as castrate levels are not reached in 30% of patients. Alternative therapy includes the use of analogs of the hypothalamic luteinizing hormone releasing hormone (LHRH). These occupy the receptors of LHRH in the pituitary, initially stimulating the release of luteinizing hormone and then blocking the subsequent stimulation of the receptors by the endogenous pulsatile secretion of luteinizing hormone.

Finally, synthetic antiandrogens are also being used. These all act by competing with androgen receptors in the hormone-sensitive prostatic cells, benign or malignant. In the late 1980s, total androgen blockade was advocated to prevent the effect of the non-testicular circulating testosterone formation by the adrenals. After initial enthusiasm, recent studies have failed to show any survival advantage in patients treated with maximum androgen blockade[3,4]. Approximately 15% of patients will not respond to hormonal manipulation, and the majority will relapse within 2–3 years from initiation of treatment. Chemotherapy is ineffective. Radiotherapy can be given as a palliative measure, either as hemibody irradiation, or as 'spot-welding' to treat painful metastatic foci in bone. Strontium-89 can be administered intravenously and appears to have similar efficacy to external beam irradiation. Simple and complex analgesic regimens can be used, including combinations of non-steroidal anti-inflammatory agents and opiates. In addition, bisphosphonate compounds appear to have a beneficial analgesic effect. More recently, the compounds have been tested in clinical trials prophylactically, in an attempt to delay/prevent the appearance of bone lesions in patients with locally advanced disease. Despite these various treatment strategies, the morbidity caused by hormone-resistant disease remains considerable. In order to improve our management of advanced prostate cancer, it is important to understand the pathophysiology and molecular mechanisms of androgen sensitivity and resistance, which develop almost invariably in the late stages of the disease.

Androgen regulation of the prostate

Androgens are important male sex hormones which, in addition to being essential for the growth and differentiation of all male sex accessory organs, are strongly associated with the development and progression of prostate cancer. Androgen action in the prostate is mediated through the androgen receptor, a ligand-dependent transcription factor which is a member of the steroid/thyroid hormone receptor gene superfamily. The mitogenic effects of androgens on prostatic growth appear to be mediated through the action of soluble peptide growth factors, acting in either an autocrine or a paracrine manner. For androgen blockade to be effective in prolonging disease-free survival, it has to rely, at least initially, on the presence of a majority of androgen-dependent cells. However, this treatment is only palliative since androgen-independent clones of cancer cells expand and progress. This observation has been made in almost every case of prostate cancer. The origin of androgen-independent prostate cancer cells remains unclear. It has been stipulated that either they may originate directly from basal stem cells, and eventually outgrow cells monoclonally derived from androgen-sensitive amplifying basal cells, or they are derived directly from initially androgen-dependent glandular cells. Subsequent changes in the cancer cell phenotype may result from a combination of structural, regulatory and genetic changes, some of which are described below. These androgen-independent cells acquire the ability to proliferate in the absence of androgen through genetic mutations. Some of the proposed mechanisms include ligand-independent activation of the androgen receptor through 'cross-talk' with other signal transduction pathways, overexpression of androgen receptor co-activators and alterations in androgen receptor binding. Mutations may result in changes in the function/expression of androgen receptor protein or growth factors and their receptors. A better understanding of the structure of the androgen receptor is essential in order to investigate the molecular factors involved in hormonal escape.

The androgen receptor

The androgen receptor can be structurally divided into three domains: a transcriptional activation domain, a DNA-binding domain and a ligand-binding domain (Figure 1). Cellular signalling occurs following androgen binding to the androgen receptor and translocation to the nucleus. This activated complex associates with

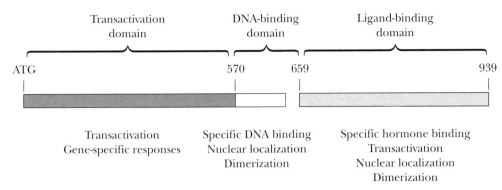

Figure 1 The androgen receptor

androgen-responsive elements contained in the DNA sequence of a number of target genes to affect their transcriptional activity. The possible presence *in vivo* of alternative androgen receptor isoforms, the extent of androgen receptor phosphorylation, the association with other proteins and the presence of polymorphic glutamine and glycine regions may provide additional levels of control for androgen receptor action.

Radioligand-binding studies and immuno-histochemistry have been used to detect androgen receptor protein expression. Both primary and metastatic prostate cancer show elevated androgen receptors by ligand-binding assays when compared to non-malignant prostate tissue. Immunohistochemistry supports elevated androgen receptors in prostate cancer with strong nuclear staining, mostly of a heterogeneous nature in hormone-relapsed and in primary and metastatic hormone-refractory prostate cancer.

Androgen receptor abnormalities

A number of studies suggest a high frequency of amino acid substitutions in the androgen receptor protein (25–50%) for untreated advanced prostate cancer and in hormone-relapsed tumors from primary and metastatic sites. Functional analysis of these mutations reveal alterations in ligand binding and transcriptional activation. Additionally, androgen receptor gene amplification has been identified in 30% of recurrent prostate tumors.

Examination of the corresponding primary tumor prior to initiation of hormone therapy showed no evidence of amplification, suggesting that amplification occurred during androgen deprivation, conferring a growth advantage on the prostate cancer cells. Variation in the length of a polyglutamine stretch in the N-terminal domain of the androgen receptor protein, causing an alteration in androgen receptor function, has been suggested as a contributory factor towards an increased lifetime risk for the development of prostate cancer. More recently, a double missense mutation of the androgen receptor in a patient with androgen-insensitive prostate cancer appeared to function as a high-affinity cortisol receptor. This led to the promotion of androgen-independent growth of prostate cancer by circulating glucocorticoids. This information paves the way to potential novel therapeutic manipulations in patients with hormone-resistant disease[5].

Apoptosis-regulating genes

Hormone ablation in prostate cancer achieves its effect by activation of apoptosis (programmed cell death)[6,7], which is a distinct mode of cell death occurring in both normal physiological conditions as well as in disease including cancer[8]. Apoptosis is an active process characterized by distinct morphological changes in single cells, with compaction and margination of nuclear chromatin, cytoplasmic condensation and convolution of nuclear and cell outlines. Later changes involve nuclear fragmentation and budding of the cell with the development of membrane-bound apoptotic bodies, which are removed by phagocytosis. In contrast to necrosis, which is a passive process, there is no associated inflammation. A number of genes are involved in the control of apoptosis including the proto-oncogene Bcl-2 on chromosome 18 region 18q21[9,10] and the tumor suppressor gene p53 on chromosome 17 region 17p13[11].

Bcl-2

The bcl-2 gene was initially identified in B-cell lymphomas[12], and the gene product acts by inhibiting apoptosis, but has no direct effect on cell proliferation[9]. A rapidly expanding group of genes showing homology to bcl-2 have been described and named the bcl-2 gene family, forming two functionally antagonistic groups controlling the balance between cell death and survival. Bax accelerates apoptotic cell death by forming heterodimers with bcl-2 leading to suppression of apoptosis[13]. The molecular mechanisms by which the bcl-2 protein suppresses apoptosis remain unresolved. In the prostate, bcl-2 is normally expressed in basal epithelial cells, seminal vesicles and ejaculatory ducts. In primary prostate cancer, bcl-2 is expressed in around 25% of cases[14]. Bcl-2 overexpression is associated with increasing tumor stage and the development of hormone-refractory disease[15,16]. In high-grade prostatic intraepithelial neoplasia (HGPIN), the reported expression of bcl-2 has shown a wide variation from 0 to 100%[14,17,18]. The largest study reported bcl-2 expression in 4/24 (17%) cases of HGPIN[17].

p53

Inactivation of the tumor suppressor gene p53 is presently the most common mutation identified in human cancers[11]. Functional (wild type) p53 protein has DNA-binding properties and forms a key part of the mechanism by which mammalian cells undergo growth arrest or apoptosis in response to DNA damage.

Mutation of p53 may result in loss of its normal function[19]. Mutations in the p53 gene commonly occur in the highly conserved exons 5, 6, 7 and 8. In most cases, one allele is completely deleted with a missense mutation in the remaining allele[20]. Mutant p53 protein has a prolonged half-life compared to the wild type p53 protein, and its nuclear accumulation is detectable by immunohistochemistry.

In benign prostatic epithelium, p53 positivity is absent. In primary prostate cancer, p53 nuclear positivity is present in around 20% of cases[21-23]. Accumulation of p53 protein appears to be a late event being associated with advanced stage, high Gleason tumor grade, hormonal resistance, poor survival DNA aneuploidy and high cell proliferation rate[23-26]. A good correlation is seen between p53 immuno-reactivity in prostate cancer and direct evidence of gene mutation using the polymerase chain reaction (PCR) and single-strand conformational polymorphism (SSCP) and direct sequencing[27]. p53 positivity is infrequent in HGPIN, the largest study showing strong nuclear staining in 14%[28].

Wild type p53 may participate with bcl-2 and Bax in a common pathway regulating cell death by decreasing the expression of bcl-2 while simultaneously increasing the expression of Bax, resulting in apoptosis[29]. The combination of Bcl-2 overexpression and p53 nuclear protein accumulation in human prostate cancer has been shown to correlate with the development of hormone-refractory disease[16] and are independent prognostic markers for post-radical prostatectomy recurrence[30].

Peptide growth factors

Peptide growth factors can have a regulatory effect on prostate growth through either a paracrine or an autocrine mechanism. Stromal cells can be induced to secrete growth factors (paracrine effect), with subsequent re-programming of cancer cells to produce their own factors. Alternatively, androgen may bind with androgen receptors in the glandular cells independently from the stromal cells. Androgen action induces glandular cells to produce and secrete peptide growth factors, thus inducing an autocrine stimulation.

Fibroblast growth factors

The fibroblast growth factor (FGF) family of polypeptide growth factors have diverse physiological and pathological functions including development, wound healing, angiogenesis and tumorigenesis[31]. In man, the FGFs comprise at least ten genes and the receptor family comprises four members. Multiple ligands and receptors allow interaction between a single receptor and several ligands, and between different receptor monomers through heterodimerization following activation by FGF[32]. Basic FGF (FGF-2) is secreted by prostatic fibroblasts in response to androgen and acts in an autocrine fashion to stimulate fibroblast cell growth[33]. Stroma-derived keratinocyte growth factor (KGF/FGF-7) is up-regulated in hormone-resistant prostate cancer and has a role as a potential paracrine growth factor on epithelial cells[34]. KGF has a potent mitogenic action on epithelial cells and has been proposed to act as an androgen-regulated mediator of epithelial cell growth[35]. A similar paracrine action applies to FGF-8 (androgen-induced growth factor), which is secreted in response to androgens and can stimulate growth of epithelial and fibroblast cells.

Insulin-like growth factors

Insulin-like growth factor (IGF)-1 and -2 are important mitogens that mediate normal and neoplastic cell growth. The IGFs bind to specific receptors, designated type I and II IGF receptors (IGFR). Type I IGFR is a transmembrane heterotetramer tyrosine kinase which primarily mediates the mitogenic actions of IGFs. IGFs are two of the most abundant growth factors in bone[36], the preferential site for metastatic prostate cancer. Type I IGFR is expressed by prostate cancer cells which could facilitate the development of bone metastases.

IGFs also have high affinity for a family of at least six IGF-binding proteins (IGFBPs) which act to regulate their bioavailability[37]. The levels of circulating IGFBPs are regulated by endocrine factors and by specific proteases that cleave IGFBPs to small inactive peptides. IGFBPs are believed to modulate proliferative and mitogenic effects of IGFs as well as modulating cell growth independently of IGFs. Although all IGFBPs have high affinity for IGFs, IGFBP-3 is the major transporter of IGFs in serum. A number of studies have suggested that IGFBPs may be involved in growth modulation of prostate malignancy. One study showed elevated IGFBP-2 and decreased IGFBP-3 in patients with prostate cancer[38]. More recently, using cDNA microarray technology Bubendorf and colleagues[39] compared hormone-sensitive xenografts (CWR22R) with hormone-insensitive xenografts (CWR22), and surveyed 5184 genes. Of those, 37 genes (0.7%) were increased more than two-fold in hormone-resistant (HR) cells compared with hormone-sensitive (HS) xenografts. IGFBP-2 + HSP27 (27 kDa heat shock protein) were consistently overexpressed in CWR22R. Investigation of 208 primary prostate cancers, 30 hormone-resistant cases, and 26 benign prostatic hyperplastic specimens by tissue microarray showed high expression of IGFBP-2 protein in all cancers, 36% of primary tumors, 0% of benign prostatic hyperplasia (BPH), and increased HSP27 in 31% of HR tumors, 5% of primary cancers and no expression in BPH. This exemplifies the way forward in rapidly investigating a large number of candidate genes *in vitro*, substantiated by the study of large cohorts of patient material.

Epidermal growth factor

Binding of epidermal growth factor (EGF) to the extracellular domain of its receptor, EGFR, results in activation of the receptor's cytoplasmic tyrosine kinase, phosphorylation of substrate proteins and stimulation of cell proliferation. Members of the EGF family play a role in modulation of prostatic growth. Withdrawal of androgen from the rodent prostate leads to reduced expression of EGF, which is a potent mitogen for epithelial cells[40]. Thus the continued presence of androgens within the prostate helps maintain epithelial cell proliferation mediated through the expression of EGF. HER-2/neu, a member of the EGF tyrosine kinases, is known to interact with estrogen receptor signalling in breast cancer, and predicts anti-estrogen resistance. Forced expression leads to estrogen-independent growth. HER-2/neu is normally expressed in prostate epithelial cells, overexpressed and/or amplified in some prostate cancer patients. Elevated serum levels correlate with hormone-refractory disease, and forced expression leads to hormone independence in castrated animals. HER-2/neu appears to activate androgen receptor signaling in the absence of ligand, enhancing the androgen receptor response in the presence of low androgen levels[41,42].

Understanding these various mechanisms, and their clinical relevance in the development of hormone-resistant disease in prostate cancer, remains a challenge for scientists and clinicians alike. Further research can only pave the way to design novel therapeutic strategies in the management of this ubiquitous disease.

References

1. Møller Jensen O, Estève J, Møller H, *et al.* Cancer in the European community and its member states. *Eur J Cancer* 1990;26:1167–256
2. Huggins C, Hodges CV. Studies on prostate cancer. The effect of castration, of oestrogen and of androgen injection on serum phosphatase in metastatic carcinoma of the prostate. *Cancer Res* 1941;1:293–7
3. Prostate Cancer Trialists' Collaborative Group. Maximum androgen blockade in advanced prostate cancer: an overview of 22 randomised trials with 3283 deaths in 5710 patients. *Lancet* 1995;346:265–9
4. Caubet JF, Tosteson TD, Dong EW, *et al.* Maximum androgen blockade in advanced prostate cancer: a meta-analysis of published randomized controlled trials using nonsteroidal antiandrogens. *Urology* 1997;49:71–8
5. Zhao X-Y, Malloy PJ, Krishnan AV, *et al.* Glucocorticoids can promote androgen-independent growth of prostate cancer cells through a mutated androgen receptor. *Nature Med* 2000;6:703–6
6. Kyprianou N, English HF, Isaacs JT. Programmed cell death during regression of PC-82 human prostate cancer following androgen ablation. *Cancer Res* 1990;50:3748–53
7. Colombel M, Symmans F, Gil S, *et al.* Detection of the apoptosis-suppressing oncoprotein bcl-2 in hormone-refractory human prostate cancers. *Am J Pathol* 1993;143:390–400
8. Kerr JFR, Winterford CM, Harmon BV. Apoptosis. Its significance in cancer and cancer therapy. *Cancer* 1994;27:2013–26
9. Hockenbery D, Nunez G, Milliman C, *et al.* Bcl-2 is an inner mitochondrial membrane protein that blocks programmed cell death. *Nature (London)* 1990;348:334–6
10. Lu QL, Abel P, Foster CS, *et al.* bcl-2: role in epithelial differentiation and oncogenesis. *Hum Pathol* 1996;27:102–10
11. Lane DP. p53, guardian of the genome. *Nature (London)* 1992;358:15–16
12. Kroemer G. The proto-oncogene Bcl-2 and its role in regulating apoptosis. *Nature Med* 1997;3:614–20
13. Bostwick DG. Prospective origins of prostate carcinoma. Prostatic intraepithelial neoplasia and atypical adenomatous hyperplasia. *Cancer* 1996;78:330–6
14. Bauer JJ, Sesterhenn IA, Mostofi FK, *et al.* Elevated levels of apoptosis regulator proteins p53 and bcl-2 are independent prognostic biomarkers in surgically treated clinically localised prostate cancer. *J Urol* 1996;156:1511–16
15. McDonnell TJ, Troncoso P, Brisbay SM, *et al.* Expression of the proto-oncogene bcl-2 in the prostate and its association with emergence of androgen-independent prostate cancer. *Cancer Res* 1992;52:6940–4
16. Apakama I, Robinson MC, Walter NM, *et al.* bcl-2 overexpression combined with p53 protein accumulation correlates with hormone-refractory prostate cancer. *Br J Cancer* 1996;74:1258–62
17. Krajewski M, Krajewski S, Epstein JI, *et al.* Immunohistochemical analysis of bcl-2, bax,

bcl-X and mcl-1 expression in prostate cancers. *Am J Pathol* 1996;148:1567–76

18. Stattin P, Damber J-E, Karlberg L, *et al.* Bcl-2 immunoreactivity in prostate tumourigenesis in relation to prostatic intraepithelial neoplasia, grade, hormonal status, metastatic growth and survival. *Urol Res* 1996;24:257–64

19. Vogelstein B, Kinzler KW. p53 function and dysfunction. *Cell* 1992;70:523–6

20. Levine AJ, Momand J, Finlay CA. The p53 tumour suppressor gene. *Nature (London)* 1991;351:453–6

21. Mellon K, Thompson S, Charlton RG, *et al.* p53, c-erbB-2 and the epidermal growth factor receptor in the benign and malignant prostate. *J Urol* 1992;147:496–9

22. Thomas DJ, Robinson M, King P, *et al.* p53 expression and clinical outcome in prostate cancer. *Br J Urol* 1993;72:778–81

23. Visakorpi T, Kallioniemi OP, Heikkinen A, *et al.* Small subgroup of aggressive, highly proliferative prostatic carcinomas defined by p53 accumulation. *J Natl Cancer Inst* 1992;84:883–7

24. Aprikian AG, Sarkis AS, Fair WR, *et al.* Immunohistochemical determination of p53 protein nuclear accumulation in prostatic adenocarcinoma. *J Urol* 1994;151:1276–80

25. Kallakury BV, Figge J, Ross JS, *et al.* Association of p53 immunoreactivity with high gleason tumor grade in prostatic adenocarcinoma. *Hum Pathol* 1994;25:92–7

26. Heidenberg HB, Sesterhenn JP, Gaddipati JP, *et al.* Alteration of the tumour suppressor gene p53 in a high fraction of hormone refractory prostate cancer. *J Urol* 1995;154:414–21

27. Navone NM, Troncoso P, Pisters LL, *et al.* p53 protein accumulation and gene mutation in the progression of human prostate carcinoma. *J Natl Cancer Inst* 1993;85:1657–69

28. Humphrey PA, Swanson PE. Immunoreactive p53 protein in high-grade prostatic intraepithelial neoplasia. *Pathol Res Pract* 1995;191:881–7

29. Miyashita T, Reed JC. Tumor suppressor p53 is a direct transcriptional activator of the human bax gene. *Cell* 1995;80:293–9

30. Moul JW, Bettencourt M-C, Sesterhenn IA, *et al.* Protein expression of p53, bcl-2 and KI-67 (MIB-1) as prognostic biomarkers in patients with surgically treated, clinically localized prostate cancer. *Surgery* 1996;120:159–66

31. Basilico C, Moscatelli D. The FGF family of growth factors and oncogenes. *Adv Cancer Res* 1992;59:115–65

32. Leung HY, Hughes CM, Kloppel G, *et al.* Expression and functional activity of fibroblast growth factors and their receptors in human pancreatic cancer. *Int J Oncol* 1994;4:1219–23

33. Story MT. Regulation of prostate growth by fibroblast growth factors. *World J Urol* 1995;13:297–305

34. Leung HY, Mehta P, Gray LB, *et al.* Keratinocyte growth factor expression in hormone insensitive prostate cancer. *Oncogene* 1997;15:1115–20

35. Tanaka A, Miyamoto K, Matsuo H, *et al.* Human androgen-induced growth factor in prostate and breast cancer cells: its molecular cloning and growth properties. *FEBS Lett* 1995;363:226–30

36. Yoneda T, Sasaki A, Mundy GR. Osteolytic bone metastasis in breast cancer. *Breast Cancer Res Treatm* 1994;32:73–84

37. Jones JI, Clemmons DR. Insulin-like growth factors and their binding proteins: biological actions. *Endocr Rev* 1995;16:3–34

38. Kanety H, Madjar Y, Dagan Y, *et al.* Serum insulin-like growth factor-binding protein-2 (IGFBP-2) is increased and IGFBP-3 is decreased in patients with prostate cancer: correlation with serum prostate-specific antigen. *J Clin Endocrinol Metab* 1993;77:229–33

39. Bubendorf L, Kolmer M, Kononen J, *et al.* Hormone therapy failure in human prostate cancer: analysis by complementary DNA and tissue microarray. *J Natl Cancer Inst* 1999;91:1758–64

40. Denmeade SR, Lin XS, Isaacs JT. Role of programmed (apoptotic) cell death during the progression and therapy for prostate cancer. *Prostate* 1996;28:251–65

41. Craft N, Shostak Y, Carey M, *et al.* A mechanism for hormone-independent prostate cancer through modulation of androgen receptor signaling by the HER/2neu tyrosine kinase. *Nature Med* 1999;5:280–5

42. Visakorpi T. New pieces to the prostate cancer puzzle. *Nature Med* 1999;5:264–5

Early versus delayed endocrine therapy

19

P. Iversen

Introduction

In the years following the introduction of hormonal therapy for prostate cancer by Huggins and Hodges[1], early institution of such treatment was recommended based on comparison with historical controls[2]. Later, initial interpretations of the VACURG (Veterans Administration Cooperative Urological Research Group) studies[3] made the pendulum swing in the opposite direction, and it became common practice to defer hormonal therapy until symptomatic progression. It is important to recognize that the VACURG studies were not designed specifically to answer the question of timing of endocrine therapy. Moreover, their results were influenced by the significant cardiovascular effects of diethylstilbestrol (DES) 5 mg, which was used as one of the hormonal therapies employed in the studies. The increased risk of cardiovascular death associated with DES 5 mg outbalanced an apparent benefit of early endocrine therapy in terms of progression-free and overall survival. With regard to the optimal timing of therapy, a later review of the data by the VACURG statistician, David Byar, confirmed that early endocrine therapy delayed progression from stage III to stage IV, and, furthermore, a survival benefit was suggested, particularly for younger patients with high-grade tumors[4].

A number of non-controlled and non-randomized studies have indicated longer progression-free and overall survival to result from early institution of endocrine therapy[5,6]. In one retrospective study, two comparable groups of patients with lymph node metastases were identified and followed for outcome. One group received immediate endocrine therapy, while treatment was deferred in the other until development of distant metastases. Remarkable differences in outcome were observed: the median time to distant metastasis and median time to death were 100 and 150 months in the immediate group versus 43 and 90 months in the deferred group[7].

At the Mayo Clinic, 370 patients underwent radical prostatectomy between 1966 and 1985 and were found to have lymph node metastasis (stage D1). Eighty per cent of patients received, based on the surgeon's decision, immediate adjuvant hormonal treatment, while 20% did not. Immediate hormonal treatment resulted in significant prolonged progression-free survival in all ploidy classes (diploid, tetraploid and aneuploid), while significant improvement of survival was seen only in patients with diploid tumors[8]. While this study also suggested a beneficial effect of early endocrine therapy in node-positive disease, at least in selected groups of patients, it was rightfully criticised for not being randomized.

There is an experimental rationale for early endocrine therapy in the mangement of prostate cancer. With the Dunning R3327H rat prostatic adenocarcinoma as a model test system, Isaacs demonstrated that the earlier castration is performed, the more effective is the therapy with regard to survival. Further, in the same model, it was shown that the use of additional chemotherapy (cyclophosphamide) was most effective when both therapies (castration and chemo) were begun simultaneously and as early as possible[9].

In recent years, the old controversy of appropriate timing of androgen deprivation therapy has gained new and stronger momentum. Contributing to this is a change in stage distribution at diagnosis, with more early cancers being detected. Also, a growing interest in multi-modal therapy and the advent of prostate-specific antigen (PSA), enabling a better monitoring of the disease, have led to revived interest in early endocrine therapy. Further, the introduction of less toxic and well-tolerated pharmaceutical agents, like luteinizing hormone releasing hormone (LHRH) agonists and antiandrogens, has served to shift the delicate balance between anti-tumor efficacy and loss of quality of life caused by side-effects of treatment in a more favorable direction.

Randomized studies

Recently, randomized clinical studies, specifically designed to address the issue of timing of hormonal treatment, have matured.

In the study conducted by the Medical Research Council of Great Britain (MRC), 938 patients were randomized between immediate and deferred endocrine therapy[10]. Included patients were M0, asymptomatic M1, and also patients where metastatic status was not assessed (Mx). Nodal status was not known. In the vast majority of patients, endocrine treatment was bilateral orchidectomy or LHRH agonist therapy.

One important question was answered by the study. How long will patients in the deferred group be saved the side-effects of treatment before they eventually commence endocrine therapy? The median time from randomization to initiation of endocrine therapy in the deferred group was approximately 1 year among metastatic patients and approximately 2 years in M0 patients.

The study showed that immediate endocrine therapy delays disease progression: in M0 patients, progression to M1 was significantly delayed. In M1 patients, appearance of bone pain was delayed; local progression with need for transurethral resection occurred less frequently, and also the incidence of ureteric obstruction was reduced following immediate therapy, compared with deferred therapy.

Of major clinical importance was the observation that the incidence of spinal compression was significantly higher in the group of patients receiving deferred therapy. A total of 23 patients in the deferred group developed this serious manifestation of metastatic disease, as compared to nine in the immediate group. Nineteen of the 23 had already started endocrine therapy for another indication when spinal compression occurred. This observation strongly indicates that the event of spinal compression was not a consequence of failure to diagnose and institute relevant endocrine therapy, but rather a failure of deferred endocrine therapy as a concept[11].

For all patients randomized, both cause-specific and overall survival of those patients treated with immediate endocrine therapy were superior to those receiving deferred therapy. Stratifying by metastatic status at entry, this benefit was clear and significant in M0 patients, while no statistically significant difference could be established among M1 patients.

The major criticism of the MRC study related to the protocolled follow-up of patients which required only an annual clinical report form. Perhaps reflecting this, 26 patients apparently died of prostate cancer without ever receiving any endocrine therapy. Still, the conclusions of the study seem well founded and appear difficult to disregard: immediate endocrine therapy improves survival, particularly in M0 patients, and the incidence of serious and feared manifestations of disseminated disease is significantly reduced in M1 patients.

A randomized, prospective trial (EORTC 22863) compared external radiotherapy (50 + 20 Gy) with external radiotherapy plus immediate hormone therapy continued for 3 years (LHRH agonist goserelin 3.6 mg/4 weeks plus cyproterone acetate 150 mg for the 1st month) in patients with locally advanced prostate cancer[12]. When the study was analyzed, the median follow-up was 45 months. Kaplan–Meier estimates of 5-year overall survival and 5 years free of disease strongly favored the combination of radiotherapy and adjuvant endocrine therapy. Five-year survival rates were

62 and 79%, respectively, and the proportion of patients surviving 5 years free of disease was 48 versus 85%, respectively. These differences were highly significant. Analysis of sites of progression revealed that the major difference between the two groups was caused by a marked reduction in incidence of distant metastases. Out of a total of 78 clinical progressions in the radiotherapy-only group, 65 involved distant failure, as opposed to only 17 out of 20 clinical progressions in the combination arm. This finding suggests that the superiority of the combination is not only explained by improved local control due to synergism between radiotherapy and hormonal therapy, but probably more so by immediate endocrine suppression of distant micro-metastases already present at the time of randomization.

Thus, from a strict scientific point of view, the results of the EORTC 22863 trial should be interpreted as only supporting the use of immediate endocrine therapy in locally advanced prostate cancer. Whether combining endocrine therapy with radiotherapy improves outcome further logically will have to await the results of ongoing studies randomizing patients with locally advanced prostate cancer between endocrine therapy alone and the combination of endocrine therapy and radiotherapy.

In contrast to the EORTC 22863 study, where no information was available about lymph node status, a Swedish study surgically lymph node staged 91 M_0 patients with T_{1-4} prostatic tumors before randomizing them between radiotherapy alone and orchidectomy plus radiotherapy 3–4 weeks after castration[13]. When the study was reported, it was mature with a median follow-up of more than 9 years. Sixty-one per cent had clinically progressed in the radiotherapy group, as opposed to only 31% in the combination group ($p = 0.005$). Almost all progressions were distant failures. Similarly, the overall mortality was 61% versus 38% ($p = 0.02$). It is noteworthy that the large difference was almost exclusively caused by patients who were node-positive at entry (19/46 and 20/45, respectively). Among patients with negative nodes at entry, no statistical differences could be found in time to progression and

survival. However, as the authors point out, the study had insufficient statistical power to demonstrate a modest advantage for immediate endocrine therapy in node-negative patients. Thus, in agreement with the EORTC 22863 study, although being more specific in terms of disease stage, the authors concluded that immediate endocrine therapy significantly improves progression-free and overall survival in lymph node-positive patients who are treated with radiotherapy.

The Eastern Cooperative Oncology Group (ECOG) randomized 98 patients, who underwent radical prostatectomy and pelvic lymphadenectomy and who were found to have nodal metastases, to either immediate endocrine treatment (LHRH agonist therapy or surgical castration) or deferred therapy instituted at progression[14]. At the time of randomization, following prostatectomy, 80% of included patients had non-detectable PSA, reflecting a small tumor burden. The median follow-up was 7.1 years. In this study, marked differences in mortality were observed. Seven out of 47 receiving immediate endocrine therapy had died, only three from prostate cancer (one of these never accepted endocrine therapy, but was included in the intention-to-treat analysis). In the deferred therapy group, 18 of 51 had died, 16 of these from prostate cancer (the two dying of other causes had positive bone scans). These differences in overall and cancer-specific mortality are highly statistically significant ($p = 0.02$ and $p < 0.01$, respectively). Likewise, a significant difference in risk of progression was observed in favor of immediate endocrine therapy. The conclusion, that immediate endocrine treatment after radical prostatectomy and lymphadenectomy improves survival and reduces the risk of recurrence, is based on convincing data. On the other hand, the cancer-specific mortality after 7.1 years in the deferred group (where 81% had non-detectable PSA at randomization) is remarkably high ($16/51 = 31\%$), compared with similar series.

Another study, the EORTC 30846, also randomized node-positive patients between immediate and deferred endocrine therapy[15]. However, patients in this study did not undergo radical prostatectomy. A preliminary analysis of time to progression, defined as development of metastasis, in a subgroup of 84 patients, demonstrated a marked and highly significant difference ($p = 0.0001$) in favor of immediate therapy. From Kaplan–Meier curves, the 5-year progression rate in the two groups can be calculated as 50% versus 100%, respectively. However, according to a subsequent survival analysis of 91 patients from the same study, the marked difference in time to progression has not yet translated into a survival difference. In fact, in this analysis, where the selection of the 91 included patients remains unclear, a significant survival benefit for the deferred treatment group was reported[16]. Even though the final analysis of this study with more than 300 included patients is not yet available and one has to be cautious with interpretations of these preliminary results, the apparent discrepancy between results from this study and those from the above discussed ECOG trial[14] is striking. It may be speculated whether the 'debulking' effect of radical prostatectomy, performed in all included patients in the ECOG trial as opposed to the EORTC trial, where prostatectomy was not performed when patients were found to be node-positive, may be part of the explanation for the apparent discrepancy in the results.

A large ongoing trial program, the Early Prostate Cancer (EPC) program, was designed to compare the efficacy of bicalutamide 150 mg daily with placebo in non-metastatic prostatic cancer, as an adjuvant to therapy with primary curative intent, or as immediate hormonal therapy[17]. The study program, consisting of three individual trials (0023 in North America, 0025 in Nordic countries and 0024 in Europe, Australia, South Africa, Israel and Mexico) has completed recruitment of 8113 patients. Patients eligible for the study included those undergoing watchful waiting as well as those who had undergone curatively intended therapy (radical prostatectomy or radiation therapy). The trials have been protocolled for a combined analysis examining time to objective progression and overall survival. Approximately 54% of included patients have undergone radical prostatectomy and receive the study medication (bicalutamide or placebo) as an adjuvant therapy. Eighteen per cent have received curative radiotherapy, and approximately 28% were included as watchful waiting patients, i.e. they had not received any therapy for their prostate cancer before inclusion[18]. Median follow-up is currently 3 years. Results are eagerly awaited and are expected to provide crucial information on the role of early endocrine therapy. Because of the huge size of the study program, there will be sufficient statistical power to allow meaningful analysis of various subgroups.

Concluding remarks

With regard to efficacy, a strong case is building up for early or immediate endocrine therapy. Several of the studies discussed in this review have found immediate therapy to result in a statistically significant survival advantage in locally advanced and/or node-positive prostate cancer. Further, in metastatic patients, where the actual delay of endocrine therapy is short, and a potential survival difference therefore will be harder to recognize, a significant reduction in incidence of serious manifestations of disseminated disease has been demonstrated in the MRC trial[10].

Still, the decision to initiate early endocrine therapy continues to be a delicate balance between anti-tumor efficacy and side-effects associated with endocrine treatment. Castration therapy, either as orchidectomy or treatment with LHRH agonists, is associated with loss of sexual interest and function, loss of muscle mass, and a feeling of less energy and drive, all of which have obvious implications for quality of life[19–21]. Recently, studies have emphasized the risk for osteoporosis and osteoporotic fractures in patients enduring long-standing castration therapy. If conventional therapy is to be used to pursue the potential benefits of early endocrine therapy, ways to eliminate/significantly reduce side-effects must be explored. New treatment modalities, like antiandrogen monotherapy and intermittent androgen suppression, have interesting potentials in early and long-duration therapy because of their apparent quality-of-life benefits[22]. Moreover, both modalities seem to be especially effective relative to conventional therapy in early, non-metastatic disease.

Further to the aspect of toxicity and side-effects, both tumor-associated prognostic factors, as well as patient factors like age and preference, must be taken into consideration when deciding whether an individual patient is best served with early endocrine therapy. An elderly patient with a well-differentiated locally advanced non-metastatic prostatic tumor with slowly rising PSA may still be better served without endocrine therapy. Thus, individualized management of prostate cancer patients still leaves room for watchful waiting.

If a therapeutic strategy of immediate endocrine therapy is adopted, it will mean that a large number of asymptomatic prostate cancer patients will be treated for a much longer time. This will have obvious implications for cost. Nonetheless, the side-effects associated with hormonal therapy and their impact on quality of life remain the most important and relevant issues for the individual patient and make the decision to initiate immediate hormonal treatment an individualized trade-off between advantages and disadvantages, thereby adding itself to the long list of difficult informed treatment choices for prostate cancer patients.

References

1. Huggins C, Hodges CV. Studies on prostatic cancer. I. The effect of castration, estrogen and androgen injection on serum phosphatases in metastatic carcinoma of the prostate. *Cancer Res* 1941;1:293–7
2. Nesbit RM, Baum WC. Endocrine control of prostatic carcinoma. Clinical and statistical survey of 1,818 cases. *J Am Med Assoc* 1950;143:1317–20
3. Byar DP. The Veterans Administration Cooperative Urological Research Group's studies of cancer of the prostate. *Cancer* 1973;32:1126–30
4. Byar DP, Corle DK. Hormone therapy for prostate cancer. Results of the Veterans Administration Cooperative Urological Research Group studies. *Natl Cancer Inst Monogr* 1988;7:165–70
5. Kozlowski JM, Ellis WJ, Grayhack JT. Advanced prostatic carcinoma. Early versus late endocrine therapy. *Urol Clin North Am* 1991;18:15–24
6. van Aubel OGJM, Hoekstra WJ, Schröder FH. Early orchiectomy for patients with stage D1 prostatic carcinoma. *J Urol* 1985;134:292–4
7. Kramolowsky EV. The value of testosterone deprivation in stage D1 carcinoma of the prostate. *J Urol* 1988;139:1242–4
8. Zincke H, Bergstralh EJ, Larson-Keller JJ, *et al.* Stage D1 prostate cancer treated by radical prostatectomy and adjuvant hormonal treat-

ment. Evidence for favorable survival in patients with DNA diploid tumors. *Cancer* 1992;70 (Suppl 1): 311–23
9. Isaacs JT. The timing of androgen ablation therapy and/or chemotherapy in the treatment of prostatic cancer. *Prostate* 1984;5:1–17
10. Medical Research Council Prostate Cancer Working Party Investigators Group. Immediate versus deferred treatment for advanced prostatic cancer: initial results of the Medical Research Council trial. *Br J Urol* 1997;79:235–46
11. Kirk D. MRC study: when to commence treatment in advanced prostate cancer. *Prost Cancer Prost Dis* 1997;1:11–15
12. Bolla M, Gonzalez D, Warde P, *et al.* Improved survival in patients with locally advanced prostate cancer treated with radiotherapy and goserelin. *N Engl J Med* 1997;337:295–300
13. Granfors T, Modig H, Damber J-E, Tomic R. Combined orchiectomy and external radiotherapy versus radiotherapy alone for non-metastatic prostate cancer with or without pelvic lymph node involvement: a prospective randomized study. *J Urol* 1998;159:2030–4
14. Messing EM, Manola J, Sarosdy M, *et al.* Immediate hormonal therapy compared with observation after radical prostatectomy and pelvic lymphadenectomy in men with node-positive prostate cancer. *N Engl J Med* 1999;341:1781–8

15. Van den Ouden D, Tribukait B, *et al.* and The European Organization for Research and Treatment of Cancer Genitourinary Group. Deoxyribonucleic acid ploidy of core biopsies and metastatic lymph nodes of prostate cancer patients: impact on time to progression. *J Urol* 1993;150:400–6

16. Wijburg C, Boeken Kruger AE, van der Cruijsse I, *et al.* Immediate or delayed endocrine treatment for lymph node metastasized prostate cancer, is there a best choice? *J Urol* 1999;161 (Suppl 4):299 (abstr 1149)

17. Fourcade RO, McLeod D, Iversen P, *et al.* Can hormonal treatment be beneficial for non-metastatic prostate cancer patients? Initiation of a world-wide study. In Murphy G, Griffiths K, Denis L, *et al.*, eds. *Proceedings of First International Consultation on Prostate Cancer*, Monaco, 1996. Scientific Communication International Ltd, 1997:267–303

18. Wirth MP, Iversen P, McLeod D, *et al.* Bicalutamide (Casodex) early prostate cancer (EPC) programme – final demographic data from over 8000 randomised patients. *Eur Urol* 1999;35(Suppl 2):13 (abstr 52)

19. Herr HW, Kornblith AB, Ofman U. A comparison of the quality of life of patients with metastatic prostate cancer who received or did not receive hormonal therapy. *Cancer* 1993;71: 1143–50

20. Lucas MD, Strijdom SC, Berk M, *et al.* Quality of life, sexual functioning and sex role identity after surgical orchidectomy in patients with prostatic cancer. *Scand J Urol Nephrol* 1995; 29:497

21. Iversen P. Quality of life issues relating to endocrine treatment options. *Eur Urol* 1999;36 (Suppl 2):20–6

22. Daniell HW, Dunn SR, Ferguson DW, *et al.* Progressive osteoporosis during androgen deprivation therapy for prostate cancer. *J Urol* 2000;163:181

Antiandrogen monotherapy – better quality of life?

20

F. H. Schröder

Antiandrogen monotherapy is one of the treatment options for endocrine treatment of prostate cancer. There are two types of commercially available substances: steroidal antiandrogens of the type cyproterone acetate and non-steroidal or pure antiandrogens of the type flutamide, bicalutamide and nilutamide. Steroidal and non-steroidal antiandrogens differ fundamentally in their mechanism of action. Reviews are available[1,2]. All anti-androgens have in common is their ability to block the action of androgens at the target cell level, by interacting with their binding to the androgen receptor. Obviously, target cells are not only prostate or prostate cancer cells but also other androgen-responsive cells such as those which are responsible for the feedback mechanism with luteinizing hormone releasing hormone (LHRH) in the diencephalon. Pure antiandrogens are gonadotropic; their use leads to an elevation of plasma testosterone, which is self-limiting, probably because of the anti-gonadotropic effect of the elevated estrogen levels which result from aromatization of the increased plasma levels of testosterone. The frequently encountered gynecomastia with this form of treatment in monotherapy is also due to the same mechanism. Steroidal antiandrogens of the cyproterone acetate type are gestagenic, in addition to being antiandrogenic. Because of their gestagenic activity, they are anti-gonadotropic and, in recommended dosages, lead to a reduction of plasma testosterone about half-way between normal and castration levels. The differential mechanisms of flutamide, as an example of a pure antiandrogen, and cypro-terone acetate are well demonstrated in a short-term study of young healthy volunteers[3].

In considering the potential side-effects of different forms of endocrine treatment, an understanding of the mechanism of action is essential. For example, osteoporosis, as measured by bone mineral density, is induced by reducing testosterone and, as a result of that, male estradiol production to castration levels[4,5]. Antiandrogens will block the action of the remaining androgens at the androgen receptors in the osteoblasts just as well as in the prostate. However, antiandrogens will not interfere with the effect of increasing estrogen levels, which is likely to counteract the osteoporotic process. In a similar way, anemia may be prevented or ameliorated with the use of antiandrogens, in comparison to castration[6].

Why worry about the quality of life?

Traditionally, endocrine treatment is applied to patients with prostate cancer who suffer from metastatic disease. In these patients, the median time to clinical progression was found to be in the range of 1.5 years, while median survival is in the range of 2.5–3 years[7]. Patients with metastatic disease often have an impaired performance status, may suffer pain, experience a severe psychological impact from the know-ledge of the disease status and its potential outcome, and will usually not have much interest in libido, potency and sexual activity. For these patients, the prospect of delaying progression and of prolongation of life by endocrine treatment is a top priority. Many of the side-effects of endocrine treatment increase or show their full impact only after prolonged periods of time. Such prolonged treatment periods will result from the application of endocrine treatment to locally extensive ($T_3N \times M_0$) disease[8,9] or to patients with lymph node-positive disease. In these situations, median treatment periods of 6–8 years have been described. Early endocrine treatment, which may be the future treatment of choice if presently available data are confirmed[10,11], will usually be applied to asymptomatic men who are younger and to whom the maintenance of libido and potency is of importance. Other side-effects, such as mood changes, depression, tiredness, anemia, osteoporosis and spontaneous fractures, can be expected to increase in proportion and severity with such long treatment periods. This problem may be even further enlarged if very early endocrine treatment, such as in the management of rising levels of prostate-specific antigen (PSA) after potentially curative treatment measures, is applied.

Changing indications and changing patient populations

As elaborated above, considering the short time from diagnosis of metastatic disease to metastatic progression and to death, as well as the impact of the disease, quality-of-life considerations are of lesser importance for this group of patients. Also, the age at the occurrence of metastatic disease, as evidenced by a large number of trials, usually amounts to 70 years and older[12]. With earlier diagnosis, earlier onset of treatment and the resulting longer treatment periods, the impact on the quality of life may be expected to be of much greater importance. Future trials in these disease categories will certainly be evaluated not only with respect to overall survival, which is the obvious main endpoint of randomized clinical trials (RCT) but also with respect to quality adjusted life years (QUALYs).

What is standard endocrine treatment?

Since the mid-1980s, it was claimed that maximal androgen blockade (MAB) was the standard endocrine treatment of prostate cancer. It was expected that simultaneous testicular and adrenal androgen suppression would lead to a statistically and clinically significant advantage in overall survival. Recent data[13,14], however, clearly indicate that this is not the case. Subgroups which may benefit from this aggressive form of treatment have not been clearly and conclusively identified. Since the comparisons of MAB were performed with castration or chemical castration with LHRH analogs, these forms of treatment must now be considered standard endocrine management. Can this be considered true also for the situation of very prolonged endocrine treatment, in which quality of life has to be factored in as an endpoint? This will obviously depend on comparisons of the side-effect profiles of different forms of endocrine treatment. Patients suffering from locally extensive disease, having to anticipate endocrine treatment periods of 6–8 years, may happily accept a trade in life-time for improvements in quality of life. We may, therefore, need different definitions of standard endocrine treatment: one that applies to the management of patients with metastatic disease, in which prolongation of survival should be the main goal, and another that applies to patients with other stages of disease, in which very long treatment and survival periods are to be expected. In this situation, standard treatment should be based on survival and quality-of-life parameters. This obviously poses new challenges for clinical investigations and also for current clinical practice.

Patient populations eligible for endocrine treatment are changing rapidly. With the increased use of PSA-driven early diagnostic measures, the incidence of prostate cancer in the US and in many other countries of the world has increased drastically[15]. While this increase may be temporary, the level of incidence that will be reached as an equilibrium with yearly or less frequent but regular screening efforts is not known at this time. Under the controlled situation of the European Randomized Study of Screening for Prostate Cancer (ERSPC), section Rotterdam, the ratio between prevalence in the screening arm and incidence in the control arm amounts to 6.2. In the screening arm, the prevalence of metastatic disease is about 13-fold less than in the control arm. Eighty per cent of all diagnosed cases are locally confined and eligible for potentially curative management. In the long term, 20–30% of these men will experience a rise of PSA in spite of aggressive management and may become candidates for early endocrine management for periods of time that may be expected to exceed 10 years[16,17]. Increasing evidence suggests that early endocrine treatment may be superior to delayed endocrine treatment[8–10]. Walsh has given a recent comprehensive review of these developments[18]. This review stresses, together with other publications, the weakness of present evidence for early endocrine treatment. Consensus exists with respect to metastatic disease, where no differences between early and delayed treatment can be stated with reasonable certainty. On the other hand, all evidence with respect to possible advantages of early endocrine treatment relates to locally advanced disease or lymph node-positive disease. PSA progression after potentially curative management represents a totally different group of patients who have never been studied with respect to the early versus delayed application of endocrine management.

Side-effects and their mechanisms

Loss of libido and potency is inevitable with any form of endocrine management. However, about 20% of men under castration or antiandrogen treatment seem to remain potent and sexually active after prolonged periods of time[19,20]. Furthermore, in men with metastatic disease who were potent at the time of the initiation of endocrine treatment, it was shown that the median time to loss of sexual functions amounted to about 1 year. This opens a window for the use of either steroidal or non-steroidal antiandrogens in intermittent endocrine treatment regimens, which will be addressed later. The Kaplan–Meier projections of loss of potency in the EORTC protocol 30892, which compares, in patients with good prognostic factor metastatic disease, flutamide to cyproterone acetate monotherapy, are shown in Figure 1.

The effect of castration versus the use of estrogens in the management of prostate cancer on bone mineral density has recently been evaluated in a Scandinavian study[21]. Castration and other treatment options were also compared with respect to the occurrence of osteoporosis[4,5,22]. Available data are compatible with the possibility that normal or elevated levels of estrogens, as they are seen with estrogen treatment or with the use of pure or steroidal antiandrogens, will have a preventive effect on this important long-term side-effect. Similar mechanisms probably apply to the occurrence of anemia, which was only recently realized to be a relevant side-effect of endocrine treatment[6,23]. Anemia may be related to the frequently reported side-effect of fatigue and mood changes. The same mechanism may be applicable also to the decrease of muscle mass (muscle wasting)[24,25]. Decrease of muscle mass has been identified as the major reason for frailty associated with andropause and old age in males.

At present, we are far from understanding completely the mechanism of all the side-effects of endocrine management. Even more so, documentation of the possible prevention of given side-effects, by the application of management strategies that do not decrease testosterone to castrate levels, are largely unknown. These issues represent a research priority for future clinical studies. In the meantime, the impact on the quality of life of these side-effects can be studied and has to be described in terms of using validated questionnaires in a multicenter setting.

Antiandrogen monotherapy

As elaborated above, castration at this time must be considered standard management for metastatic prostate cancer. Early application of endocrine treatment, such as with lymph node-positive disease or $T_3N_xM_0$ disease, with or without nodal metastases, will lead to very prolonged treatment periods, and quality-of-life impact has to be factored in as an endpoint. This is even more the case if endocrine treatment is considered in the situation of rising PSA after

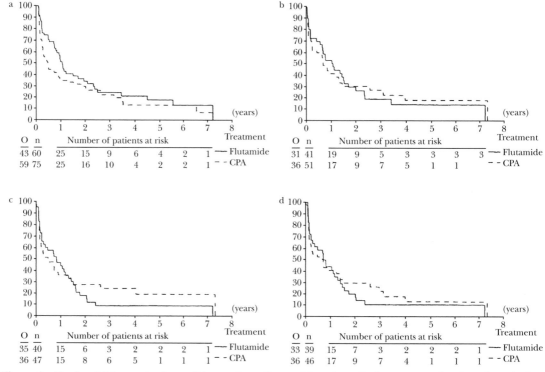

Figure 1 Kaplan–Meier projections of time to loss of sexual functions. Patients recovering functions during treatment are included. (a) Morning/night erections, $p = 0.154$; (b) sexual activity, $p = 0.907$; (c) erections with sexual excitement, $p = 0.684$; (d) orgasm, $p = 0.616$. CPA, cyproterone acetate. Reproduced with permission from *Br J Cancer* 2000;82:283–90[20]

potentially curative management. These situations will occur much more frequently than the diagnosis of metastatic disease in present and future clinical practice. However, PSA-driven early detection regimens are used.

Antiandrogen monotherapy in metastatic disease

Cyproterone acetate has never been compared head on with castration. Cyproterone acetate can be considered as standard treatment for metastatic disease because similar results were obtained in two major studies comparing this drug to either 3 mg of diethylstilbestrol or ethinylestradiol at standard dosages[26,27]. Recently, flutamide was compared head on to cyproterone acetate in monotherapy; no differences in the respective endpoints of disease-specific survival and overall survival were seen[28]. Nilutamide has not been studied adequately in

monotherapy. Bicalutamide was shown to be inferior to castration with respect to cancer-specific and overall survival in patients with metastatic disease. However, in locally extensive N_xM_0 disease, no differences in the respective endpoints are seen and advantages with respect to parameters of quality of life have been established[9].

Potentials for the use of antiandrogens in monotherapy

Antiandrogens are candidate treatments for all situations where quality-of-life considerations can be matched against survival and where survival time may be traded by patient preference against improved quality of life. This statement mainly relates to those situations where prolonged treatment periods are to be expected. Table 1 gives a comparison of side-effects encountered with the use of cyproterone

Table 1   Toxicity of flutamide, Cyproterone acetate and bicalutamide

	Flutamide (n = 154) n (%)	Cyproterone acetate (n = 156) n (%)	Bicalutamide (n = 576)* n (%)
No toxicity	34 (22.1)	89 (57.1)	
Gynecomastia and pain	65 (42.2)	11 (7.1)	224 (39.5)
Gynecomastia, all	99 (64.3)	46 (29.5)	230 (40.5)
Nausea	24 (16.8)	11 (7.7)	
Diarrhea	44 (22.6)	19 (12.2)	33 (5.8)†
ALAT and/or ASAT‡ d 2.5x	16 (10.4)	10 (6.4)	
Bilirubin 2.5x	5 (3.3)	2 (1.3)	

Other side-effects seen in > 10% of cases and in excess of castration: hot flushes (13.2%), asthenia (10.4%) *Zeneca trial 307, Tyrell et al.[29]; † nausea *and* diarrhea; ‡ALAT, alanine aminotransferase; ASAT, aspartate aminotransferase

acetate, flutamide or bicalutamide in mono-therapy. It is evident that gynecomastia, painful or not painful, is a very frequent adverse effect of antiandrogen monotherapy[29]. Flutamide has important gastrointestinal side-effects which are not seen with either cyproterone acetate or bicalutamide. In EORTC protocol 30892, a head-on comparison of cyproterone acetate and flutamide toxicity led to patients being taken off study under flutamide in 15.6%, under cyproterone acetate in 5.8% and under nilutamide in 5.8% of the study populations of 154, 156 and 576 patients, respectively. Further details are given in Chapter 21 of this issue which summarizes the results of EORTC protocol 30892.

Antiandrogens may be useful in the future use of intermittent and 'step-up' treatment schemes if their value is proven in the ongoing randomized clinical trials. In these schemes, antiandrogen monotherapy would be followed by castrations or by the use of an LHRH agonist. Considering the data shown in Figure 1, where 50% of patients remained potent and sexually active under either flutamide or cyproterone acetate, antiandrogen monotherapy may be par-ticularly useful in intermittent schemes, because, in 50% of cases, sexual functioning may be preserved continuously, independently of the duration of the on-and-off treatment periods. In these situations, antiandrogens also have the advantage of an immediate effect and also an immediate recovery from androgen suppression at the time of discontinuation of treatment.

Conclusions

The use of antiandrogen monotherapy may have advantages with respect to quality of life, especially temporary preservation of sexual functions in those patients who are treated for potentially very long periods of time. Some of the relevant side-effects, such as osteoporosis, spontaneous fractures, anemia, fatigue and loss of muscle mass, may be favorably influenced because of the elevated levels of estrogens seen with non-steroidal antiandrogen monotherapy and the maintenance of intermediate estrogen levels encountered with the use of steroidal antiandrogens. These parameters should be evaluated in prospective randomized trials. If these potential advantages in quality of life can be substantiated, antiandrogen monotherapy may develop into standard treatment in all situations where early endocrine management turns out to be applicable. Considering the mechanism of action, the quick effectiveness and the fast relief of endocrine suppression with the discontinuation of antiandrogens, this form of treatment seems to be particularly useful in intermittent treatment regimens. Ongoing studies on this issue will also have to confirm whether the use of castration or of an LHRH agonist/antagonist leads to remission whenever progression under antiandrogen monotherapy occurs. The same information will become available from ongoing randomized clinical trials studying 'step-up' schemes, where minimally invasive endocrine treatment is followed by castration or the use of LHRH agonists. These trials will also show what the value of second-line antiandrogen use may be. Evidence with respect to this issue is anecdotal at this time[30].

References

1. Schröder FH. Cyproterone acetate – mechanism of action and clinical effectiveness in prostate cancer treatment. *Cancer* 1993;72:3810–15
2. Furr BJA. The case for pure antiandrogens. *Ballières Clin Oncol* 1988;2:581–90
3. Knuth UA, Hano R, Nieschlag E. Effect of flutamide or cyproterone acetate on pituitary and testicular hormones in normal men. *J Clin Endocrinol Metab* 1984;59:963–9
4. Daniell HW. Osteoporosis after orchiectomy for prostate cancer. *J Urol* 1997;157:439–44
5. Daniell HW, Dunn SR, Ferguson DW, Lomas G, Niazi Z, Stratte PT. Progressive osteoporosis during androgen deprivation therapy for prostate cancer. *J Urol* 2000;163:181–6
6. Strum SB, McDermed JE, Scholz MC, Johnson H, Tisman G. Anaemia associated with androgen deprivation in patients with prostate cancer receiving combined hormone blockade. *Br J Urol* 1997;79:933
7. Robinson MRG, Smith PH, Richards B, Newling DWW, Pauw M de, Sylvester R. The final analysis of the EORTC Genito-Urinary Group Phase III clinical trial (Protocol 30805) comparing orchidectomy, orchidectomy plus cyproterone acetate and low dose stilboestrol in the management of metastatic carcinoma of the prostate. *Eur Urol* 1995;28:273–83
8. Bolla M, Gonzalez D, Warde P, *et al.* Improved survival in patients with locally advanced prostate cancer treated with radiotherapy and goserelin. *N Engl J Med* 1997;337:295–300
9. Iversen P, Tyrrell CJ, Kaisary AV, *et al.* Casodex (bicalutamide) 150-mg monotherapy compared with castration in patients with previously untreated nonmetastatic prostate cancer: results from two multicenter randomized trials at a median follow-up of 4 years. *Urology* 1998;51:389–96
10. Messing EM, Manola J, Sarosdy M, *et al.* Immediate hormonal therapy compared with observation after radical prostatectomy and pelvic lymphadenectomy in men with node-positive prostate cancer. *N Engl J Med* 1999;341:1781–8
11. The Medical Research Council Prostate Cancer Working Party Investigators Group. Immediate versus deferred treatment for advanced prostatic cancer: initial results of the Medical Research Council Trial. *Br J Urol* 1997;79:235–46
12. Prostate Cancer Trialists' Collaborative Group (PCTCG). Maximum androgen blockade in advanced prostate cancer: an overview of 22 randomised trials with 3283 deaths in 5710 patients. *Lancet* 1995;346:265–9
13. Prostate Cancer Trialists' Collaborative Group. Maximum androgen blockade in advanced prostate cancer: an overview of the randomised trials. *Lancet* 2000;355:1491–8
14. Eisenberger MA, Blumenstein BA, Crawford ED, *et al.* Bilateral orchiectomy with or without flutamide for metastatic prostate cancer. *N Engl J Med* 1998;339:1036–42
15. Stanford JL, Stephenson RA, Coyle LM, *et al. Prostate Cancer Trends 1973–1995, SEER Program National Cancer Institute.* National Cancer Institute Monograph 1998. *http://www.seer.img. nci.nih.gov*
16. Pound CR, Partin AW, Eisenberger MA, *et al.* Natural history of progression after PSA elevation following radical prostatectomy. *J Am Med Assoc* 1999;281:1591–7
17. Ouden D van den, Bentvelsen FM, Boevé ER, Schröder FH. Positive margins after radical prostatectomy: correlation with local recurrence and distant progression. *Br J Urol* 1993;72:489–94

18. Walsh PC, De Weese TL, Eisenberger MA. Immediate versus deferred androgen suppression in prostate cancer: evidence for deferred treatment. A structured debate. *J Urol* 2001; in press

19. Ellis WJ, Grayhack JT. Sexual function in aging males after orchiectomy and estrogen therapy. *J Urol* 1963;89:895–9

20. Schröder FH, Colette L, De Reijke TM, Whelan P and members of the EORTC Genitourinary Group. Prostate cancer treated by anti-androgens: is sexual function preserved? *Br J Cancer* 2000;82:283–90

21. Eriksson S, Eriksson A, Stege R, Carlström K. Bone mineral density in patients with prostatic cancer treated with orchidectomy and with estrogens. *Calcif Tissue Int* 1995;57:97–9

22. Wei JT, Gross M, Jaffe CA, *et al.* Androgen deprivation therapy for prostate cancer results in significant loss of bone density. *Urology* 1999;54:607–11

23. Weber JP, Walsh PC, Peters CA, Spivak JL. Effect of reversible androgen deprivation on hemoglobin and serum immunoreactive erythropoietin in men. *Am J Hematol* 1991;36:190–4

24. Bhasin S, Storer TW, Berman N, *et al.* The effects of supraphysiologic doses of testosterone on muscle size and strength in normal men. *N Engl J Med* 1996;335:1–7

25. Lamberts SW, van den Beld AW, van der Lely AJ. Endocrinology of aging. *Science* 1997;278:419–24

26. Jacobi GH. Intramuscular cyproterone acetate treatment for advanced prostatic carcinoma: results of the first multicentric randomized trial. *Proceedings Androgens and Antiandrogens,* International Symposium, Utrecht, 1982:161–9

27. Pavone-Macaluso M, Voogt HJ de, Viggiano G, *et al.* Comparison of diethylstilbestrol, cyproterone acetate and medroxyprogesterone acetate in the treatment of advanced prostatic cancer: final analysis of a randomized phase III trial of the European Organization for Research on Treatment of Cancer Urological Group. *J Urol* 1986;136:624–31

28. Schröder FH, Whelan P, De Reijke Th, Pavone-Macaluso M, Mattelaer J, Van Velthoven RF, Collette L, and members of the EORTC Genitourinary Group. Metastatic prostate cancer treated by flutamide versus cyproterone acetate. Final analysis of the European Organization for Research and Treatment of Cancer (EORTC protocol 30892). Submitted

29. Tyrrell CJ, Kaisary AV, Iversen P, *et al.* A randomised comparison of 'Casodex' (bicalutamide) 150 mg monotherapy versus castration in the treatment of metastatic and locally advanced prostate cancer. *Eur Urol* 1998;33:447–56

30. Schröder FH. Total androgen suppression in the management of prostatic cancer. A critical review. In Schröder FH, Richards B, eds. *Progress in Clinical and Biological Research,* Volume 185A. EORTC GU Group Monograph 2, Part A. *Therapeutic Principles in Metastatic Prostatic Cancer.* New York: Alan R. Liss Inc, 1985:307–17

Metastatic prostate cancer – a randomized study of cyproterone acetate versus flutamide: summary of results

21

F. H. Schröder and members of the European Organization for Research and Treatment of Cancer (EORTC) Genitourinary Group

Introduction and objectives

Prostatic cancer (PC), one of the main causes of cancer death in men, can be treated by endocrine therapy using anti-androgens. There are two classes of anti-androgens: pure, non-steroidal anti-androgens such as flutamide and steroidal anti-androgens such as cyproterone acetate[1]. In a previous study[2], it was found that men treated with flutamide monotherapy maintained libido and potency, important aspects of quality of life, over a period of a year. Cyproterone acetate, however, has been shown to be effective in reducing libido and sexual performance in sexual delinquents[3].

At present, there is clear evidence of the limited clinical value of maximal androgen blockade in the treatment of metastatic prostate cancer[4,5]. Members of the EORTC Genitourinary Group considered that it was important that a regimen was used which had the potential to conserve quality of life by preserving libido and potency for at least some of the time. It was, therefore, decided to carry out a comparative study of flutamide versus cyproterone acetate as standard treatment in previously untreated patients with metastatic prostate cancer and favorable prognostic factors.

The main objective of the study was to detect a difference of 50% in median duration of survival between the two treatments, with a power of 80%. Secondary objectives were the comparison of disease-specific survival, and time to progression and toxicity, especially with respect to the loss of libido and sexual function.

This chapter presents a summary of data which are submitted for publication[6].

Materials and methods

In a multicenter, randomized trial, patients ($n = 310$) were randomly allocated to first-line monotherapy of either flutamide (250 mg three times per day orally) or cyproterone acetate (100 mg three times per day orally). Only men with previously endocrine untreated, painless, metastatic prostate cancer and favorable prognostic factors and an absence of a recent history of active cardiovascular disease were eligible. In addition, two of the following three criteria had to be met: World Health Organization (WHO) performance status 0; alkaline phosphatase, < 2.5 times normal; $T < T_4$. The treatment scheme is shown in Figure 1.

The endpoints were survival, disease-specific survival and progression/progressive disease (PD). Using a two-sided log rank test at the 5% significance level, it was estimated that 192 events (deaths) needed to be observed to meet the main objective. Objective progression was defined as the appearance of new soft tissue or bone metastases. Subjective progression was defined as the presence of two out of three of the following parameters:

(1) An increase of acid phosphatase, alkaline phosphatase or prostate-specific antigen (PSA) to more than 2.5 times normal levels;

(2) An increase of pain by two scores;

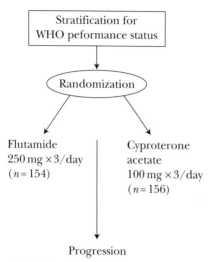

Figure 1 Study treatment scheme

(3) A worsening of the performance status by two scores.

Quality of life was evaluated using a physician-administered sexual function questionnaire, WHO performance status and pain score. Side-effects were also evaluated.

Results

Of the 310 randomized patients (154 to flutamide and 156 to cyproterone acetate), 12 (3.9%) were ineligible. Prognostic factors at entry were not balanced between the two arms with respect to age, respiratory disease, transurethral resection (TUR) prior to entry, T and G categories, ureteric obstruction and visceral metastases (differences > 2%).

The median follow-up was 5.1 years; 205 patients have died, 135 of them from prostate cancer. Median survival on flutamide versus cyproterone acetate was 3.5 years (95% confidence interval (CI) 2.7–4.3) versus 3.0 years, respectively (95% CI 2.4–3.7), translating into a hazard ratio of death of 1.26 for cyproterone acetate versus flutamide (95% CI 0.96–1.66), $p = 0.0997$. After correction for the imbalance of prognostic factors, a hazard ratio for survival of flutamide/cyproterone acetate of 1.02 (95% CI 0.73–1.41, $p = 0.9178$) was found.

Toxicity

No toxicity was seen in 34 (22.1%) patients treated with flutamide or in 89 (57.1%) patients treated with cyproterone acetate. Side-effects such as painful gynecomastia, diarrhea, nausea and liver function deterioration were significantly more frequent with flutamide than with cyproterone acetate and led more often to discontinuation of treatment (24 versus nine patients). The most frequent adverse event was painful gynecomastia, but this was only rarely a reason for discontinuing treatment.

No significant differences in time to progression, disease-specific survival and time to treatment failure have been seen so far and this includes patients who discontinued treatment for side-effects. Table 1 shows the median times and relative risk estimates for overall, disease-specific survival and first objective progression for the two treatment arms flutamide and cyproterone acetate.

The trend for superiority of flutamide in survival and disease-specific survival disappears after correction for imbalance of prognostic factors at entry (Table 2).

There were no significant differences for the parameters of sexual activity and loss of sexual functions under study. The median time to loss of spontaneous erections was about 12 months.

Discussion

This study has shown that there is no significant difference in overall survival between the two treatment arms after the required estimate of 192 events (deaths) necessary for evaluation was fulfilled. This is not, however, cancer-specific survival. Approximately one-third of all the patients are still alive. Of those who died, 65.9% died of prostate cancer, and the remainder of non-disease-related mortality, the latter being almost equal between the two treatment arms. It is, therefore, possible that disease-specific and overall survival between the two arms may change. Independent evaluation of the causes of deaths within the study may lead to a more valid analysis of prostate-cancer-specific survival.

Table 1 Median times and relative risk estimates per treatment arm for overall, disease-specific survival and first objective progression (not adjusted in imbalance for prognostic factors at entry)

Endpoint	O/N*	Median (years)	Relative risk estimates (95% CI)	p Value
Duration of survival				
Flutamide[†]	98/154	3.5		
Cyproterone acetate	107/156	3.0	1.26 (0.96–1.66)	0.0997
Disease-specific survival				
Flutamide[†]	98/154	5.1		
Cyproterone acetate	107/156	4.1	1.37 (0.97–1.92)	0.0698
Time to first objective/subjective progression				
Flutamide[†]	64/154	3.5		
Cyproterone acetate	62/156	4.5	0.90 (0.63–1.28)	0.5520
Time to first PD leading to go off study (including non-protocol PD)				
Flutamide[†]	81/154	2.5		
Cyproterone acetate	76/156	3.1	0.89 (0.65–1.22)	0.4757

*O/N, observed number of events/number of patients; [†]reference category; PD, progressive disease

Table 2 Relative risk of death adjusted for imbalance at entry

Prognostic factors	Relative risk estimate	95% CI	p Value
Treatment	1.02	(0.73–1.41)	0.9178
Age	1.39	(0.99–1.94)	0.0567
Respiratory disease	1.62	(0.89–2.95)	0.1112
G category	1.22	(0.97–1.53)	0.0944
Ureteral obstruction	2.04	(1.22–3.29)	0.0060
Visceral metastases	3.30	(1.41–7.69)	0.0058

Toxicity data indicate that flutamide treatment is clearly more toxic than cyproterone acetate treatment, with painful gynecomastia being the most predominant toxic effect (42.2%). However, this was not the main cause of withdrawal from the study. Only two patients withdrew for this reason and it appears, therefore, that gynecomastia is tolerable and acceptable to men with metastatic prostate cancer. Liver toxicity and diarrhea were the main causes of withdrawal from the study for patients treated with flutamide. The elevation of estrogen concentrations prevents a continuous rise of testosterone production and this allows sufficient growth control by androgen blockade at the receptor level. The increase in estrogen concentrations may be the cause of gynecomastia, with or without pain.

The data on sexual function are fully reported elsewhere[7] and show that there is no difference between the two treatment arms. The median time to loss of sexual activity for both drugs is approximately 1 year.

Conclusions

This trial shows no significant differences with respect to study endpoints between the treatment arms. Toxicity is more pronounced with flutamide and thus cyproterone acetate has a more favorable safety profile. Erectile function and sexual activity are not preserved with flutamide but decay slowly with both antiandrogens. While the study is mature and satisfies the criteria required (192 events necessary to evaluate survival), further analysis of death caused by prostate cancer and of treatment after progression is mandatory and ongoing.

In 1986, Klotz and colleagues reported a pilot study of 20 patients with advanced prostate cancer who were treated with intermittent diethylstilbestrol[12]. The decision on when to stop therapy was exclusively based on clinical criteria and the authors cautiously concluded that, at least, this kind of intermittent therapy was not harmful for the patients. They also highlighted that 90% of the patients regained potency and libido after discontinuation of therapy, thus suggesting a beneficial effect in terms of patients' quality of life.

Current data indicate that 50–80% of patients will achieve a nadir PSA by 3–8 months following hormonal therapy and approximately 70% of patients will achieve PSA nadirs of 4 ng/ml or less[13,14].

Goldenberg and colleagues reported a first series of highly selected patients treated with intermittent androgen ablation[15]. For patients with stage D2 disease ($n = 14$), the median time to progression and median overall survival were 108 and 166 weeks, respectively, and the patients spent about 40% of the treatment period off therapy. At first sight, these results look similar to those we would expect in patients with advanced prostate cancer, treated conventionally. However, we must be aware that patients entered in intermittent protocols are positively selected in that only those patients who reach a PSA nadir of less than 4 ng/ml after 6–8 months of continuous androgen withdrawal are treated intermittently. These patients, however, are expected to progress only after 3–3.5 years when treated continuously[13].

Nevertheless, these results indicate that, while testing an exciting scientific hypothesis, this approach can also provide adequate palliation of this group of incurable patients with advanced prostate cancer, with a potential for prolonged therapy-free intervals, resulting in improved quality of life, delay in progression to androgen independence, and reduced cost of therapy.

Several authors[13,14] have reported a significant correlation between PSA response after hormone suppression and survival and interval to progression. The actual mechanism that accounts for the fall in PSA level after hormone therapy is complex. Evidence suggests that PSA expression may be under hormonal control and changes in serum levels may be independent of tumor response[2]. Nonetheless, prognostic significance has been demonstrated for a decrease in PSA level after hormone therapy and is worth further study.

Preliminary results of studies on intermittent androgen suppression

After the initial experimental and clinical data on intermittent androgen suppression, a number of prospective randomized trials were initiated in centers and cooperative groups around the world. Some of these studies have been closed to accrual and their results are available, while others are ongoing.

All these trials share a common basic design. After registration, there is an induction period of maximal androgen blockade with anti-androgen and LHRH agonist, at the end of which those patients who have achieved a satisfactory PSA nadir are randomized to either the continuous or intermittent treatment groups. Patients in the intermittent group restart treatment when their serum PSA levels rise above a pre-established value and stop when the PSA again falls to an acceptable level. Such on–off treatment cycles are then continued until maximum androgen blockade no longer produces the desired PSA response or until progression. Since the literature contains no clear indication on the optimal length of the induction period or on the best PSA response criteria to adopt, these vary from study to study.

The European Organization for Research and Treatment of Cancer (EORTC) Genito-Urinary Group conducted a phase II feasibility trial on intermittent androgen suppression[15]. A total of 114 patients with previously untreated metastatic prostate cancer, with PSA levels above 20 ng/ml, were recruited by 15 centers over an 18-month period. Treatment consisted of bicalutamide 50 mg/day and goserelin acetate 3.6 mg every 4 weeks. Treatment was stopped if the serum PSA level declined by at least 80% of baseline values within 9 months and was restarted when the PSA level rose by 50% or more with respect to its most recent nadir value. One to seven cycles of treatment were administered, with a median of two cycles per patient. Of the patients, 77% achieved a 1st nadir after a median period of 19 weeks of treatment, and 71% of the patients, who began a second cycle of treatment, achieved a 2nd nadir after a median of 13.6 weeks of treatment. The median durations of the first and second off-treatment periods were 14.3 and 16 weeks, respectively. Up to seven cycles of treatment were administered. Quality-of-life evaluation was included in the study design and was slightly better during the off-treatment periods, even though the limited number of patients precluded definitive conclusions.

The Portuguese Cooperative Group conducted the SEUG 9401 study[16]. A total of 750 patients with newly diagnosed clinical stage T_3 and T_4 prostate cancer, with serum PSA levels between 4 and 100 ng/ml, were enrolled, of which 590 were randomized and 57 were ineligible. The induction period was 14 weeks, during which maximum androgen blockade consisting of cyproterone acetate and an LHRH agonist was administered. Patients were randomized if, at the end of the induction period, the serum PSA level had fallen to normal levels (< 4 ng/ml) or by at least 80% of baseline levels. Patients randomized to the intermittent group, whose PSA had normalized, restarted treatment when the PSA level rose to 10 ng/ml or greater in the symptomatic patient or 20 ng/ml or greater in the asymptomatic patient. Intermittent patients whose PSAs had not fallen to normal levels restarted treatment when the PSA increase was 80% of the nadir level. After a median follow-up period of 24 months, it was found that the median off-treatment period in the intermittent arm was 39 weeks and that patients with PSA nadirs ≤ 4 ng/ml remained off treatment for approximately 12 months (range 9–18 months).

Another randomized trial (TULP study protocol) included 282 previously untreated patients with T_2–T_4 N_0 M_1 or T_2–T_4 N_{1-3} M_{0-1} prostate cancer and PSA > 10 ng/ml. Maximum androgen blockade consisted of nilutamide and buserelin. Patients whose PSA levels decreased to normal after 6 months of treatment were randomized to the intermittent or continuous treatment arm. The criteria for treatment restart differed according to disease status. Patients with distant metastases restarted treatment when the serum PSA level rose to 10 ng/ml or greater and those with only lymph node metastases were replaced on treatment when the PSA level rose to 20 ng/ml or higher. Of the 282 patients entered into the study, 193 were randomized. Of the 97 patients who were assigned to the intermittent androgen suppression arm, 48 have had to restart treatment and 15 have been switched to continuous maximum androgen blockade due to failure to reach secondary PSA nadirs. The mean period off treatment was 14 months. Thirteen patients in the continuous arm and eight in the intermittent androgen suppression arm had disease progression during follow-up.

Ongoing trials

One of the largest ongoing trials on intermittent androgen suppression is the cooperative SWOG–EORTC trial which includes patients with stage D2 prostate cancer. Patients are evaluated after 7 months of maximum androgen blockade with bicalutamide and goserelin, and those with normalized PSA levels are randomized to receive either intermittent or continuous treatment. Patients on the intermittent arm restart treatment when the PSA level rises to 20 ng/ml and may again stop treatment only after 7 months of maximum androgen blockade if serum PSA levels at months 6 and 7 are normal. In this manner, intermittent patients may repeat treatment cycles until clinical progression or until failure to reach PSA normalization. The primary endpoint of this study is to determine whether patients on the intermittent androgen suppression arm have survival that is not substantially worse than those on the continuous treatment arm.

The concept of intermittent treatment is also being tested in patients with biochemical relapse after radical prostatectomy. In the industry-funded 'Relapse' trial, patients with undetectable postoperative PSA levels whose PSA level then rises to > 1 ng/ml are randomized to receive either continuous or intermittent LHRH agonist. The objectives of the study are to compare the incidence of subsequent androgen independence in the two groups and to compare side-effects and toxicity.

The Portuguese Cooperative Group is running an international study to test a novel form of intermittent treatment. Patients with T_3–T_4, M_0 and T_1–T_4, M_1 disease receive maximum androgen blockade for 14 weeks, and those who achieve PSA normalization are randomized to receive either continuous maximum androgen blockade or intermittent antiandrogen alone (cyproterone acetate 300 mg/day). The primary endpoints of this study are time to PSA failure, time to clinical progression, quality of life and survival (Study SEUG 9901).

Conclusions

Intermittent androgen suppression for the treatment of prostate cancer is one of the most interesting current areas of clinical research. The results of the more recent studies seem to indicate that intermittent treatment is feasible and provides results similar to those of continuous androgen blockade in terms of improvement of symptoms. Prolonged periods of no treatment are possible which, in addition to saving costs, theoretically lead to an improvement in quality of life. The latter needs confirmation on a large number of patients, using a formal quality-of-life evaluation.

The urological community will be anxiously waiting for the long-term results of randomized trials to see what impact intermittent androgen suppression has on disease progression and survival. If patients receiving intermittent treatment fare at least as well as those on continuous treatment, while improving quality of life and reducing costs, intermittent androgen suppression may become a standard treatment modality.

References

1. Jacobi GH. Hormonal treatment of metastatic carcinoma of the prostate. In Fitzpatrick JM, ed. *The Prostate*. Edinburgh: Churchill Livingstone, 1989:389–95
2. Leo ME, Bilhartz DL, Bergstralh EJ, *et al.* Prostate specific antigen in hormonally treated stage D2 prostate cancer: is it always an accurate indicator of disease status? *J Urol* 1991;145:802–6
3. Denis L, Murphy GP. Overview of phase III trial on combined androgen treatment in patients with metastatic prostate cancer. *Cancer* 1993;72 (Suppl):3888–95
4. Denis L. Prostate cancer. Primary hormonal treatment. *Cancer* 1993;71S:1050–8
5. Denis LJ, Griffiths K. Endocrine treatment in prostate cancer. *Semin Surg Oncol* 2000;18:52–74
6. Bruchovsky N, Rennie PS, Coldman AJ, Goldenberg SL, To M, Lawson D. Effects of androgen withdrawal on the stem cell composition of the Shionogi carcinoma. *Cancer Res* 1990;50:2275–82
7. De Marzio AM, Nelson WG, Meeker AK, Coffey DS. Stem cell features of benign and malignant prostate epithelial cells. *J Urol* 1998; 160:2381–92
8. Akakura K, Bruchovsky N, Goldenberg SL, Rennie PS, Buckley AR, Sullivan LD. Effects of intermittent androgen suppression on androgen-dependent tumors. Apoptosis and serum prostate specific antigen. *Cancer* 1993; 71:2782–90
9. Trachtenberg J. Experimental treatment of prostatic cancer by intermittent hormonal therapy. *J Urol* 1987;137:785–8

10. Noble RL. Hormonal control of growth and progression in tumors of Nb rats and a theory of action. *Cancer Res* 1977;37:82–94

11. Russo P, Liguori G, Heston WDW, *et al*. Effects of intermittent diethylstilbestrol diphosphate administration on the R3327 rat prostatic carcinoma. *Cancer Res* 1987;47:5967–70

12. Klotz LH, Herr HW, Morse MH, Whitmore WF. Intermittent endocrine therapy for advanced prostate cancer. *Cancer* 1986;58:2546–50

13. Miller JI, Ahmann FR, Drach GW, Emerson SS, Bottacchini MR. The clinical usefulness of serum prostate specific antigen after hormonal therapy of metastatic prostate cancer. *J Urol* 1992; 147:956–61

14. Matzkin H, Eber P, Todd B, Van der Zwaag R, Soloway MS. Prognostic significance of changes in prostate-specific markers after endocrine treatment of Stage D2 prostatic cancer. *Cancer* 1992;70:2302–9

15. Albrecht W, Collette L, Fava C, *et al*. Intermittent maximal androgen blockade in patients with metastatic prostate cancer – an EORTC feasibility study. In press

16. Calais da Silva F, Bono AV, Whelan P, *et al*. Phase III study of intermittent MAB versus continuous MAB: international cooperative study. *Eur Urol* 1999; 35S:54A

Section VI

Prostate cancer: advanced

Adjuvant and neoadjuvant treatment of prostate cancer

23

M. P. Wirth, M. Froehner and O. W. Hakenberg

Introduction

The cure rates, especially in patients with locally advanced prostate cancer or lymph node-positive prostate cancer, are unfavorable both after radical prostatectomy and after radiotherapy. In a multicenter study of 298 patients with clinical stage T_3 prostate cancer, the tumor-specific 10-year survival rate after pelvic lymphadenectomy with or without radical prostatectomy was only 57%[1]. Similarly, results after treatment by radiotherapy only are equally disappointing in locally advanced tumor stages[2]. Even in patients with clinically localized disease, biochemical relapse is observed in about 35% within 10 years following radical prostatectomy[3]. In stage cT_2 tumors treated with external beam radiotherapy, Pollack and Zagars[4] reported a biochemical failure rate of 30% after only 4 years. These data show that additional treatment is required in patients with a high risk of tumor recurrence in order to improve outcome after local curative treatment.

One possible treatment strategy under these circumstances consists of the so-called neoadjuvant treatment which is applied before definitive treatment with curative intent[5–8]. The intention of neoadjuvant therapy is to reduce tumor size as well as to induce apoptosis of micrometastatic cells. A different approach which has been investigated consists of an adjuvant treatment applied after potentially curative local treatment by surgery or radiotherapy. Since the primary treatment is potentially curative, studies of adjuvant therapy look at the extent to which additional, adjuvant treatment increases progression-free and overall survival.

Possibilities for adjuvant treatment modalities can be endocrine, chemotherapeutic or radiotherapeutic. The modern forms of endocrine treatment of prostate cancer offer acceptable and well-tolerated substances which also allow transient androgen withdrawal. These substances such as the luleinizing hormone (LHRH) releasing hormone analogs and the antiandrogens do not constitute an irreversible androgen withdrawal as orchidectomy does. Nor do they have the potentially life-threatening side-effects of estrogen treatment as demonstrated by the Veterans' Administration Cooperative Urological Research Group (VACURG) study[9]. Estrogen treatment has largely been abandoned for this reason. Chemotherapy was in the past shown to be of limited value in prostate cancer. Nevertheless, also in this field, studies have been undertaken to assess its value in the neoadjuvant setting prior to radical prostatectomy[10].

Since a number of new studies looking at neoadjuvant and adjuvant treatment have been published, it seems of interest to review the current concept of these two modes of additional therapy in the treatment of prostate cancer.

Neoadjuvant therapy before radical prostatectomy

In 1964, Scott[11] reported his experience with neoadjuvant orchidectomy before radical prostatectomy in 31 patients. He offered radical prostatectomy only to patients who showed a clinical response to orchidectomy and, based on his results at the time, proposed this strategy as the standard treatment for prostate cancer. In more modern times, a multitude of clinical studies have dealt with neoadjuvant treatment of localized prostate cancer in the stages T_1 and T_2. In the majority of these studies, pharmacological maximal androgen blockade was given for 3 months before radical prostatectomy was performed. Consistently, a reduction in prostate size by 30–50% and a reduction in the incidence of positive margins by 18–37%, as well as a downstaging in about 30% (Table 1), was seen[5]. However, except for one study that showed a slight delay of prostate-specific antigan (PSA) progression after neoadjuvant treatment[12], the clinical effects of neoadjuvant hormonal treatment are disappointing in the radical prostatectomy setting. Whether much longer follow-up periods will add further knowledge remains to be seen. However, at present it seems clear that neoadjuvant treatment of T_1/T_2 prostate cancer has a role only in prospective randomized trials.

For the neoadjuvant treatment of locally advanced T_3 stages before radical prostatectomy, there are only a few studies with a limited number of cases. Only one group reported a reduced incidence of positive surgical margins after neodjuvant treatment for stage cT_3 prostate cancer[13]. In one randomized study, there was a trend towards a lower clinical relapse rate in stage C prostate cancer patients treated with both neoadjuvant and adjuvant endocrine treatment, compared with those treated only with adjuvant treatment; however, the follow-up of only 2 years was too short to assess survival[14]. Altogether, it must be concluded that, at present, there is no valid

Table 1 Probability of the downstaging of locally advanced prostate cancer after neoadjuvant hormonal therapy (literature review modified according to reference 34)

Authors	n	Downstaged to $pT_1/_2(\%)$
Hellström et al. (1999)[36]	35	50
Pummer et al. (1994)[37]	25	4
Labrie et al. (1994)[38]	15	73
Schulman et al. (1994)[39]	15	27
Fair et al. (1993)[40]	55	26–40
Kennedy et al. (1992)[41]	7	29
Flamm et al. (1991)[42]	21	33
Morgan et al. (1991)[43]	36	11
Thompson et al. (1991)[44]	24	13

evidence for a beneficial role of neoadjuvant treatment before radical prostatectomy for clinical stage T_3 prostate cancer.

The protagonists of neoadjuvant hormonal treatment argue that the reason for the poor results lies in the short duration of neoadjuvant treatment of, usually, 3 months. Since a PSA decrease can be observed for up to 8 months, it is believed that neoadjuvant treatment of more than 3 months' duration might have a better effect[15,16]. This, however, is speculative and it can be concluded that at present no advantage of neoadjuvant treatment before radical prostatectomy has been consistently and convincingly demonstrated[5–7]. This also applies to any potential effect of neoadjuvant treatment on surgery; no study has demonstrated that neoadjuvant treatment reduces the complications of radical prostatectomy[6,17].

Neoadjuvant treatment before radiotherapy

Neoadjuvant hormonal therapy reduces, as already mentioned, the volume of the prostate by 30–50%. This volume reduction allows a reduction of field size and dose distribution in radiotherapy for prostate cancer thus reducing the radiation exposure of the bladder, rectum and other adjacent organs. This leads to a significant reduction of radiation-related side-effects and complications[5,18]. Similar effects of neoadjuvant treatment before permanent brachytherapy for prostate cancer have been reported[19]. However, despite these significant advantages of neoadjuvant hormonal treatment in target volume reduction and decrease in side-effects[5,19], there is, so far, no evidence that this treatment strategy improves patient survival. Significant advantages have been seen only in local tumor control[20].

Adjuvant treatment

It is the aim of adjuvant treatment after potentially curative local treatment (radical prostatectomy, radiotherapy) to improve the patients' prognosis. Adjuvant treatment strategies after surgery or radiotherapy offer the possibility of treating only those patients who are at a high risk of tumor progression. Independent risk factors for tumor progression after radical prostatectomy are the Gleason score of the prostatectomy specimen, the degree of capsular penetration and the presence of positive surgical margins[21]. According to a review by Wieder and Soloway[22], the mean risk of progression in stage T_2 prostate cancer with positive surgical margins after radical prostatectomy is around 29% with a range of 0–71%. In stage T_3 prostate cancer, the risk of progression after radical prostatectomy increases to 53% with a range of 25–90%[22]. Adjuvant treatment options after radical prostatectomy are local radiotherapy and androgen withdrawal. After primary radiotherapy, adjuvant treatment can consist only of systemic treatment.

Adjuvant treatment after radical prostatectomy

A number of studies looking at the results of adjuvant treatment in lymph node-positive patients after radical prostatectomy have been published, in particular by the group working at the Mayo Clinic in the USA. Thus, Zincke and co-workers[23] could show in a retrospective analysis that adjuvant hormonal treatment in D_1 patients significantly reduced the progression rate after radical prostatectomy. However, an improvement in overall survival was not seen. In a later publication by the same group[24], a retrospective analysis showed that only patients with diploid tumors gained a significant survival advantage from immediate versus delayed adjuvant hormonal treatment.

Recently, Messing and co-workers[25] showed in a prospective randomized trial that both progression-free and overall survival could be significantly improved in D_1 prostate cancer patients after radical prostatectomy with immediate androgen withdrawal. Conflicting data, however, have been reported by other authors[26].

The available data are much more scarce for adjuvant treatment of locally advanced prostate cancer. In our own multicentric prospective randomized trial on adjuvant treatment after radical prostatectomy for stage pT_3 prostate cancer, 139 evaluable patients underwent adjuvant treatment with flutamide and were compared with 144 controls. There was a significantly improved progression-free survival (Figure 1); the data were, however, not mature enough for the calculation of survival statistics[27]. It was noticeable, however, that a high percentage (20.1%) of the patients in the treatment arm discontinued medication owing to side-effects (Table 2).

In conclusion, it can be stated that, to date, there have been relatively few studies which demonstrate a benefit of adjuvant hormonal treatment after radical prostatectomy. Therefore, the Early Prostate Cancer Programme is of special importance. More than 8000 patients with prostate cancer have been recruited into this study (Figure 2)[28]. This study represents the largest prospective, randomized, hormonal treatment study on prostate cancer undertaken so far. The first results of patients treated in an adjuvant fashion with bicalutamide following radical prostatectomy or radiotherapy can be expected in 2001.

Adjuvant radiotherapy after radical prostatectomy

There are no prospective randomized studies investigating the results of adjuvant radiotherapy after radical prostatectomy. However, it has been shown by retrospective analyses that local recurrence can almost always be prevented by adjuvant radiotherapy[29]. In a matched-pair analysis, Valicenti and Gomella[30] found that the application of adjuvant radiotherapy to patients with adverse prognostic criteria after radical prostatectomy (high Gleason score, PSA > 10 ng/ml, seminal vesicle involvement) resulted in a significantly improved biochemical disease-free 5-year survival rate (89% versus 55%, $p = 0.002$). Improved disease control was observed above a level of 61.2 Gy[30]. However, the available non-randomized clinical trials, to date, do not show that adjuvant radiotherapy improves overall survival. There are prospective trials being undertaken at present which can be

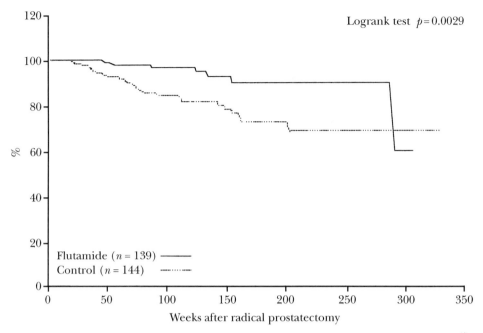

Figure 1 Tumor progression during adjuvant treatment with flutamide versus the control group[27]

Table 2 Side-effects and discontinuation of treatment: flutamide versus the control group[27]

Side-effect	Flutamide (n = 144)		Control (n = 144)	
	n	%	n	%
Gynecomastia	29	20.8	—	—
Hepatic toxicity	4	2.9	—	—
Nausea/vomiting	10	7.2	2	1.4
Discontinuation because of side-effects	28	20.1	1	0.7

expected to answer this question[31]. In the meantime, adjuvant radiotherapy after radical prostatectomy cannot be considered a standard treatment. It remains to be seen whether or not delayed secondary radiotherapy, applied when local recurrence appears, is equally effective. This approach would spare patients with positive surgical margins who might develop metastases rather than local recurrence, and those who do not develop recurrence at all, the potential complications of radiotherapy.

Adjuvant hormonal treatment after radiotherapy

The most reliable data available from prospective randomized studies concerning the role of adjuvant hormonal treatment are for patients treated primarily with radiotherapy. Bolla and co-workers[2] showed a highly significant survival advantage for adjuvant treatment with LHRH agonists after radiotherapy. Similarly, Granfors and colleagues[32] using 10-year survival data demonstrated that patients with $T_{1-4}N_{0-1}$ prostate cancer treated by radiotherapy and orchidectomy have a highly significant survival advantage over patients without adjuvant orchidectomy. However, the survival advantage was largely demonstrable for patients with lymph node metastases, while in lymph node-negative patients – possibly due to the small number of cases – this advantage could not be seen. In another prospective randomized trial published by Pilepich and co-workers[33] it was shown that patients with C and D_1 disease had a significantly better disease-specific survival with adjuvant LHRH treatment although there was no demonstrable influence

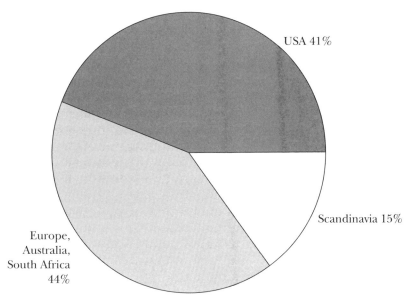

Figure 2 Distribution of recruited patients over the three trials of the Bicalutamide Early Prostate Cancer Programme[7]

on overall survival. However, subgroup analysis showed a significant survival benefit in patients with Gleason score ≥ 8 with adjuvant hormonal treatment.

It thus seems clear that adjuvant hormonal treatment after primary radiotherapy in patients at risk of progression (stages C and D_1) is beneficial[2,33–35]. It has not, however, been clearly demonstrated which role hormone therapy has on its own, as there are no studies comparing radiotherapy with hormone therapy. It is conceivable that the survival advantage of patients with adjuvant hormonal therapy after radiotherapy might be largely due to the treatment benefit of androgen withdrawal on its own.

References

1. Gerber GS, Thisted RA, Chodack GW, *et al.* Results of radical prostatectomy in men with locally advanced prostate cancer: multi-institutional pooled analysis. *Eur Urol* 1997;32: 385–90

2. Bolla M, Gonzalez D, Warde P, *et al.* Improved survival in patients with locally advanced prostate cancer treated with radiotherapy and goserelin. *N Engl J Med* 1997;337:295–300

3. Pound CR, Partin AW, Eisenberger MA, *et al.* Natural history of progression after PSA elevation following radical prostatectomy. *J Am Med Assoc* 1999;281:1591–7

4. Pollack A, Zagars GK. External beam radiotherapy for stage T1/2 prostate cancer: how does it stack up? *Urology* 1998;51:258–64

5. Tyrrell CJ. Adjuvant and neoadjuvant hormonal therapy for prostate cancer. *Eur Urol* 1999;36: 549–58

6. Scolieri MJ, Altman A, Resnick ML. Neoadjuvant hormonal ablative therapy before radical prostatectomy: a review. Is it indicated? *J Urol* 2000;164:1465–72

7. Wirth M, Froehner M. A review of studies of hormonal adjuvant therapy in prostate cancer. *Eur Urol* 1999; 36(Suppl 2):14–19

8. Lee HHK, Warde P, Jewett MAS. Neoadjuvant hormonal therapy in carcinoma of the prostate. *BJU Int* 1999;83:438–48

9. Byar DP. VACURG studies of conservative treatment. *Scand J Urol Nephrol* 1980;55(Suppl): 99–102

10. Pettaway CA, Pisters LL, Troncoso P, *et al.* Neoadjuvant chemotherapy and hormonal therapy followed by radical prostatectomy: feasibility and preliminary results. *J Clin Oncol* 2000;18:1050–7

11. Scott WW. An evaluation of endocrine therapy plus radical prostatectomy in the treatment of advanced carcinoma of the prostate. *J Urol* 1964;91:97–102

12. Aus G, Abrahamsson, PA, Ahlgren G, *et al.* Hormonal treatment before radical prostatectomy: a 3-year follow up. *J Urol* 1998;159:2013–16

13. Lee F, Siders DB, McHugh TA, *et al.* Neoadjuvant androgen ablation therapy prior to radical prostatectomy: results of a 3-year follow-up. *Endocr Relat Cancer* 1996;3:171–7

14. Homma Y, Akaza H, Okada K, *et al.* Early results of radical prostatectomy and adjuvant endocrine therapy for prostate cancer with or without preoperative androgen deprivation. The Prostate Cancer Study Group. *Int J Urol* 1999;6: 229–37

15. Gleave ME, La Bianca SE, Goldenberg SL, *et al.* Long-term neoadjuvant hormone therapy prior to radical prostatectomy: evaluation of risk for biochemical recurrence at 5-year follow-up. *Urology* 2000;56:289–94

16. Ditonno P, Battaglia M, Montironi R, *et al.* Prosit Study Group. Multicenter randomized comparative study of radical prostatectomy versus 3 and 6 months of neoadjuvant hormonal therapy (NHT) prior to radical prostatectomy (RP) in stage B and C prostate cancer. *J Urol* 2000;163(Suppl):292,A1296 (abstr)

17. Witjes WP, Schulman CC, Debruyne FM. Preliminary results of a prospective randomized study comparing radical prostatectomy versus radical prostatectomy associated with neoadjuvant hormonal combination therapy in T2–3 N0 M0 prostatic carcinoma. The European Study Group on Neoadjuvant Treatment of Prostate Cancer. *Urology* 1997;49(Suppl 3A):65–9

18. Zelefsky MJ, Harrison A. Neoadjuvant androgen ablation prior to radiotherapy for prostate cancer: reducing the potential morbidity of therapy. *Urology* 1997;49(Suppl 3A):38–45

19. Blank KR, Whittington R, Arjomandy B, *et al.* Neoadjuvant androgen deprivation prior to transperineal prostate brachytherapy: smaller volumes, less morbidity. *Cancer J Sci Am* 1999; 5:370–3

20. Pilepich MV, Krall JM, al-Sarraf M, *et al.* Androgen deprivation with radiation therapy compared with radiation therapy alone for locally advanced prostatic carcinoma: a randomized comparative trial of the Radiation Therapy Oncology Group. *Urology* 1995;45:616–23

21. Epstein JI, Partin AW, Sauvageot J, *et al.* Prediction of progression following radical prostatectomy. A multivariate analysis of 721 men with long-term follow-up. *Am J Surg Pathol* 1996;20:286–92

22. Wieder JA, Soloway MS. Incidence, etiology, location, prevention and treatment of positive surgical margins after radical prostatectomy for prostate cancer. *J Urol* 1998;160:299–315

23. Zincke H, Bergstralh EJ, Larson-Keller JJ, *et al.* Stage D1 prostate cancer treated by radical prostatectomy and adjuvant hormonal treatment. *Cancer* 1992;70:311–23.

24. Seay TM, Blute ML, Zincke H. Long-term outcome in patients with pT × N+ adenocarcinoma of prostate treated with radical prostatectomy and early androgen ablation. *J Urol* 1998;159: 357–64

25. Messing EM, Manola J, Sarosdy M, *et al.* Immediate hormonal therapy compared with observation after radical prostatectomy and pelvic lymphadenectomy in men with node-positive prostate cancer. *N Engl J Med* 1999; 341:1781–8

26. Wijburg C, Boeken Kruger AE, van der Cruijsse I, *et al.* Immediate or delayed endocrine treatment for lymph node metastasized prostate cancer, is there a best choice? *J Urol* 1999;161(Suppl): A1149 (abstr)

27. Wirth M, Frohmüller H, Marx F, *et al.* for the Study Group. Adjuvant antiandrogenic treatment after radical prostatectomy in stage C prostate cancer – preliminary results of a randomized controlled trial. *J Urol* 1997; 159(Suppl):A1308 (abstr)

28. Wirth MP, Iversen P, McLeod D, for the Study Group. Bicalutamide (Casodex® early prostate cancer programme – final demographic data from over 8000 randomised patients. *Eur Urol* 1999;35(Suppl 2):A52 (abstr)

29. Paulson DF, Moul JW, Robertson JE, *et al.* Postoperative radiotherapy of the prostate for patients undergoing radical prostatectomy with positive margins, seminal vesicle involvement and/or penetration through the capsule. *J Urol* 1990;143:1178–82

30. Valicenti RK, Gomella LG. Durable efficacy of adjuvant radiation therapy for prostate cancer: will the benefit last? *Semin Urol Oncol* 2000; 18:115–20

31. Tiguert R, Forman JD. Hussain M, *et al.* Radiation therapy for a rising PSA level after radical prostatectomy. *Semin Urol Oncol* 1999;17:141–7

32. Granfors T, Modig H, Damber JE, *et al.* Combined orchiectomy and external radio-

therapy versus radiotherapy alone for non-metastatic prostate cancer with or without pelvic lymph node involvement: a prospective randomized study. *J Urol* 1998;159:2030–4

33. Pilepich MV, Caplan R, Byhardt RW, *et al.* Phase III trial of androgen suppression using goserelin in unfavorable prognosis carcinoma of the prostate treated with definitive radiotherapy – report of RTOG protocol 85-31. *J Clin Oncol* 1997;15:1013–21

34. Schröder FH, van den Ouden D. Management of locally advanced prostate cancer. 2. Radiotherapy, neoadjuvant endocrine treatment, update 1997–1999. *World J Urol* 2000;18:204–15

35. Pollack A, Zagars GK. Androgen ablation in addition to radiation therapy for prostate cancer: is there a true benefit? *Semin Radiat Oncol* 1998;8:95–106

36. Hellström M, Häggman M, Pedersen K, *et al.* A 3-year follow-up of patients with localised prostate cancer operated on with or without pre-treatment with the GnRH-agonist triptoreline. *Br J Urol* 1996;78:432–6

37. Pummer K, Crawford ED, Daneshgari F, *et al.* Hormone pre-treatment does not affect the final pathologic stage in locally advanced prostate cancer. *Urology* 1994;44:38–42

38. Labrie F, Cusan L, Gomez J, *et al.* Downstaging of early stage prostate cancer before radical prostatectomy: the first randomised trial of neoadjuvant combination therapy with flutamide and a luteinizing hormone-releasing hormone agonist. *Urology* 1994;44:29–37

39. Schulman CC. Neoadjuvant androgen blockade prior to prostatectomy: a retrospective study and critical review. *Prostate* 1994;5(Suppl):9–14

40. Fair WR, Aprikian A, Sogani P, *et al.* The role of neoadjuvant hormone manipulation in localised prostatic cancer. *Cancer* 1993;71:1031–8

41. Kennedy TJ, Sonneland AM, Marlett MM, *et al.* Luteinizing hormone-releasing hormone downstaging of clinical stage C prostate cancer. *J Urol* 1992;147:891–3

42. Flamm J, Fisher M, Holz W, *et al.* Complete androgen deprivation prior to radical prostatectomy in patients with stage T3 prostate cancer of the prostate. *Eur Urol* 1991;19:192–5

43. Morgan WR, Myers RP. Endocrine therapy prior to radical prostatectomy for clinical stage c prostate cancer: pathologic and biochemical response. *J Urol* 1991;145(Suppl):A414(abstr)

44. Thompson IM, Lowe BA, Caroll PR, *et al.* A multi-center study of hormonal 'downstaging' of clinical stage C carcinoma of the prostate followed by radical prostatectomy. *J Urol* 1991;145(Suppl):A413 (abstr)

Gene therapy in urology

24

C. H. Bangma and R. Kraaij

Introduction: gene therapy world-wide

Gene therapy is a method for introducing genetic information or material (DNA or RNA) into the cells of a host. It opens up ways for therapeutic interventions of targets at the molecular and cellular level that are not possible by current modalities of treatment. Identification of key missing or mutated genes that, when replaced, restore normal function may have a chance of clinical success.

In experimental settings, DNA has been predominantly introduced into cells by means of bacterial plasmids. The development of various other vectors has led to more preclinical and also clinical applications from the early 1990s onwards. The first successful clinical gene therapy was reported for adenosine deaminase (ADA) deficiency in 1991. Currently, approximately 425 clinical studies have been reported world-wide (*www.whiley.co.uk*), of which many are in the field of cancer therapy (in 2459 patients, i.e. 70% of all patients treated). In Europe, 97 protocols are active and include 727 patients, i.e. more than 20% of the gene therapy effort world-wide. Up to March 2000, five of these protocols have been conducted in The Netherlands.

There are numerous vehicles used to introduce genetic material into cells. Most clinical trials use retroviral (38%) or adenoviral (20%) vectors, while in 18% of trials liposomes are included. Also, the choice of the therapeutic gene varies considerably. Suicide genes play an important role, especially for the treatment of cancer. In 16% of all patients treated with gene therapy (576 out of 3476), a cytotoxic prodrug system is or has been used in a total number of 12 trials. In 18% of patients, cytokines are the therapeutic gene, while in 26% antigens are introduced. World-wide, 77% of the gene therapy trials are in phase I or I–II, while only two trials have reached a phase III status.

The various strategies used for the application of gene therapy in the battle against cancer are also reflected in the ongoing clinical trials for urological tumors. In other words, urological tumors offer a wide range of possibilities for gene therapy.

Immunological strategies

The human immune system offers various possibilities for eliminating cells from the body that are recognized as foreign and intruding, in the context of major histocompatibility complex (MHC) I and II antigens. Protein antigens are presented to cytotoxic T-lymphocytes as small peptides (approximately 9–10 amino acids long) bound to class I molecules of the MHC. Presentation of antigens is effectively done by antigen-presenting cells or dendritic cells. Although cancer cells are autologous, and may resemble the cells from which they originate, most of them have been altered in a way that might become subjected to an immune response. The identification of tumor-associated antigens (TAAs) and specific peptide epitopes (i.e. antigenic determinants) may be useful in the development of anticancer vaccines.

In the absence of a definite set of tumor-specific antigens as a target for prostate cancer-specific immunotherapy, prostate cancer cells may serve as a basis for the production of prostate cancer vaccines. Whole-cell allogeneic vaccines combined with a strong immunological adjuvant have shown an immunological response to unknown antigens after intradermal injection[1]. In order to enhance an immunological response against autologous prostate cancer cells, tumor cells were modulated to produce cytokines, and applied as vaccines. Retroviral transfection with potent cytokines such as granulocyte–macrophage colony stimulating factor (GM-CSF)[2] or interleukin (IL)-2 prior to lethal irradiation of the tumor cells, contributed to the induction of cytotoxic T-lymphocytes in tumor models of renal cell cancer[3]. Immunological adverse reactions in the direct surroundings of malignant cells bearing (unknown) tumor antigens have been observed, and have led to the application of autologous intradermal vaccines in metastatic renal cell cancer (Food and Drug Administration (FDA) approved trials by Simons, 1993) and metastatic prostate cancer (1994)[4]. Similarly, IL-2-infected autologous vaccines against prostate cancer have been made and applied (FDA-approved trial by Paulson 1995).

Instead of an *ex vivo* approach, removing the cancer cells from the patient and infecting them with cytokine-producing vectors, the local production of cytokines by direct intratumoral injection of gene therapeutic vectors coding for these cytokines has been attempted. For prostate cancer, adenoviral vectors coding for IL-2 have been applied in studies by Beldegrun[4] and by Trachtenberg[4]. Other cytokines, like IL-12, appear to be promising in an experimental setting for adenovirus-based gene therapy, resulting in tumor rejection and regression of established metastases[5].

The immune response is mediated by antigen-presenting cells, such as dendritic cells, and effector cells, such as tumor-infiltrating and cytotoxic lymphocytes. Modulating these cells may result in efficient tumor reduction. The enhancement of the immunological response by IL-2 is being used to stimulate tumor-infiltrating lymphocytes (TILs), as was done for renal cell cancer by infecting TILs with adenoviral IL-2[6]. An adoptive immunological approach with activated lymphocytes expressing human leukocyte antigen (HLA)-B7 after priming with anti-CD3 (FDA-approved trial by Fox, 1995) has been initiated for renal cell cancer. HLA-B7 has also been introduced in

renal cell cancers as a plasmid, and combined with low-dose IL-2[7] (FDA-approved trial by Figlin 1995).

To target antigen-presenting dendritic cells to tumor-associated antigens and to initiate a tumor-specific immunological response, dendritic cells have been transfected with viral vectors coding for TAAs. Although these antigens might not be disease-specific, their tissue specificity might induce the warranted effect of reducing tumor load. For prostate cancer, antigens such as prostatic acid phosphatase (PAP) and prostate-specific antigen (PSA) have been used to target the cellular immune response by T-lymphocytes towards prostatic cells[8,9]. A vaccinia virus coding for PSA was injected intradermally in patients with prostate cancer in order to have PSA epitopes (oligopeptides) presented by dermal dendritic cells (FDA-approved trials[4] in patients with biochemical recurrence after radical prostatectomy by Chen 1995, Kufe 1996, Sanda 1997). For prostate-specific membrane antigen (PSMA) pulsed dendritic cell experiments led to the conduction of a clinical phase I trial in men with hormone-refractory prostate cancer[10]. Although these antigens may present on various non-prostatic cells, no significant toxicity was observed. Immune reactivity against two PSMA-derived oligopeptides was detected in HLA-A2-positive patients infused with pulsed dendritic cells. In some patients, a PSA decrease was observed, as well as a partial response. These results have initiated a phase II clinical study. For renal cell cancer, a phase I study is anticipated based on the tumor-associated antigen G-250[11].

Various other TAAs have been postulated as immunological targets for prostate cancer, and in a panel of prostatic and non-prostatic benign and malignant tissues, various antigens have been screened for their possible application in the context of immunotherapy[12]. From the 30 antigens screened, GM-2, Thompson–Friedenreich (TF), Tn, sTn, human chorionic gonadotrapin (hCG)-β, MUC-1, MUC-2, Kallikrein specific antigen (KSA) and PSMA were selected as the best candidates based on the intensity and the specificity of expression on primary and metastatic prostate cancer cells.

T-cells would have to be triggered by antigen-presenting cells that offer these prostatic antigens in the context of MHC class I antigens. Unfortunately, especially poorly differentiated cells may lose their MHC expression, resulting in an escape from the immune system. Upregulation of these and related co-stimulatory antigens, and of TAAs by cytokines, provides a possibility for restoring immune recognition[13]. A combination of antigen presentation with cytokine expression has been shown in a trial of an intramuscular vaccination with a vaccinia virus coding MUC-1 (a previously mentioned prostate cancer antigen, Figlin 1998) and IL-2 in patients with prostate cancer cells expressing the antigen MUC-1.

Correction of missing or mutated genes: repair

The repair of genetic alterations found in tumor cells is considered a target especially restricted to gene therapy. Mutated genes have been identified as the basis for many metabolic diseases, and have been identified in the histological sequence from dysplasia to tumor. Various tumor suppressor genes and oncogenes have also been described for urological cancers. The absence of the *p53* tumor-suppressor gene, which codes for a key molecule in the apoptotic pathway, has been detected in up to 50% of prostate[14] and bladder cancers[15]. Replacement of this gene by vectors coding for its wild type by intratumoral injection for prostate cancer (FDA-approved trial[4] by Logothetis 1997) is ongoing. For bladder cancer, studies with the instillation of adenoviral vectors coding for *p53* (FDA-approved trial[4] by Pagliaro 1997) and retinoblastoma gene (FDA-approved trial[4] by Small 1996) in patients with locally advanced and metastatic bladder cancer are ongoing. For the oncogene c-*myc*, an antisense RNA approach was chosen in a clinical phase I trial for prostate cancer (Steiner, 1995)[4]. The antisense RNA stretch, intratumorally delivered by means of a retroviral vector, blocks the translation of the oncogene RNA.

Numerous genetic alterations have been identified in prostate cancer tissues, and the choice to correct for one or more genetic changes is difficult, and may ultimately not bring the expected success. In clinical prostate cancer, the absence of the tumor-suppressor gene *PTEN* is regularly found in up to 50% of cells (similar to *p53*), especially in poorly differentiated tumors. *PTEN* is located on chromosome 10, q23.3. In Cowden disease, germline mutations of *PTEN* lead to hamartomas at multiple sites, and predisposition to various sporadic tumors (neuroblastomas, endometrial and prostate carcinomas). *PTEN* mutations and deletions have also been reported in four out of 11 xenografts available in our institute (deletions in PC-133, PC-324, PC-295 and PC-EW, nonsense mutations in PC-82 and PC-346, and a frame shift mutation in PC-374[16]. The function of *PTEN* is not completely known, but it is involved in a novel phospholipid signal-transducing pathway that plays a role in apoptosis and cell-cycle regulation. *PTEN* is also involved in cell adhesion, migration and differentiation. *PTEN* is a protein phosphatase, dephosphorylating inositol phospholipids (PtdIns-3-P). It is linked to two oncogenes, *PI-3-K* that can phosphorylate PtdIns, and AKT/PKB, which is a downstream target of PtdIns-3-P[17]. In Rotterdam, research on adenovirus-delivered *PTEN* (Adv-*PTEN*) in human prostate cancer cells *in vitro* showed a reduction in survival and an increase in apoptosis compared to Adv-*p53* and control vector Adv-*EGFP* (Figure 1a). *Ex vivo* infected prostate cancer cells with identical vectors, and orthotopically injected into the prostates of nude mice, showed a delayed tumor growth for Adv-*PTEN* compared to Adv-*p53* (Figure 1b), as measured by transrectal ultrasonography.

An interesting approach for the application of 'repair' genes for the treatment of urological cancers is the introduction of the multiple drug resistance gene by retroviral vectors in blood stem cells in patients undergoing chemotherapy in order to protect the bone marrow against toxicity and to increase the chemotherapeutic dose. This has been performed for germ cell tumors (FDA-approved trial[4] by Cornetta 1997), and for bladder tumors in Rotterdam (Mickisch 1995[4]).

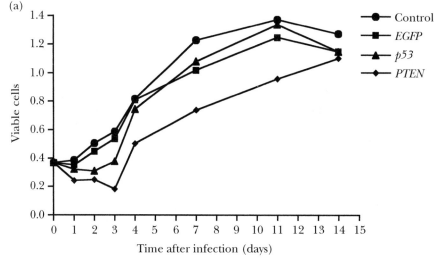

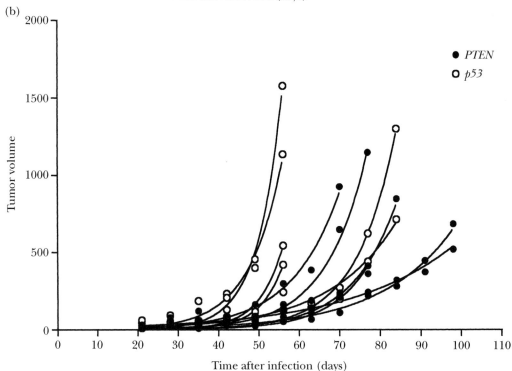

Figure 1 (a) *In vitro* cell survival of PC-346C human prostate cancer cells after infection (MOI 50) by adenoviral vectors coding for *PTEN* (Adv-*PTEN*) compared to Adv-*p53* and control vector Adv-*EGFP*. (b) *In vivo* tumor growth of PC-346C human prostate cancer cells after *ex vivo* infection with identical vectors and orthotopic injection in nude mice

Suicide genes

The concept of the application of suicide genes in a prodrug system has been the subject of extended research, and has led to the local introduction of adenoviral vectors coding for thymidine kinase (Adv-*tk*), followed by an intravenous course of ganciclovir (GCV). After transcription of the *tk* gene, thymidine kinase converts GCV in a toxic phosphorylated nucleotide analog, which subsequently blocks the transcription of DNA. An important advantage of such systems is the presence of a so-called bystander effect, in which toxic metabolites are transferred to neighboring cells resulting in cell death. This compensates for the relatively restricted number of virally infected cells after local injection into the prostate. A phase I study was performed in patients that failed locally after radiotherapy for prostate cancer (FDA-approved trial[4] by Scardino 1997). Only minimal spread was observed *in vivo*[18], and, in humans, excretion of the replication defective vector was observed in urine for a maximum of 10 days[19]. This study was followed by a second phase I–II study in which the delivery of the intraprostatically injected vector was studied in the radical prostatectomy specimens of patients with confined prostate cancer but at risk for capsular penetration of the tumor (FDA-approved[4] trial by Kadmon 1998). A similar protocol was performed in Rotterdam, in which the immunological responses, which occur due to the cytopathic effects of the vector in combination with the prodrug, were also analyzed.

In the vectors described so far, the transgene has been placed under the transcriptional control of a strong viral promoter, that of respiratory syncytial virus (RSV) or cytomegalovirus (CMV). Osteocalcin is a protein expressed and upregulated in numerous solid tumors, with its expression being further elevated in androgen-independent prostate cancers. By placing the cytotoxic *tk* under the control of the osteocalcin promoter, *tk* is transcribed especially in the cells in which osteocalcin is high. This was found to be effective in destroying prostate cancer cell lines *in vitro* and prostate tumor xenografts *in vivo* in both subcutaneous and bone sites. Via use of the osteocalcin promoter, the supporting bone stromal cells are co-targeted when the prostate cancer interdigitates with bone stroma at the metastatic skeletal sites. A phase I trial with this vector has been carried out[20].

Apart from the *tk*-GCV, various cytotoxic prodrug systems are available, and their efficacy might be variable in different tumors or models[21,22].

All of the previously discussed viral vectors have been made replication deficient by deleting the early genes of replication needed to initiate the replication pathway of the virus. In doing so, not only can the space made available in the viral genoma by the deletion be used for the insertion of therapeutic genes, but, clinically more important, this also protects the host against an overwhelming viral infection with a virus carrying a transgene. A very different approach to gene therapy, therefore, has been initiated by application of a replication-competent adenovirus, in which its replication has been made dependent on the tissue-specific PSA promoter[23] (FDA-approved trial[4] by Simons, 1998). Viral replication, and subsequent intrinsic cell death, only occurs when the natural genes for early replication are transcribed, when initiated by the PSA promoter, and, therefore, in an androgen-responsive prostate cell. The success of this method may be limited by the fact that vectors will not be active in androgen-independent, often poorly differentiated, aggressive cancer cells. On the other hand, transcription and viral replication may occur in few non-prostatic cells in which the PSA promoter is active.

Developments in experimental gene therapy

Adenoviruses have various advantages, which are the cause for their widespread use as vectors in gene therapy. The vectors are relatively easy to handle and to manipulate in an experimental setting, and can be produced in high concentrations. Importantly, adenoviruses infect cells in any phase of the cell cycle, in contrast to retroviruses that need a dividing cell. This is, theoretically, of major interest in slow-growing tumors. However, one of the disadvantages of using adenoviral vectors for the treatment of a particular cancer is their lack of specificity due to their general tropism for epithelial tissues. Therefore, efforts have been made to target these vectors in various ways to the organ or the tissue of choice. In the case of the prostate, the technique of physical targeting by intraprostatic injection under transrectal ultrasonic control is not very difficult.

Physical targeting limits the application of gene therapeutic treatment to identified and accessible foci of tumors. For systemic application of vectors, other forms of targeting to prostatic tissue are needed. To enhance prostate specificity, modification of the adenoviral vector as a vehicle and the ways of gene delivery are being studied. The current methods of targeted vector-mediated therapy can be distinguished roughly as transcriptional targeting, conditional replication and transductional targeting.

Transcriptional targeting

To improve specificity towards prostatic tissues, transcription targeting by means of therapeutic gene delivery under the control of a prostate-specific promoter has been assessed[24]. In this way, the transcription of the gene of interest will only occur under intracellular conditions in which the tissue-specific promoter is activated. For the PSA promoter this implies, for example, the presence of androgens, next to an adequate set of still marginally known transcription factors. Subsequently, this means that in androgen-independent prostate cancer cells the transcription of the gene of interest might be insufficient. Although tissue specificity has been obtained by the use of the androgen-dependent PSA promoter in PSA-transgenic mice, the expression of the gene delivered appears to be somewhat limited[25]. To enhance the expression in prostatic tissues, the PSA promoter has been successfully coupled to a yeast promoter[26]. Other specific promoters, like that of PSMA, and of human kallikrein-2 (hK2, another member of the kallikrein protease family to which PSA belongs), are currently under investigation.

Transductional targeting

Since the transport vehicle, i.e. the vector, is dependent for its entry into target cells on adhesion to specific receptors on the cell membrane, this mechanism has been identified as another possibility for targeting prostatic tumor cells.

Normally, the Coxsackie adenoviral receptor (CAR) mediates adenoviral attachment to cells, and various integrins, such as $\alpha v\beta_3$ and $\alpha v\beta_5$, play a role in internalization of the virus. Cancer cells may show a reduced receptor concentration of CAR, which may lead to a decreased infectivity, and therefore efficacy, of the virus. It would be of interest to increase the internalization of vectors into cancer cells in general or, more specifically, into prostate cancer cells by a higher transduction efficacy.

The number of CARs is reduced in primary prostate cancer cells, and may be completely absent in flow cytometric analysis of poorly differentiated, metastatic cell lines. Results from our laboratory show that expression of adenovirus-mediated reporter genes was greatly reduced in these cell lines, in contrast to well-differentiated prostate cancer cells *in vitro*. In order to enhance infection of tumor cells with reduced CAR expression, a method was developed to direct adenoviruses to other receptors that might be more available on the surface of these cells. Theoretically, these might be receptors that are upregulated on cancer cells in general or, preferably, on prostate cancer cells. One method used to accomplish this retargeting by transductional targeting involves the production of bispecific antibodies. The antibody blocking the viral knob (normally directed at CAR) is conjugated to an antibody that is directed at a membrane receptor of choice. The fibroblast growth factor receptor (FGFR) was used successfully to retarget the adenoviral vector with bispecific antibodies to Kaposi cells *in vitro*[27], and in an ovarian tumor model equivalent survival rates were achieved with a 10-fold lower dose of the FGF2 redirected Ad/CMV/tk compared with the unmodified vector[28]. The epidermal growth factor receptor (EGFR) appeared to be an adequate target for adenoviral retargeting in glioma cells[29]. EGFR is present on most epithelial cells, but seems to be enhanced in concentration on tumor cells, including prostate cancer cells. The number of binding sites on androgen-independent DU-145 prostate cancer cells was 10-fold higher compared to the androgen-dependent LnCAP cells. In adenocarcinoma of the colon, retargeting of the adenoviral vector to the pan-carcinoma epidermal cellular adhesion molecule (EpCAM) membrane antigen by a conjugate made from α-323 antibody was successful in increasing expression of a reporter gene compared to controls[30]. In our laboratory, transductional targeting of an adenoviral vector coding for *EGFP* with EpCAM conjugate showed an increased transgene expression in especially poorly differentiated prostate cancer cells, PC-3, compared to non-targeted adenoviral vectors (Figure 2a). Retargeting by bispecific antibodies to PSMA with the PSMA antibody J-591 (kindly obtained from Dr N.H. Bander, Cornell University, New York, USA) showed that the specificity of adenoviral vectors to well-differentiated prostatic cells might be enhanced, but the expression of the transgene *EGFP* was decreased compared to non-targeted vectors (Figure 2b).

A different way to alter the target of the adenoviral vehicle is by changing the adenoviral coat protein. This penton base contains the peptide motif RGD that mediates binding to the integrin cell surface receptors $\alpha v\beta_3$ and $\alpha v\beta_5$. These integrins then mediate adenovirus internalization. In order to target tissue-specific integrin receptors, wild-type viral RGD peptide motifs were replaced by newly developed penton base chimeras that recognized $\alpha v\beta_3$ and $\alpha 4\beta 1$-specific peptide motifs[31]. For prostate cancer, no applications have been published so far.

It remains to be seen whether the integral membrane proteins like PSMA or prostate-specific stem cell antigen will be adequate not only as targets for transductional targeting, but, at the same time, also for organ-specific targeting. It is likely that soon methods will be available to genetically modify the adenoviral knob in order to produce vectors, which stably express a target molecule on their surface, avoiding the need for a chemical conjugate.

Immunological limitations

Next to its lack of cell specificity, a further disadvantage of the clinical use of adenoviral vectors is the presence of circulating adenoviral antibodies in humans against the most commonly used vector Adv 5. Although, so far, no limitations to the efficiency of the sole or repeated local injection of the vector have been reported in clinical studies[32], it is expected that the efficiency of systemic injections will be reduced, owing to a rapid inactivation of the vector by the immune system.

The search for a (initially) less immunogenic vector continues, and various candidates might be at hand. The family of adenoviridae contains several members that do not show human tropism, and therefore lack a specific antibody. Immunogenicity can be reduced by the reduction of viral genes in 'gutless' vectors that lack most genes coding for the capsid proteins. Other non-human viruses might become candidates for gene therapy in order to avoid the inactivating effects of circulating antibodies on first application.

Conclusion

It is obvious that there is no general, uniform, method for approaching urological cancers. Initially, the emphasis of clinical trials has been in the field of renal cell cancer, since hardly any treatment, except surgery, can be expected to be successful in localized disease. The unique tissue-specific properties of prostate cancer offer a means of continuing research into targeted approaches.

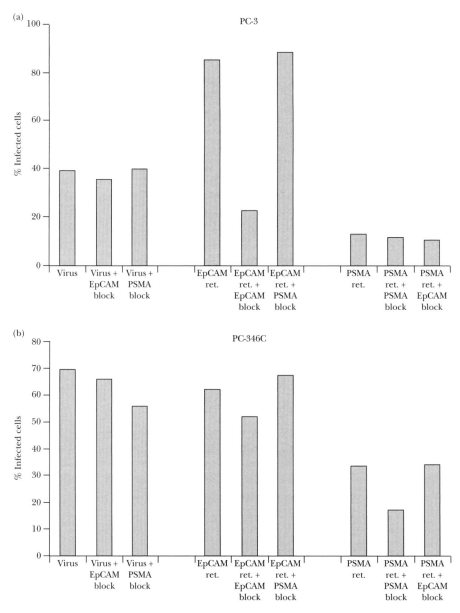

Figure 2 Percentage of infected cells by FACS analysis of *EGFP*; transductional targeting with epidermal cellular adhesion molecule (EpCAM)- or prostate-specific membrane antigen (PSMA)-conjugate of an adenoviral vector coding for *EGFP*. An increased transgene expression is seen after retargeting to EpCAM in especially poorly differentiated prostate cancer cells PC-3 compared to non-targeted adenoviral vectors (a, lane 4 versus lane 1). The retargeted (ret.) vectors show specificity for the targeted surface receptors, as illustrated by the specific blocks with antibodies. PSMA-retargeted vectors do not show increased transduction in well-differentiated PC-346C cells (b, lane 7 versus lane 1) but the retargeting may enhance prostate specificity

References

1. Hrouda D, Baban B, Dunsmuir WD, *et al.* Immunotherapy of advanced prostate cancer: a phase I/II trial using Mycobacterium vaccae (SRL172). *Br J Urol* 1998;82:568–73

2. Nigam A, Yacavone RF, Zahurak ML, *et al.* Immunomodulatory properties of antineoplastic drugs administered in conjunction with GM-CSF-secreting cancer cell vaccines. *Int J Oncol* 1998;12:161–70

3. Dranoff G, Jaffee E, Lazenby A, *et al.* Vaccination with irradiated tumor cells engineered to secrete murine granulocyte–macrophage colony-stimulating factor stimulates potent, specific, and long-lasting anti-tumor immunity. *Proc Natl Acad Sci USA* 1993;90:3539–43

4. Office of Biotechnology Activities of the National Institute of Health. www.4.od.nih.gov

5. Nasu Y, Bangma CH, Hull GW, *et al.* Adenovirus-mediated interleukin-12 gene therapy for prostate cancer: suppression of orthotopic tumor growth and pre-established lung metastases in an orthotopic model. *Gene Ther* 1999;6:338–49

6. Mulders P, Tso CL, Pang S, *et al.* Adenovirus-mediated interleukin-2 production by tumors induces growth of cytotoxic tumor-infiltrating lymphocytes against human renal cell carcinoma. *J Immunother* 1998;21:170–80

7. Rini BI, Selk LM, Vogelzang NJ. Phase I study of direct intralesional gene transfer of HLA-B7 into metastatic renal carcinoma lesions. *Clin Cancer Res* 1999;5:2766–72

8. Peshwa MV, Shi JD, Ruegg C, *et al.* Induction of prostate tumor-specific CD8(+) cytotoxic T-lymphocytes *in vitro* using antigen-presenting cells pulsed with prostatic acid phosphatase peptide. *Prostate* 1998;36:129–38

9. Correale P, Walmsley K, Nieroda C, *et al. In vitro* generation of human cytotoxic T lymphocytes specific for peptides derived from prostate-specific antigen [see comments]. *J Natl Cancer Inst* 1997;89:293–300

10. Salgaller ML, Tjoa BA, Lodge PA, *et al.* Dendritic cell-based immunotherapy of prostate cancer. *Crit Rev Immunol* 1998;18:109–19

11. Bolhuis RL, Willemsen RA, Lamers CH, *et al.* Preparation for a phase I/II study using autologous gene modified T lymphocytes for treatment of metastatic renal cancer patients. *Adv Exp Med Biol* 1998;451:547–55

12. Zhang S, Zhang HS, Reuter VE, *et al.* Expression of potential target antigens for immunotherapy on primary and metastatic prostate cancers. *Clin Cancer Res* 1998;4:295–302

13. Bander NH, Yao D, Liu H, *et al.* MHC class I and II expression in prostate carcinoma and modulation by interferon-alpha and -gamma. *Prostate* 1997;33:233–9

14. Eastham JA, Stapleton AMF, Gousse AE, *et al.* Association of p53 mutations with metastatic prostate cancer. *Clin Cancer Res* 1995;1:1111–18

15. Van Brussel JP, Mickisch GH. Prognostic factors in renal cell and bladder cancer. *BJU Int* 1999;83:902–8, quiz 908–9

16. Vlietstra RJ, van Alewijk DC, Hermans KG, *et al.* Frequent inactivation of PTEN in prostate cancer cell lines and xenografts. *Cancer Res* 1998;58:2720–3

17. Cantley LC, Neel BG. New insights into tumor suppression: PTEN suppresses tumor formation by restraining the phosphoinositide 3-kinase/AKT pathway. *Proc Natl Acad Sci USA* 1999;96:4240–5

18. Timme TL, Hall SJ, Barrios R, *et al.* Local inflammatory response and vector spread after direct intraprostatic injection of a recombinant adenovirus containing the herpes simplex virus thymidine kinase gene and ganciclovir therapy in mice. *Cancer Gene Ther* 1998;5:74–82

19. Herman JR, Adler HL, Aguilar-Cordova E, *et al. In situ* gene therapy for adenocarcinoma of the prostate: a phase I clinical trial. *Hum Gene Ther* 1999;10:1239–49

20. Koeneman KS, Kao C, Ko SC, *et al.* Osteocalcin-directed gene therapy for prostate-cancer bone metastasis. *World J Urol* 2000;18:102–10

21. Shirakawa T, Gardner TA, Ko SC, *et al.* Cytotoxicity of adenoviral-mediated cytosine deaminase plus 5-fluorocytosine gene therapy is superior to thymidine kinase plus acyclovir in a human renal cell carcinoma model. *J Urol* 1999;162:949–54

22. Aghi M, Hochberg F, Breakefield XO. Prodrug activation enzymes in cancer gene therapy. *J Gene Med* 2000;2:148–64

23. Rodriguez R, Schuur ER, Lim HY, *et al.* Prostate attenuated replication competent adenovirus (ARCA) CN706: a selective cytotoxic for prostate-specific antigen-positive prostate cancer cells. *Cancer Res* 1997;57:2559–63

24. Gotoh A, Ko SC, Shirakawa T, *et al.* Development of prostate-specific antigen promoter-based gene therapy for androgen-independent human prostate cancer. *J Urol* 1998;160:220–9

25. Cleutjens KB, van der Korput HA, Ehren-van Eekelen CC, *et al.* A 6-kb promoter fragment mimics in transgenic mice the prostate-specific and androgen-regulated expression of the

endogenous prostate-specific antigen gene in humans. *Mol Endocrinol* 1997;11:1256–65

26. Segawa T, Takebayashi H, Kakehi Y, *et al.* Prostate-specific amplification of expanded polyglutamine expression: a novel approach for cancer gene therapy. *Cancer Res* 1998;58:2282–7

27. Goldman CK, Rogers BE, Douglas JT, *et al.* Targeted gene delivery to Kaposi's sarcoma cells via the fibroblast growth factor receptor. *Cancer Res* 1997;57:1447–51

28. Rancourt C, Rogers BE, Sosnowski BA, *et al.* Basic fibroblast growth factor enhancement of adenovirus-mediated delivery of the herpes simplex virus thymidine kinase gene results in augmented therapeutic benefit in a murine model of ovarian cancer. *Clin Cancer Res* 1998; 4:2455–61

29. Miller CR, Buchsbaum DJ, Reynolds PN, *et al.* Differential susceptibility of primary and established human glioma cells to adenovirus infection: targeting via the epidermal growth factor receptor achieves fiber receptor-independent gene transfer. *Cancer Res* 1998; 58:5738–48

30. Haisma HJ, Pinedo HM, Rijswijk A, *et al.* Tumor-specific gene transfer via an adenoviral vector targeted to the pan-carcinoma antigen EpCAM. *Gene Ther* 1999;6:1469–74

31. Wickham TJ, Carrion ME, Kovesdi I. Targeting of adenovirus penton base to new receptors through replacement of its RGD motif with other receptor-specific peptide motifs. *Gene Ther* 1995;2:750–6

32. Shalev M, Kadmon D, Teh BS, *et al.* Suicide gene therapy toxicity after multiple and repeat injections in patients with localized prostate cancer. *J Urol* 2000;163:1747–50

Non-endocrine systemic approaches for prostate cancer: current status and future directions

25

M. A. Eisenberger

Introduction

Over the past few years, the experience with chemotherapy in androgen-independent prostate cancer strongly suggests that this is not a highly chemoresistant disease. Response rates are now consistently reported in the range of 40–70% with various chemotherapeutic regimens. Ongoing phase III trials evaluating the effects on survival of some of the most promising regimens are in progress. In addition, an increased understanding of the biology of cancer has provided the opportunity for the discovery of new agents specifically designed to target various distinct, critical biological mechanisms involved in cancer progression and metastasis. Furthermore, the increased understanding of molecular mechanisms involved in the complexities of cancer cell proliferation and differentiation has resulted in several new compounds, which target important molecular steps and which are in active clinical development at the present time. Tumor vaccines, acting as tumor-specific immune stimulants or designed to replace critical molecularly altered genes or gene products identified under the umbrella of 'gene therapy', have been shown to be feasible treatments, which are in active development in patients with various malignancies, including prostate cancer.

As such new modalities of treatment are identified, it is becoming increasingly clear that their development constitutes a major challenge to clinical investigators. Among the various issues is to establish the most appropriate clinical setting for testing, selection of adequate dose/schedules of treatment and

identification of feasible endpoints to quantify treatment effects. For example, agents classified broadly as anti-metastatic drugs are more likely to be effective before the establishment of clinically evident metastasis. Similarly, appropriate doses may not necessarily represent the highest tolerable dose (as with cytotoxics) and prolonged drug administration schedules make better sense from the biological point of view. It is also likely that the most adequate endpoints to evaluate treatment effects with anti-metastatic compounds are better expressed as delay in tumor progression as opposed to the standard approach with conventional cytotoxic agents, which involves the evaluation of tumor shrinkage. In this review, we summarize the experience with some of the most active conventional cytotoxic regimens and outline some of the most promising new approaches currently in clinical development.

Current experience with cytotoxic chemotherapy

Table 1 summarizes the recent experience with some of the most commonly used chemotherapeutic regimens. Current data demonstrate that taxanes are the most active compounds for the treatment of prostate cancer, either in combination with other compounds or as single agents, and represent the critical component of the most active treatment regimens. In view of the fact that the initial studies conducted with these compounds employed mostly combination regimens, the single-agent experience has only evolved more

Table 1   Recent experience with taxane-based regimens

Regimen	PSA response	Measurable responses
Taxotere[34] 75 mg/m^2 every 3 weeks	25/35	7/25
Taxotere[40] 75 mg/m^2 every 21 days	5/12	Unclear
EMCYT 280 mg q.6 × 5 doses (1 day) + Taxotere 70 mg/m^2 every 21days[35]	12/27	2/11
EMCYT 10 mg/kg/day × 5 days[36] + Taxotere + 70 mg/m^2 + low-dose hydrocortisone every 21 days	11/19	5/9
EMCYT 10 mg/kg/day × 5 days + Taxotere 60–80 mg/m^2 every 21 days[37]	21/33	5/28
Taxol 150 mg/m^2 in 1 hour weekly × 6 weeks every 8 weeks[41]	6/12	2/4
EMCYT 10 mg/kg days 1–14 + Taxol 135 mg/m^2 over 1 hour on day 2 + Etoposide 100 mg days 1–7[38]	26/37	10/22
EMCYT 600 mg/m^2 daily + Taxol 120 mg/m^2/96 hours[39]	17/32	4/9

EMCYT, estramustine phosphate

recently. Initial studies employed estramustine phosphate in combination with various chemotherapeutic agents. Estramustine phosphate is a nitrogen mustard derivative of estradiol-17-β phosphate which has demonstrated limited single-agent activity in this disease. This drug has been shown in preclinical evaluation to exert its cytotoxic activity through microtubular inhibition[1] and binding to nuclear matrix[2]. In an attempt to enhance the cytotoxicity of estramustine phosphate, investigators combined this agent with other drugs which also exert their cytotoxic effects at the level of the microtubule, such as vinblastine and taxol (Table 1). Similarly, it has been shown that etoposide acts synergistically with estramustine phosphate by affecting the nuclear matrix[3]. Indeed, initial clinical trials testing the combination of estramustine plus vinblastine or etoposide, conducted approximately one decade ago, have some level of consistent clinical activity. While response rates of 30–40% with these two combinations were consistently reported by various groups, phase III trials failed to demonstrate major survival benefits in patients with hormone refractory disease. More recent experience with newer combinations primarily introducing taxanes has resulted in promising evidence of antitumor activity in phase II studies. As with estramustine phosphate, etoposide, vinblastine and taxol have

minimal activity in patients with hormone-resistant prostate cancer, while taxotere has shown significant single-agent activity to a level higher than any other single agent evaluated in this disease over the past several years.

While current data may suggest that combinations are superior to combination regimens in terms of response rates, the overall duration of clinical benefits and duration of survival observed with single agents and combinations appear quite similar in an across-trials evaluation. As expected, estramustine-containing combinations show a higher prostate-specific antigen (PSA) response proportion than non-estramustine-containing combinations or single agents, primarily in view of a likely hormonal effect on PSA by this hybrid compound. This is obviously an important issue that requires proper attention in prospective randomized trials, in view of the major toxicity difference between single agents and combination regimens. Ongoing phase III trials will hopefully answer some of the questions regarding the differences in toxicity, response and survival between single agents at different schedules and more standard and intensive combinations.

The usefulness of the serum PSA as a surrogate endpoint for clinical trials (i.e. relationship between changes in PSA and therapeutic benefits) remains an issue of major debate[4]. Various reports suggest that PSA changes with treatment indeed reflect a prognostically important finding; however, the surrogate value, with regard to survival and subjective benefits of a PSA decline following treatment, require proper evaluation in specifically designed phase III trials. More recently, a consensus report by various investigators recommended specific guidelines for clinical trials in patients with advanced prostate cancer (Table 2)[5]. It has been suggested that the interpretation of therapeutic results on the basis of PSA decreases need to be cautiously undertaken because various drugs have been shown to reduce PSA secretion without changing tumor growth[4].

New treatment approaches

Targets related to tumor growth invasion and metastasis

This broad field is emerging as one of the major focuses for development of new compounds to treat human cancer. With our increasing understanding of the molecular mechanisms of cancer invasion and metastasis, we begin to characterize the metastatic phenotype, select new targets for therapeutic interventions and design new compounds accordingly. The extracellular matrix represents a well-organized biological structure which is important for various critical functions including growth, migration, differentiation and angiogenesis[6].

Matrix metalloproteinases (MMPs) are a family of enzymes that are responsible for remodelling of the extracellular matrix in processes of growth and morphogenesis. These enzymes, collectively, are capable of degrading all of the components of the extracellular matrix, such as collagens, fibronectin, laminin, elastin and basement membrane glycoproteins[6,7]. These enzymes have been shown to be over-expressed in a number of human cancers, including adenocarcinoma of the prostate[6,7]. Based on initial preclinical information, it has been hypothesized that MMPs play an important role in the process of tumor invasion, metastatic spread and angiogenesis, and a number of potent inhibitors of these enzymes (MMPIs) have been developed for clinical testing. Among those in active development are Marimastat (British Biotech) and AG3340 (Auguron)[8,9]. These orally administered compounds have been demonstrated to be safe and suitable for long-term administration without the need for significant monitoring; however, it appears that dose-limiting musculoskeletal toxicity may be a more significant problem with Marimastat, which represents a broader inhibitor of MMPs[8].

Other compounds with antiangiogenesis activity, including TNP-470[10], CM-101[11], thalidomide[12], tecogalan[13], angiostatin[14], endostatin[15], anti-VEGF antibodies, small molecules designed to block important signal transduction steps of various growth factors such as VEGF, FGF, EGF and PDGF and anti-integrin therapies (small molecules or

Table 2 Summary of consensus guidelines for clinical trials in patients[5]

Patient eligibility	Response outcome
Increase in size and number of measurable sites	*Responses* (All should be separately reported) (a) objective (measurable responses) (b) PSA decline by $\geq 50\%$ confirmed ≥ 4 weeks later
New bone scan lesions (at least one)	
PSA of 5 ng/ml or higher for patients with no measurable disease	*Progression* (a) one or more new lesions on bone scan
Two consecutive rises in PSA at least 1 week apart	(b) increase on new measurable lesions (c) 25% increase of PSA over the baseline
Progression after antiandrogen withdrawal	(d) increase of PSA by 50% over the nadir
Evidence of gonadal suppression in the castrate range	

humanized antibodies), are actively undergoing preclinical and clinical testing. Suramin, which has known activity against prostate cancer, has been shown to inhibit binding of b-FGF and also significant anti-angiogenesis properties[16].

Differentiation treatment

Differentiation therapy involves the use of different drugs that are able to affect the proliferation of tumor cells. Among agents with significant differentiating activity *in vitro* are the retinoids[17], vitamin D derivatives[18] and butyrates[19]. Among promising agents are phenylbutyrate, an aromatic fatty acid with potent differentiating properties in tumor cell lines. The drug is well-absorbed orally and has demonstrated a reasonable safety profile in phase I trials[20]. As with other differentiating agents, phenylbutyrate has been shown to upregulate the PSA expression, which confounds the evaluation of antitumor effects in phase II trials and the development of this drug in prostate cancer. Evaluation of conventional disease progression (not PSA-based) is a more adequate methodological way to assess the efficacy of these compounds. Retinoids act primarily as nuclear transcription regulators which promote tumor cell maturation and inhibition of growth[17]. These agents have demonstrated activity in cell lines when combined with interferon, and some clinical responses in patients with hormone-refractory prostate cancer have been reported in early phase I–II trials[21].

Treatment targeted at the intracellular vitamin D receptor, which is a member of the steroid and retinoid receptor superfamily, represents a strategy under current investigation. Calcitriol (1,25 (OH)2 vitamin D) remains under careful clinical testing as well as other non-calcemic vitamin D analogs[22–24]. Toxicity in general has been mild; however, hypercalcemia may be dose-limiting. A more recent compound shown to interact with a specific member of the nuclear receptor superfamily, which heterodimerizes the retinoid receptor, is troglitazone. Troglitazone acts as an agonist of the peroxisome proliferator-activated receptor γ which induces growth inhibition and differentiation of prostate cancer *in vitro*[25]. Clinical trials with this compound are in progress.

Inhibition of signal transduction and cell–cell interaction mechanisms

Various biological agents have been directed to these critical signalling pathways of cell growth. Among those in active development are those which inhibit farnesyl transferase activity, specifically involving the *Ras* oncogene, which has been shown to contribute to the metastatic potential of various tumors[26,27]. Agents capable of inhibiting *Ras* farnesylation have shown activity against cell lines with the wild type or mutant *Ras* oncogene and are currently undergoing trials in solid tumors and leukemias. The HER-2 system has been targeted primarily in breast cancer with a humanized monoclonal antibody, trastuzumab, which has been approved by the US Food and Drug Administration for the treatment of breast cancer[28]. This compound is currently being developed clinically in prostate cancer in combination with other active compounds.

Anti-sense compounds

These drugs are synthetic oligonucleotides essentially targeted at the mRNA which results in cleavage and subsequent degradation of DNA. Among anti-sense drugs currently in development are those aiming at Bcl-2 and other proteins which may have a role in the mediation of apoptotic events[29]. Bcl-2 anti-sense compounds are particularly attractive for use in combination with chemotherapeutic agents which induce phosphorylation of Bcl-2, such as taxanes and vinca alkaloids[30].

Tumor vaccines and gene therapy

Molecular medicine has resulted in the identification of numerous antigens associated with several cancers, including adenocarcinoma of the prostate. Induction of antitumor immune responses after immunization has been demonstrated in preclinical studies. Specific immune cells responsible for tumor killing in the laboratory have been shown to detect target cells by recognizing major histocompatibility complex proteins in the membrane of these cells, and evidence of antitumor activity has been detected *in vivo*. Among the most potent antigen-presenting cells are dentritic cells, which have been used as vehicles for tumor-specific antigens, such as prostate-specific membrane antibody, and this constitutes the background for immuno-stimulatory strategies against prostate cancer[31]. Initial phase I studies with a dendritic cell vaccine have demonstrated safety in patients with advanced hormone refractory disease, and additional trials are in process to evaluate

the efficacy of this approach. Cytoreductive approaches include the use of granulocyte–macrophage colony stimulating growth factor-transduced allogeneic prostate cancer cells[32]. Tumor-specific immune responses have been reported, along with evidence of safety in patients with advanced disease, and clinical trials are in process to further define the efficacy in prostate cancer[33]. Other approaches include the transduction of suicide genes, such as the thymidine kinase gene, which can be activated by agents such as gancyclovir, toxins such as diphtheria and pseudomonas, and targeting against critical cellular promoters such as adhesion molecules and various other mechanisms involved in tumor cell-specific cell kill.

References

1. Hudes G, Greenberg R, Krigel R. Phase-II study of estramustine and vinblastine, two microtubule inhibitors, in hormone-refractory prostate cancer. *J Clin Oncol* 1992;10:1754–61
2. Hartley ASPB, Kruse E. Nuclear protein matrix as a target for estramustine-induced cell death. *Prostate* 1986;9:387–95
3. Pienta K, Redman B, Hussain M. Phase-II study of estramustine and oral etoposide in hormone-refractory adenocarcinoma of the prostate. *J Clin Oncol* 1994;12:2005–12
4. Eisenberger MA, Nelson WG. How much can we rely on PSA level as an endpoint to evaluate clinical trials in prostate cancer? A word of caution! *J Natl Cancer Inst* 1996;88:779–80
5. Bubley G, Carducci M, Dahut W, *et al*. Eligibility and response guidelines for phase II clinical trials in androgen independent prostate cancer: recommendations of the PSA working group. *J Clin Oncol* 1999;17:3461–7
6. Chambers AF, Matrisian LM. Changing views of the role of matrix metalloproteinase in metastasis. *J Natl Cancer Inst* 1997;89:1260–70
7. Bauer K, Rudek M, Lush R, *et al*. Novel targets in cancer therapy: angiogenesis, matrix metalloproteinases, cycline dependent kinases, and signal transduction. *Highlights Oncol Pract* 1998;16:3–11
8. Boasberg P, Harbaugh N, Eisenberger M, *et al*. Marimastat in patients with hormone refractory

prostate cancer: a dose finding study. *Proc Am Soc Clin Oncol* 1997;16:316a (abstr 1126)
9. Wilding G. *Noncytotoxic Approaches to Advanced Prostate Cancer*. American Society of Clinical Oncology, Educational Book, 1998:373–84
10. Ingber D, Fugita T, Kushimoto S. Synthetic analogues of fumagillin that inhibit angiogenesis and suppress tumor growth. *Nature* 1990;348: 555–7
11. Hellerqvist C, Thurman G, Page D, *et al*. Antitumor effects of GBS toxin: a polysaccharide exotoxin from group B hemolytic streptococcus. *J Cancer Res Clin Oncol* 1993; 120:63–70
12. Bauer K, Dixon S, Figg W. Inhibition of angiogenesis by thalidomide requires activation which is species specific. *Biochem Pharmacol* 1998;55:1827–34
13. Tulpule A, Espina B, Higashi L, *et al*. A phase-I study of tecogalan, a novel angiogenesis inhibitor in the treatment of AIDS related sarcoma and solid tumors. *New Cancer Strategies: Angiogenesis Inhibitors*. Washington DC, 1995
14. O'Reilly MS, Holmgrem S, Singh Y, *et al*. Angiostatin: a novel angiogenesis inhibitor that mediates the suppression of metastasis by a Lewis lung carcinoma. *Cell* 1994;79:315–28
15. O'Reilly MS, Boehm T, Singh Y, *et al*. Endostatin: an endogenous inhibitor of angiogenesis and tumor growth. *Cell* 1997;88:277–85

16. Braddock PS, Hu DE, Fan TP. A structure activity analysis of antagonism of the growth factor and angiogenesis activity of basic fibroblast growth factor by suramin and related polyanions. *Br J Cancer* 1994;69:890–8

17. Pienta KJ, Nguyen NM, Lehr JE. Treatment in prostate cancer in rat with the synthetic retinoid fenretinide. *Cancer Res* 1993;53:224–6

18. Schwartz GG, Oelert A, Uskokovic MR. Human prostate cancer cells: inhibition of proliferation by vitamin D analogues. *Anticancer Res* 1994; 14:1077–82

19. Schak S, Miller A, Liu L. Vulnerability of multidrug resistant tumor cells to the aromatic fatty acids phenylacetate and phenylbutyrate. *Clin Cancer Res* 1996;2:865–72

20. Carducci M, Nelson JB, Chan-Tak KM. Phenylbutyrate induces apoptosis in human prostate cancer and is more potent than phenylacetate. *Clin Cancer Res* 1996;2:379–87

21. DiPaola RS, Weiss R, Goodin S. The clinical and biological effects of 13-cis-retinoic acid and plasma interferon in patients with prostatic specific antigen progression after initial local therapy for prostate cancer. *Proc Am Soc Clin Oncol* 1997;16:A1185

22. Peehl DM, Skowronski RJ, Leung GK, Wong ST, Stamey TA, Feldman D. Antiproliferative effects of 1,25-dihydroxyvitamin D3 on primary cultures of human prostatic carcinoma cells. *Cancer Res* 1994;54:805–10

23. Gross C, Stamey T, Hancock S, Feldman D. Treatment of early recurrent prostate cancer with 1,25-dihydroxyvitamin D3 (calcitriol). *J Urol* 1998;161:2035–40

24. Kubota T, Koshizuka K, Koike M, Uskokovic M, Miyoshi I, Koeffler HP. 19-nor-26,27,bishomo-vitamin D3 analogs: a unique class of potent inhibitors of proliferation of prostate, breast, and hematopoietic cancer cells. *Cancer Res* 1998; 58:3370–5

25. Tontonoz P, Singer S, Forman BM. Terminal differentiation of human liposarcoma cells induced by ligands for peroxisome proliferator-activated receptor γ and the retinoid X receptor. *Proc Natl Acad Sci USA* 1997;94:237–1

26. Carter BS, Epstein JI, Isaacs WB. Ras gene mutations in human prostate cancer. *Cancer Res* 1990;50:6830–2

27. Sepp-Lorenzino L, Ma Z, Rands E. A peptidomimetic inhibitor of farnesyl-protein transferase blocks the anchorage-dependent and independent growth of human tumor cell lines. *Cancer Res* 1995;55:5302–9

28. Agus DB, Scher HI, Higgins B. Response of prostate cancer to anti-Her-2/neu antibody in androgen independent human xenograft models. *Cancer Res* 1999;59:4761–4

29. Lipponem P, Vesalainen S. Expresssion of the apoptosis suppressing protein bcl–2 in prostatic adenocarcinoma is related to tumor malignancy. *Prostate* 1997;32:9–15

30. Morris MJ, Tong W, Osman I. A phase I/IIa dose escalating trial of Bcl–2 antisense treatment (G3139) by 14-day continuous intravenous infusion for patients with androgen-independent prostate cancer or other advanced solid tumor malignancies. *Proc Am Soc Clin Oncol* 1999;16:323a

31. Israeli RS, Miller Wh Jr, Su SL. Sensitive detection of prostatic hematogenous tumor cell dissemination using prostate specific-membrane derived primers in the polymerase chain reaction. *J Urol* 1995;153:573–7

32. Sanda M, Ayyagari SR, Jaffee EM, *et al.* Demonstration of a rational strategy for human prostate cancer gene therapy. *J Urol* 1994;151: 622–8

33. Simmons JW, Carducci MA, Weber E, *et al.* Bioactivity of autologous radiated prostate cancer vaccines generated by *ex vivo* GM-CSF gene transfer. *Proc Am Soc Clin Oncol* 1998;17:313a (abstr 1205)

34. Picus J, Schultz M. Docetaxel as monotherapy in the treatment of hormone refractory prostate cancer. *Semin Oncol* 1999;26:14–18

35. Sinibaldi VJ, Carducci M, Laufer M, *et al.* Preliminary evaluation of a short course of estramustine phosphate and docetaxe (Taxotere) in the treatment of hormone-refractory prostate cancer. *Semin Oncol* 1999;26(5 Suppl 17):45–8

36. Savarese D, Taplin ME, Halabi S. A phase II study of docetaxel, estramustine and low dose hydrocortisone in men with hormone refractory prostate cancer. *Semin Oncol* 1999;26:39–44

37. Petrylak D, Macarthur RB, O'Connor J. Phase I trial of docetaxel and oral estramustine in patients with androgen independent prostate cancer. *J Clin Oncol* 1999;17:958–67

38. Smith DC, Esper P, Strawderman M. Phase II trial of oral estramustine, oral etoposide and intravenous paclitaxel in hormone refractory prostate cancer. *J Clin Oncol* 1999;17:1664–71

39. Hudes GR, Nathan F, Khater C, *et al.* Phase II trial of 96-hour paclitaxel plus oral estramustine phosphate in metastatic hormone-refractory prostate cancer. *J Clin Oncol* 1997;15:3156–63

40. Friedland D, Cohen J, Miller R, *et al.* A phase-II trial of taxofene in hormone refractory prostate cancer: correlation of antitumor activity to phosphorylation of BCL_2. *Proc Am Soc Clin Oncol* 1999;18:322 (abstr 1237)

41. Trivedi C, Redman B, Flaherty LE, *et al.* Weekly 1-hour infusion of paclitaxel. Clinical feasibility and efficacy in patients with hormone refractory prostate carcinoma. *Cancer* 2000;89:431–6

Section VII

Bladder cancer

Novel detection strategies for transitional cell carcinoma

26

C. S. Stewart, K. C. Halling and M. M. Lieber

Introduction

There has been an explosion of new tests for diagnosing transitional cell carcinoma (TCC) over the past 10 years. Any of the major urological journals in a given month will include a new detection strategy for bladder cancer. The majority of these tests use a patient's urine sample to screen for either tumor-related antigens or genetic alterations. Since Papanicolaou and Marshall described the importance of urine cytology in 1945[1], it has been considered the gold standard for detecting TCC in urine samples. The advantages of this test are numerous; it has a proven track record, it is a non-invasive test which is relatively inexpensive compared to newer point-of-service commercial tests and it demonstrates a high degree of specificity. The main disadvantages are low sensitivity, particularly in lower-grade tumors, and a moderate degree of interobserver variability.

Numerous urothelial cancer-related proteins have been actively investigated with the development of commercial assays for many of these compounds. Collectively these proteins are known as biomarkers and the bulk of recent investigations have centered around a few of the commercial assays, namely bladder tumor analyte (BTA), nuclear matrix protein (NMP22), and fibrin degradation products (FDP). These biomarkers have all shown variable degrees of improvement in the sensitivity of detecting TCC compared to standard cytology. Detection of some of these biomarkers can be carried out using point-of-service kits in a physician's office, while others must be performed in a clinical laboratory.

The discovery of genetic changes commonly associated with TCC have made the development of genetic tests for urothelial cancer attractive. Modern theories of tumorigenesis suggest a systematic series of genetic changes, which lead to loss of regulation of cell growth and subsequent overproliferation. Methods for detecting these genetic changes can be divided into cytogenetic versus molecular genetic studies. Cytogenetic studies focus on numerical and structural abnormalities of chromosomes and include karyotyping, flow cytometry, DNA image analysis (DIA) and fluorescence *in situ* hybridization (FISH) analysis.

Molecular genetic studies focus on polymerase chain reaction (PCR) and Southern blot analysis for the detection of polymorphic microsatellite sequences and restriction fragment length polymorphisms associated with TCC. Most of these genetic tests provide an improvement compared to cytology in the sensitivity of detecting bladder cancer, while offering similar specificities.

Conventional cytology

Conventional cytology has long been considered the gold standard test for detecting TCC from urine. One of the greatest benefits of cytology is its consistently reported high specificity, $> 95\%$. However, the sensitivity of cytology is highly variable, with the majority of studies showing an overall sensitivity of 40–60%[2,3]. The sensitivity of cytology increases with increasing grade of the tumor.

Methods for improving the sensitivity of cytology have centered on the collection method, number of samples and reappraisal of current grading systems (especially for grade 1 pT_a tumors). Voided samples generally have the lowest sensitivity, owing to their relative hypocellularity, but the technique is non-invasive and the samples are easy to collect. Badalament and colleagues demonstrated a 41% overall sensitivity for one voided urine sample but an increase by 19%, to 60%, if three voided samples were collected[4]. Catheterized specimens increase the sensitivity of cytology and have less contamination from epithelial cells but the technique is invasive and requires a trained individual to collect the sample. Similarly, barbotage and bladder washings increased the sensitivity to 61% in detecting TCC[4,5]. These samples are significantly more cellular than voided specimens but there is a risk of instrument artifact. Catheterizing the urethra and bladder often results in the denudation of benign transitional cell clusters, which can be difficult or impossible to distinguish from low-grade papillary tumors[6].

Grading of urine cytology specimens is subjective and this often results in significant interobserver variability. Attempts to unify diagnosis and grading of cytological specimens have resulted in the establishment of several classification systems, including the World Health Organization (WHO) grading system. Generally these schemes rely on an increase in cellular pleomorphism, nuclear-to-cytoplasmic ratios and nuclear hyperchromasia with increasing grade. It is well known that cytology has the poorest sensitivity in low-grade TCCs of 4–34%[7,8]. Some authors have suggested that it is the grading of these tumors that is at fault and that by liberalizing and incorporating more cytological features than the WHO criteria allow, we can increase our yield of detecting grade 1 tumors. However, this incorporates more false-positive results and risks decreasing the excellent specificity enjoyed by cytology[9–13]. Recently, multimodal approaches to diagnosing TCC have utilized both conventional cytology and adjuvant tumor marker tests to improve the detection rate of TCC compared to cytology alone[14–16].

Novel tumor markers

The search for a unique and ubiquitously expressed substance by urothelial carcinomas has, to this date, been unfruitful. However, there have been several protein and tumor by-products discovered which have increased the sensitivity of detecting TCC in voided urine compared to cytology. Table 1 shows these markers and other modalities segregated by method of TCC detection.

Assays to detect these biomarkers have been developed, with some available as commercial kits. Detection of these proteins and by-products relies on the consistent production of these substances by tumor cells in contact with urine, and the biomarkers may be present in minute amounts necessitating either ultra-sensitive assays or amplification techniques. This illustrates two major drawbacks of these tests: reliance on consistent production of biomarkers by the tumor and, often, under-detection of early and small-volume disease. In general, while these antigen-based tests have an improved sensitivity in detecting TCC, it is at the expense of a decreased specificity. The same shortcomings of cytology in detecting low-grade

Table 1 Biomarker assays for the detection of transitional cell carcinoma

Category	Test
Tumor-associated antigens	bladder tumor analyte (BTA) *stat*, p53, nuclear matrix protein (NMP) 22, Lewis blood group, antigens, hyaluronic acid, vascular endothelial growth factor (VEGF), fibrin degradation products (FDP)
Tumor-associated enzymes	telomerase
Cytogenetics	fluorescence *in situ* hybridization (FISH), flow cytometry, digital image analysis (DIA)
Molecular genetics	restriction fragment length polymorphisms (RFLPs), polymorphic microsatellite sequences

tumors also plague many of these biomarker assays. It appears that these low-grade tumors are not de-differentiated and abnormal enough to result in consistent biomarker production.

Tumor proteins

Mutations which inactivate the *P53* tumor suppressor gene are common in invasive bladder cancer. Typically, inactivation of the *P53* gene occurs by deletion of one of the alleles and a missense mutation of the other allele. The allele with the missense mutation leads to the synthesis of an inactive p53 protein with a prolonged half-life, resulting in cellular accumulation of p53. Immunohistochemistry can detect cells with an abnormal accumulation of mutant p53 protein, and correlates strongly with the presence of *P53* mutations at the DNA level and, thus, serves as a very good surrogate marker for the presence of *P53* mutations. However, *P53* has primarily been used as a prognostic indicator and not for the detection of recurrent TCC[16–18].

Bladder tumor analyte

The first-generation bladder tumor analyte (BTA) test was a latex-agglutination test for by-products of tumor-related enzymatic action on bladder urothelium. This showed an increase in sensitivity over conventional cytology[19–23]. Further refinements of the BTA test occurred with the development of monoclonal antibody assays for human complement factor H-related protein (hCFHrp), which has been shown to be increased in patients with TCC. The BTA *stat* and BTA TRAK tests (Polymedco, Cortlandt Manor, NY, USA) are qualitative and quantitative assays, respectively, for hCFHrp. The BTA *stat* test is a convenient point-of-service kit with improved detection of TCC compared to the original BTA test[24]. The sensitivity of BTA *stat* for monitoring TCC recurrence has ranged from 57% to 83%[19,24–29]. The specificity of the BTA *stat* assay in patients with non-neoplastic genitourinary disorders (such as benign prostatic hyperplasia (BPH), prostatitis, urinary tract infection and urolithiasis, etc.) ranges from 68% to 82% (Table 2)[19,24–30]. Most of the studies reporting specificities close to 100% for BTA *stat* used normal controls without coexisting non-cancerous bladder and/or prostate pathology. Increased hCFHrp production may occur independently of cancer in patients with coexisting inflammatory conditions, since specificities drop to as low as 28% for patients who have recently received bacillus Calmette–Guérin (BCG)[28]. Patients with recent and/or coexistent inflammatory urinary tract disease should be evaluated cautiously with the BTA *stat* test. These limitations are not trivial; most patients being evaluated by a urologist are likely to be older patients with higher proclivities toward concurrent prostate and bladder pathology.

Table 2 Review of bladder tumor analyte (BTA) *stat*/antigen-sensitivity and specificity

Study	Number of patients	Overall sensitivity (%)	Sensitivity according to grade (%)			Sensitivity according to stage (%)				Overall specificity (%)	Year
			1	*2*	*3*	pT_a	pT_{is}	pT_1	$pT_2>$		
Raitaten[25]	151	81	63	82	100	66	100	91	96	not calculated	2000
Giannopoulos[29]	147	72	50	74	85	57	100	77	94	57	2000
Leyh[19]*	240	65	39	67	83	53	100	70	88	72	1999
Pode[28]	250	83	40	85	100	72	ND	90	100	69	1999
Ramakumar[26]	196	74	33	77	100	60	82	ND	100	73	1999
Sarosdy[24]*	220	67	42	66	83	51	61	38	88	70	1997
Wiener[27]	291	57	48	58	63	55	ND	60	58	68	1998

*Specificity calculated on patients with history of transitional cell carcinoma; ND, no data supplied for these stages

The BTA TRAK test is a quantitative assay and thus more precise, but is reserved for larger reference laboratories. The quantitative advantage that BTA TRAK enjoys over BTA *stat* may best be suited for monitoring the recurrence of TCC, rather than as an initial diagnostic test[31].

Nuclear matrix proteins

Nuclear matrix proteins (NMPs) are commonly found in all mammalian cells and play a role in DNA replication and transcription. The NMP22 test is an immunoassay which measures a unique protein inherent to mitosis, which has been shown to be elevated in patients with bladder tumors. The results are reported as a numeric value of activity per milliliter. The package insert for NMP22 gives 10 U/ml as the cut-off for normal; however, several authors have proposed different cut-offs based on receiver operating characteristic (ROC) curve analysis of their individual data[29,32]. The difficulty with comparing sensitivities and specificities across these studies is the variability in these calculated cut-off points, with ranges of 3.6–10 U/ml (Table 3)[26,29,32–37]. Giannopoulos and colleagues reported a 63% sensitivity and 74% specificity with an 8-U/ml cut-off point and concluded that this test was superior to cytology[29]. Others have shown a sensitivity of only 38% and concluded it had no advantage over conventional cytology[33].

Fibrin degration products and vascular endothelial growth factors

Transitional cell carcinomas produce vascular endothelial growth factors (VEGFs) to aid in the recruitment of new blood vessels for growth. These VEGFs aid in angiogenesis and have been isolated in urine from patients with TCC[38,39]. These vessels are often relatively permeable and promote translocation of vascular substances which result in accumulation of fibrin degradation products (FDPs) in the urine. The FDPs can be found in increased levels, with polyclonal and monoclonal antibodies, in the urine of patients with TCC compared with normal controls. Investigators have reported sensitivities ranging from 52% to 81%, with specificities of 75% to 91% (Table 4)[26,40–42]. There is some promise that FDP assays can more reliably detect low-grade tumors compared to conventional cytology, with sensitivities for pT_a and grade 1 tumors both being 61%[41].

Hyaluronic acid

Hyaluronic acid is a glycosaminoglycan found in elevated levels in the urine of patients with TCC. Hyaluronidase is an enzyme which cleaves hyaluronic acid and is thought to promote metastasis through local tissue breakdown and promotion of angiogenesis. There are several assays available for detecting increased levels of these substances in the urine with sensitivities ranging from 82% to 92% and specificities of

Table 3 Nuclear matrix protein sensitivity and specificity

Study	Number of patients	Overall sensitivity (%)	Sensitivity according to grade (%)			Sensitivity according to stage (%)				Overall specificity (%)	Test characteristics (U/ml)	Year
			1	2	3	pT_a	pT_{is}	pT_1	$pT_2>$			
Giannopoulos[29]	147	63	54	54	79	53	80	65	88	74	8	2000
Menedez[33]	92	38	14	47	50	23	NC	36	67	81	10	2000
Ramakumar[26]	193	53	44	62	62	48	45	NC	79	60	3.6	1999
Zippe[34]	330	100	NC	NC	NC	NC	NC	NC	NC	85	10	1999
Mian[35]	240	56	50	50	69	52	100	46	70	79	10	2000
Sarosdy[24]	231	68	31	74	81	61	70	100	83	80	6.4	1997
Wiener[27]	267	76	76	82	83	63	67	79	93	NC	14.6	1998
Del Nero[37]	105	83	69	94	80	66	NC	93	NC	87	10	1999

NC, not calculated

85% to 89%[43,44]. When examining both hyaluronic acid and hyaluronidase activity concomitantly, increased sensitivity is provided without compromise of specificity when compared to each individual test[43]. The sensitivity increased from 82% for the hyaluronidase ELISA assay and from 84% for the hyaluronic acid assay up to 92% for the combined study. Equally important are concerns over specificity and, in a group of 243 patients with various genitourinary conditions other than bladder cancer, Lokeshwar and co-workers found the specificity to range from 80% to 95% depending on the type of pathology present (Table 5)[44].

Telomerase

During DNA replication small fragments at the ends of chromosomes, known as telomeres, are lost and these telomeres are subsequently shortened with each cycle. This eventually results in death of the cell when these telomeres are exhausted; it is this mechanism which is postulated to be one of the 'biological clocks' of the cell. Telomerase is a complex reverse transcriptase which reconstitutes the telomeres

and provides a prolonged lifespan of the cell. It is hypothesized that the regulation of telomerase is disrupted in many malignant cells, thus rendering them immortal[26].

Urinary telomerase has been used both for cancer screening and surveillance with a high sensitivity (70%) and specificity (99%) for the detection of TCC (Table 6)[25,45,46]. However, subsequent investigators have been unable to replicate these findings. The most likely explanation for the difference between the studies is that the first study was performed on urine specimens which were rapidly analyzed after collection, while subsequent studies were performed on specimens at room temperature. Telomerase is unstable in urine and this logistical detail has limited its introduction as a commercially available test[47].

Immunocytochemistry

Lewis X antigens are not typically expressed on the surface of normal epithelium but 85–90% of tumor cells will express this blood group. Immunocytology or immunostaining with antibodies specific to either the Lewis X antigen

Table 4 Fibrin degradation product sensitivity and specificity

| Study | Number of patients | Overall sensitivity (%) | Sensitivity according to grade (%) | | | Sensitivity according to stage (%) | | | Overall specificity (%) | Year |
			1	2	3	pT_a	pT_{is}	$pT_2>$		
Ramakumar[26]	186	52	25	46	92	45	60	69	91	1999
Johnston[42]	130	81	63	88	95	74	100	85	75	1997
Schmetter[41]	192	68	61	64	86	62	67	100	80	1997

Table 5 Hyaluronic acid and hyaluronidase assays[44]

| Test | Number of patients | Overall sensitivity (%) | Sensitivity according to grade (%) | | | Sensitivity according to stage (%) | | | | Overall specificity (%) | Test characteristics | Year |
			1	2	3	pT_a	pT_{is}	pT_1	$pT_2>$			
Hyaluronic acid Hyaluronidase	513	83	80	80	85	77	87	88	86	90	500 ng/mg	2000
Hyaluronic acid-	513	82	23	83	81	43	77	88	86	84	10 mu/mg	2000
hyaluronidase*	513	91	86	96	93	88	94	94	97	84		2000

*Positive if either hyaluronic acid or hyaluronidase tests were positive

Table 6 Telomerase sensitivity and specificity

Study	Number of patients	Overall sensitivity (%)	Sensitivity according to grade (%)			Sensitivity according to stage (%)			Overall specificity (%)	Year
			1	2	3	pT_a	pT_{is}	$pT_2>$		
Ramakumar[26]	196	70	56	85	85	76	91	71	99	1999
Kavaler[45]	151	85	79	84	88	*	*	*		1998
Landman[46]	87	80	65	72	93	70	100	91	80	1998

*Did not segregate by stage

or other tumor-associated membrane-bound antigens have been reported to have sensitivities above 90%[48,49]. However, immunostaining using Lewis X antigen suffers from a low specificity as any reactive epithelium (typically epithelium subjected to mechanical trauma, chemotherapy, infection and/or radiation) will commonly express these antigens[50].

Cytogenetics

Urothelial cancers are frequently aneuploid, and the detection of these cells in urine has been exploited for TCC detection by flow cytometry and DIA. Flow cytometry allows rapid and automated analysis of a large batch of samples with reasonable detection rates for TCC. Its primary inadequacy is its inability to detect a low volume of exfoliated cancer cells and low-grade tumors. DIA attempts to maximize the detection of neoplastic cells by selecting only cells with the highest degree of cytologic atypia[51]. The major disadvantage of this test lies in the time required to analyze each sample, as compared to flow cytometry. Nonetheless, many authors have reported sensitivities from 80% to 90%[5,14].

More sophisticated methodologies exist for the screening of specific genetic alterations associated with bladder tumors. These mutations result in either the loss of function of tumor suppressor genes or increased activity of oncogenes. Recognition of a consistent set of genetic mutations, which results in carcinogenic transformation, is fundamental to early detection of neoplasms. Cytogenetic and molecular genetic analysis promises reliably to

detect known genetic alterations associated with cancer. There are several well-recognized chromosomal changes that consistently occur with TCC. Loss of part or all of chromosome 9 is the most common genetic change associated with both *in situ* carcinoma and papillary tumors[52,53]. Chromosomes 1, 7, 11, Y and 17 have also been shown to be frequently altered in patients with bladder tumors[54–57]. FISH uses fluorescently labelled DNA probes to the centromeres of various chromosomes and specific chromosomal loci (e.g. 9p21 locus, site of the *P16* gene that is frequently deleted in TCC) to detect chromosomal abnormalities that are found in urothelial cancers. Commonly seen changes are polysomy (gains of chromosomes) or hemi- or homozygous deletion of the 9p21 locus. Fluorescently labeled DNA probes bind with their corresponding centromere or chromosomal loc. and when examined with a filtered fluorescent light these probes become visible as colored dots. The finding of gains of two or more chromosomes in a cell is a very reliable indicator that the cell is neoplastic. Loss of chromosomes, as detected by loss of signal, is not as reliable an indicator of neoplasia as chromosomal gain for two reasons:

(1) Two signals can coincidentally overlap and make it appear that there is only a single signal;

(2) Inadequate hybridization of the probe to the corresponding chromosome sometimes occurs.

Only when there is a clear and consistent loss of one signal (for the centromere enumeration probe (CEP)) or both signals (for the 9p21 probe) in the potentially neoplastic cells but not in adjacent normal cells, can a loss be considered significant for neoplasia. We have used a 'cocktail' of FISH probes to the pericentromeric regions of chromosomes 3, 7, 17 and to the band 9p21 locus. These were chosen from a set of probes to 3, 8, 7, 9, 11, 18, Y and the 9p21 locus-specific probe after a statistical analysis showed that the above four combinations of probes provided the highest sensitivity and specificity in detecting TCC in patients with biopsy-proven bladder cancer[58]. A DAPI counter stain was used to help identify urothelial cells and concentrate the majority of our numeration efforts on cells with suspicious morphology by cytological criteria. In general, we focused our examination on cells with nuclear enlargement, irregular nuclear contour, and patchy and reduced DAPI staining. Urine samples were considered positive if five or more cells had gains of two or more signals or more than 20% of the cells exhibited homozygous deletion of 9p21. These criteria were developed after analysis of initial data with an ROC curve showed that these values yielded the highest combination of sensitivity and specificity[3].

After the optimal probe set for the detection of TCC and the criteria for positivity had been determined we then conducted a prospective study of 265 patients under evaluation for TCC. Urine cytology and FISH analyses were performed on specimens that were collected just prior to cystoscopy. Just over half of the patients being evaluated had a history of urothelial carcinoma. The sensitivity of FISH for grade 1, 2 and 3 tumors was 36%, 76% and 97%, respectively, and for pT_a, pT_{is} and pT_{1-4} tumors was 65%, 100% and 95%, respectively. The sensitivity for cytology for grade 1, 2 and 3 tumors was only 27%, 54% and 71%, respectively, and for pT_a, pT_{is} and pT_{1-4} tumors was 47%, 78% and 60%, respectively. The overall sensitivity of FISH was 81% with a specificity of 96%. The overall sensitivity of cytology was 58% and the specificity was 98%. Detection of TCC with FISH was significantly improved compared to cytology overall, as well

as in patients with pT_{is}, pT_{1-4} and grade 3 tumors.

FISH may improve the ability to detect recurrent TCC in patients undergoing intravesical BCG therapy. The inflammatory reaction induced by BCG treatment leads to reactive urothelial atypia and makes it difficult to distinguish reactive urothelial cells from urothelial carcinoma cells. It may even take several months for tissue biopsies of epithelium to revert back to 'normal'. Preliminary findings in our laboratory suggest that BCG inflammatory changes do not result in false-positive FISH results and do not interfere with the ability of FISH to detect malignant cells when they are present. It is possible then, that one could predict at an early stage those patients responding to intravesical therapy versus those with a minimal response so that the duration and frequency of BCG treatments can be adjusted to minimize iatrogenic morbidity from therapy. Likewise, FISH holds promise as a test which could more reliably predict which non-invasive tumors are likely to recur or progress. Further refinements of the assay may enable FISH not only to detect tumor recurrence, but also to provide prognostic information such as the likelihood of progression.

Molecular genetics

Microsatellite analysis using PCR and polymorphic microsatellite markers has shown promise as an alternative way of detecting recurrent TCC[59–61]. This method looks for loss of heterozygosity and microsatellite instability of various microsatellite markers as a way of detecting TCC. Several studies have shown that microsatellite analysis has high sensitivity and specificity for the detection of recurrent TCC. The difficulties with microsatellite analysis are:

(1) It is labor intensive (and therefore probably expensive);

(2) Theoretically it is unable to detect tumor cells when they constitute a small proportion of the total cell population (e.g. less than 5%).

Conclusion

Many of the newer bladder cancer tests increase the sensitivity of TCC detection compared to cytology but have a lower specificity than cytology. Despite their poor specificity these tests might have a role as a screening tool for the initial detection of TCC. However, in patients who are being followed for tumor recurrence a urologist often depends on urine-based studies as a confirmatory test, which necessitates a high degree of specificity. Few bladder tumor antigen tests can claim the excellent specificity enjoyed by cytology and many have a high rate of false positives in patients with genitourinary inflammatory conditions. New antigen-based tests will probably also be hindered by non-neoplastic tissue that has been injured and this lack of specificity will be unlikely to improve. Most of the studies which purport to maximize specificity often do so at the expense of sensitivity via manipulation of the cut-off points. With regard to antigen-based tests, the saying 'You can't get something for nothing' appears to be true.

Cytogenetic studies, FISH in particular, have tremendous potential in the diagnosis and surveillance of bladder carcinoma. Unlike the antigen-based assays, FISH has been shown to have both high sensitivity and specificity. As we improve the results of detecting TCC with urine-based tests, we must also develop novel strategies for localizing TCC. Currently, we rely on cystoscopy and biopsy of suspicious lesions as well as random samplings to make the 'definitive' diagnosis of TCC. It is likely that sophisticated urine-based tests will 'diagnose' urothelial cancer at an early stage which may be difficult to detect visually. In addition, the renal pelvis and the ureters are sanctuary sites from the detection of TCC by cystoscopy. Selective upper tract cytologies, nephro-ureteroscopy and imaging modalities are useful only for localizing larger volume disease. Promising work has been ongoing with fluorescence-enhanced cystoscopy to help detect microscopic involvement of tumor and field-of-change phenomena (see Chapter 27). It is imperative that, as we make progress in the detection of TCC of the urine, we complement this with the development of more sophisticated localizing techniques. Without the means to adequately localize and obtain tissue for diagnosis, the early detection and surveillance of TCC will be meritless.

References

1. Papanicolaou G, Marshall V. Urine sediment smears as a diagnostic procedure in cancers of the urinary tract. *Science* 1945;101:519
2. Brown FM. Urine cytology. It is still the gold standard for screening? *Urol Clin North Am* 2000;27:25–37
3. Halling K, King W, Sokolova I, *et al.* Comparison of cytology and fluorescence *in situ* hybridization for the detection of urothelial carcinoma. *J Urol* 2000;164:1768–75
4. Badalament RA, Hermansen DK, Kimmel M, *et al.* The sensitivity of bladder wash flow cytometry, bladder wash cytology, and voided cytology in the detection of bladder carcinoma. *Cancer* 1987;60:1423–7
5. Cajulis RS, Haines GK III, Frias-Hidvegi D, *et al.* Cytology, flow cytometry, image analysis, and interphase cytogenetics by fluorescence *in situ* hybridization in the diagnosis of transitional cell carcinoma in bladder washes: a comparative study. *Diagn Cytopathol* 1995;13:214–23, discussion 224
6. Farrow GM. Urine cytology in the detection of bladder cancer: a critical approach. *J Occup Med* 1990;32:817–21
7. Rife CC, Farrow GM, Utz DC. Urine cytology of transitional cell neoplasms. *Urol Clin North Am* 1979;6:599–612
8. Thomas L, Leyh H, Marberger M, *et al.* Multicenter trial of the quantitative BTA TRAK

assay in the detection of bladder cancer. *Clin Chem* 1999;45:472–7

9. Renshaw AA, Nappi D, Weinberg DS. Cytology of grade 1 papillary transitional cell carcinoma. A comparison of cytologic, architectural and morphometric criteria in cystoscopically obtained urine. *Acta Cytol* 1996;40:676–82.

10. Murphy WM. Current status of urinary cytology in the evaluation of bladder neoplasms. *Hum Pathol* 1990;21:886–96

11. Kannan V, Bose S. Low grade transitional cell carcinoma and instrument artifact. A challenge in urinary cytology. *Acta Cytol* 1993;37:899–902

12. Raab SS, Lenel JC, Cohen MB. Low grade transitional cell carcinoma of the bladder. Cytologic diagnosis by key features as identified by logistic regression analysis. *Cancer* 1994;74:1621–6

13. Raab SS, Slagel DD, Jensen CS, *et al.* Low-grade transitional cell carcinoma of the urinary bladder: application of select cytologic criteria to improve diagnostic accuracy. [Published erratum appears in *Mod Pathol* 1996;9:803]. *Mod Pathol* 1996;9:225–32

14. Amberson JB, Laino JP. Image cytometric deoxyribonucleic acid analysis of urine specimens as an adjunct to visual cytology in the detection of urothelial cell carcinoma. *J Urol* 1993;149:42–5

15. Hughes JH, Katz RL, Rodriguez-Villanueva J, *et al.* Urinary nuclear matrix protein 22 (NMP22): a diagnostic adjunct to urine cytologic examination for the detection of recurrent transitional-cell carcinoma of the bladder. *Diagn Cytopathol* 1999;20:285–90

16. Righi E, Rossi G, Ferrari G, *et al.* Does p53 immunostaining improve diagnostic accuracy in urine cytology? *Diagn Cytopathol* 1997;17:436–9

17. Esrig D, Elmajian D, Groshen S, *et al.* Accumulation of nuclear p53 and tumor progression in bladder cancer. *N Engl J Med* 1994;331:1259–64

18. Sidransky D, Von Eschenbach A, Tsai YC, *et al.* Identification of p53 gene mutations in bladder cancers and urine samples. *Science* 1991;252:706–9

19. Leyh H, Marberger M, Conort P, *et al.* Comparison of the BTA stat test with voided urine cytology and bladder wash cytology in the diagnosis and monitoring of bladder cancer. *Eur Urol* 1999;35:52–6

20. Sarosdy MF, deVere White RW, Soloway MS, *et al.* Results of a multicenter trial using the BTA test to monitor for and diagnose recurrent bladder cancer. *J Urol* 1995;154:379–83, discussion 383–4

21. Sarosdy MF. The use of the BTA Test in the detection of persistent or recurrent transitional-cell cancer of the bladder. *World J Urol* 1997;15:103–6

22. Kirollos MM, McDermott S, Bradbrook RA. The performance characteristics of the bladder tumour antigen test. *Br J Urol* 1997;80:30–4

23. Murphy WM, Rivera-Ramirez I, Medina CA. The bladder tumor antigen (BTA) test compared to voided urine cytology in the detection of bladder neoplasms. *J Urol* 1997;158:2102–6

24. Sarosdy MF, Hudson MA, Ellis WJ, *et al.* Improved detection of recurrent bladder cancer using the Bard BTA stat Test. *Urology* 1997;50:349–53

25. Raitanen MP, Marttila T, Kaasinen E, *et al.* Sensitivity of human complement factor H related protein (BTA stat) test and voided urine cytology in the diagnosis of bladder cancer. *J Urol* 2000;163:1689–92

26. Ramakumar S, Bhuiyan J, Besse JA, *et al.* Comparison of screening methods in the detection of bladder cancer. [Comment in *J Urol* 1999;161:447–8]. *J Urol* 1999;161:388–94

27. Wiener HG, Mian C, Haitel A, *et al.* Can urine bound diagnostic tests replace cystoscopy in the management of bladder cancer? *J Urol* 1998;159:1876–80

28. Pode D, Shapiro A, Wald M, *et al.* Noninvasive detection of bladder cancer with the BTA stat test. *J Urol* 1999;161:443–6

29. Giannopoulos A, Manousakas T, Mitropoulos D, *et al.* Comparative evaluation of the BTAstat test, NMP22, and voided urine cytology in the detection of primary and recurrent bladder tumors. *Urology* 2000;55:871–5

30. Sharma S, Zippe CD, Pandrangi L, *et al.* Exclusion criteria enhance the specificity and positive predictive value of NMP22 and BTA stat. *J Urol* 1999;162:53–7

31. Malkowicz SB. The application of human complement factor H-related protein (BTA TRAK) in monitoring patients with bladder cancer. *Urol Clin North Am* 2000;27:63–73

32. Stampfer DS, Carpinito GA, Rodriguez-Villanueva J, *et al.* Evaluation of NMP22 in the detection of transitional cell carcinoma of the bladder. [Published erratum appears in *J Urol* 1998;159:1650]. *J Urol* 1998;159:394–8

33. Menendez V, Filella X, Alcover JA, *et al.* Usefulness of urinary nuclear matrix protein 22 (NMP22) as a marker for transitional cell carcinoma of the bladder. *Anticancer Res* 2000;20:1169–72

34. Zippe C, Pandrangi L, Potts JM, *et al.* NMP22: a sensitive, cost-effective test in patients at risk for bladder cancer. *Anticancer Res* 1999;19:2621–3

35. Mian C, Lodde M, Haitel A, *et al.* Comparison of the monoclonal UBC-ELISA test and the NMP22 ELISA test for the detection of urothelial cell carcinoma of the bladder. *Urology* 2000;55:223–6

36. Sanchez-Carbayo M, Herrero E, Megias J, *et al.* Evaluation of nuclear matrix protein 22 as a tumour marker in the detection of transitional cell carcinoma of the bladder. *BJU Int* 1999; 84:706–13

37. Del Nero A, Esposito N, Curro A, *et al.* Evaluation of urinary level of NMP22 as a diagnostic marker for stage pTa-pT1 bladder cancer: comparison with urinary cytology and BTA test. *Eur Urol* 1999;35:93–7

38. O'Brien T, Cranston D, Fuggle S, *et al.* Different angiogenic pathways characterize superficial and invasive bladder cancer. *Cancer Res* 1995; 55:510–13

39. Brown LF, Berse B, Jackman RW, *et al.* Increased expression of vascular permeability factor (vascular endothelial growth factor) and its receptors in kidney and bladder carcinomas. *Am J Pathol* 1993;143:1255–62

40. Tsihlias J, Grossman HB. The utility of fibrin/fibrinogen degradation products in superficial bladder cancer. *Urol Clin North Am* 2000;27:39–46

41. Schmetter BS, Habicht KK, Lamm DL, *et al.* A multicenter trial evaluation of the fibrin/fibrinogen degradation products test for detection and monitoring of bladder cancer. *J Urol* 1997;158:801–5

42. Johnston B, Morales A, Emerson L, *et al.* Rapid detection of bladder cancer: a comparative study of point of care tests. *J Urol* 1997;158:2098–101

43. Lokeshwar VB, Block NL. HA-HAase urine test. A sensitive and specific method for detecting bladder cancer and evaluating its grade. *Urol Clin North Am* 2000;27:53–61

44. Lokeshwar VB, Obek C, Pham HT, *et al.* Urinary hyaluronic acid and hyaluronidase: markers for bladder cancer detection and evaluation of grade. *J Urol* 2000;163:348–56

45. Kavaler E, Landman J, Chang Y, *et al.* Detecting human bladder carcinoma cells in voided urine samples by assaying for the presence of telomerase activity. *Cancer* 1998;82:708–14

46. Landman J, Chang Y, Kavaler E, *et al.* Sensitivity and specificity of NMP-22, telomerase, and BTA in the detection of human bladder cancer. *Urology* 1998;52:398–402

47. Arai Y, Yajima T, Yagihashi A, *et al.* Limitations of urinary telomerase activity measurement in urothelial cancer. *Clin Chim Acta* 2000;296:35–44

48. Klan R, Huland E, Baisch H, *et al.* Sensitivity of urinary quantitative immunocytology with monoclonal antibody 486 P3/12 in 241 unselected patients with bladder carcinoma. *J Urol* 1991;145:495–7

49. Pode D, Golijanin D, Sherman Y, *et al.* Immunostaining of Lewis X in cells from voided urine, cytopathology and ultrasound for noninvasive detection of bladder tumors. *J Urol* 1998;159:389–92, discussion 393

50. Loy TS, Alexander CJ, Calaluce RD. Lewis X antigen immunostaining in the diagnosis of transitional cell carcinoma. *Mod Pathol* 1995; 8:587–90

51. Goulandris N, Karakitsos P, Georgoulakis J, *et al.* Deoxyribonucleic acid measurements in transitional cell carcinomas: comparison of flow and image cytometry techniques. *J Urol* 1996;156: 958–60

52. Tsai YC, Nichols PW, Hiti AL, *et al.* Allelic losses of chromosomes 9, 11, and 17 in human bladder cancer. *Cancer Res* 1990;50:44–7

53. Miyao N, Tsai YC, Lerner SP, *et al.* Role of chromosome 9 in human bladder cancer. *Cancer Res* 1993;53:4066–70

54. Hopman AH, Moesker O, Smeets AW, *et al.* Numerical chromosome 1, 7, 9, and 11 aberrations in bladder cancer detected by *in situ* hybridization. *Cancer Res* 1991;51:644–51

55. Matsuyama H, Bergerheim US, Nilsson I, *et al.* Nonrandom numerical aberrations of chromosomes 7, 9, and 10 in DNA-diploid bladder cancer. *Cancer Genet Cytogenet* 1994;77:118–24

56. Sauter G, Moch H, Wagner U, *et al.* Y chromosome loss detected by FISH in bladder cancer. *Cancer Genet Cytogenet* 1995;82:163–9

57. Sauter G, Moch H, Carroll P, *et al.* Chromosome-9 loss detected by fluorescence *in situ* hybridization in bladder cancer. *Int J Cancer* 1995;64:99–103

58. Sokolova I, Halling K, Jenkins R. The development of a multitarget, multicolor fluorescence *in situ* hybridization assay for the detection of urothelial carcinoma in urine. *J Molec Diagn* 2000;2:116–23

59. Mao L, Schoenberg MP, Scicchitano M, *et al.* Molecular detection of primary bladder cancer by microsatellite analysis. *Science* 1996;271: 659–62

60. Erbersdobler A, Friedrich MG, Schwaibold H, *et al.* Microsatellite alterations at chromosomes 9p, 13q, and 17p in nonmuscle-invasive transitional cell carcinomas of the urinary bladder. *Oncol Res* 1998;10:415–20

61. Mourah S, Cussenot O, Vimont V, *et al.* Assessment of microsatellite instability in urine in the detection of transitional-cell carcinoma of the bladder. *Int J Cancer* 1998;79:629–33

Transurethral resection of bladder cancer controlled by 5-aminolevulinic acid-induced fluorescence endoscopy

27

M. Kriegmair, D. Zaak, R. Knuechel, R. Baumgartner and A. Hofstetter

Introduction

5-Aminolevulinic acid (5-ALA) is a precursor of heme biosynthesis and induces an accumulation of fluorescent endogenous porphyrins, mainly protoporphyrin IX (PPIX), in tissues of epithelial origin[1]. We have been investigating 5-ALA especially for the detection of urothelial cancer since 1991 and the method was first described in 1992[2]. While the topic of photodynamic therapy with 5-ALA has been reviewed recently for oncology and specific skin disorders[3], the awareness of the organ specificity of 5-ALA and the metabolism of PPIX, as well as the exponentially increasing use of 5-ALA in urology have stimulated the summation of recent findings for the field of urology, especially for the diagnosis of bladder cancer.

Methods

5-ALA administration

A solution of 1.5 g of 5-aminolevulinic acid hydrochloride (Medac GmbH, Hamburg, Germany) in 50 ml 1.4% $NaHCO_3$ was instilled intravesically with a 14F catheter 2–3 h prior to endoscopy. The catheter was removed immediately after instillation. The pH value of the solution was 4.9. The solution was freshly prepared immediately before instillation and passed through a 0.2 μm filter to eliminate pyrogens.

Fluorescence excitation

The D-light (Storz GmbH, Tuttlingen, Germany) provides blue light (375–440 nm) for fluorescence excitation of PPIX. A yellow long-pass filter fitted into the eyepiece of the endoscope reduces the blue excitation light and enhances the fluorescence contrast. In order to keep the transmission of the blue excitation light minimal, the fiberoptic light cord was integrated into the telescope (30° lens). Switching between blue and white light is possible by means of a foot pedal.

Results and discussion

The risk of overlooking neoplastic lesions of the bladder using white-light endoscopy is significant. After transurethral resection of superficial bladder cancer, tumor remnants were found in up to 55% of the cases at repeated resection 1–2 weeks later[4–7]. Even in the case of solitary superficial bladder tumors, residual disease was found in 24% at a second transurethral resection 5 weeks later[5]. The authors emphasized the quality of their first resection by the fact that the second resection revealed infiltrative growth in only 2% of the cases. Therefore, most of the overlooked neoplasms came from positive margins or heterotopic lesions.

Klän and colleagues reported on a fractionated resection of T_1 transitional cell cancer[4]. In

28% of the patients, positive tumor margins were found, while residual disease from the tumor base was not observed in any case. A routine second resection was carried out 8–14 days later and revealed residual disease in 50% of the patients despite the surgical report of complete resection. Of the missed lesions, 76% were found to be visible tumors at repeated resection. The authors concluded that the extent of the lesions can easily be misjudged, even by experienced surgeons.

Fitzpatrick and colleagues reported on 414 newly diagnosed patients with $pT_a G_{1-2}$ tumors[8]. Patients who underwent intravesical therapy during their follow-up were excluded in this study. In one-third of the patients recurrent, or more likely residual, disease was found 3 months after the initial resection. Of these patients, 90% had further recurrences thereafter, whereas only 21% of the patients who were free of tumor 3 months after the initial resection demonstrated recurrent tumor during further follow-up. The response to the initial treatment of superficial bladder cancer[9], as well as the initial number of tumors[10], has been stressed as relevant for the outcome. In consideration of the clinical data described, a more complete removal of tumorous lesions from the bladder seems advisable. In particular, flat lesions, such as carcinoma in situ which may be concealed in the non-specific inflamed or normal-appearing mucosa, are of crucial effect for the rates of progression and recurrence, and require adequate intravesical immunotherapy without delay[11-13]. Random biopsies were found insufficient for detecting flat lesions[14,15]. In a retrospective study, Kiemeney and colleagues found no correlation between patient outcome, whether select mucosal biopsies were not performed or, if performed, were normal. However, if dysplasia or carcinoma in situ were found in patients, their risk of tumor progression was significantly higher. Therefore, random biopsies seem to be inadequate, since relevant early-stage and precancerous lesions are often missed. Cytology of voided urine or bladder washings is valuable for diagnosis, especially of high-grade lesions. However, recent prospective trials have resulted in a disappointingly low sensitivity of 54% for detecting carcinoma in situ[16].

Using white-light endoscopy, the detection of neoplasms is limited to morphological patterns. Since the 1960s, urologists have sought for methods of in vivo labelling of neoplastic lesions, in order to decrease the risk of overlooking tumors, with the help of an additional color contrast. Diagnostic methods based on detection of the fluorescence of systemically administered tetracycline, systemic porphyrin mixtures or fluorescein have only been tested in a few patients and have been abandoned. Intravesical instillation of methylene blue was also proven unsuitable, since 70% of carcinoma in situ and 84% of dysplastic lesions were not stained[17].

Following intravesical application of 5-ALA, we could demonstrate a selective accumulation of PPIX in urothelial cancer, providing an intensive color contrast between red fluorescing malignant lesions and the non-fluorescing normal blue mucosa[18]. Spectral measurements in vivo showed a more than 10-fold higher intensity of fluorescence of urothelial cancer in comparison to normal urothelium[19]. Due to the topical method of administration of 5-ALA and its fast metabolism, only minor side-effects such as urgency and algurea were observed in 7% of cases[20,21].

Initially, a krypton ion laser was used for fluorescence excitation (see below). Based on a biopsy-related evaluation, we reported a significant increase in sensitivity for the diagnosis of neoplastic urothelial lesions such as dysplasia and carcinoma in situ, as well as for papillary tumors, by the additional evaluation of the porphyrin fluorescence. In total, the procedure was marked by a sensitivity of 97% and a specificity of 65%[20].

The outstanding sensitivity of the procedure was confirmed by investigations by Jichlinski[22], Filbeck[23] and König[24] and ranges from 87% to 96%. Using this method of fluorescence detection, Jichlinski found 47 of 97 foci of carcinoma only by fluorescence marking which were invisible under white-light observation, and concluded that the sensitivity of the method appears to be twice as good as that of conventional white-light cystoscopy[22].

When large-scale laser technology was replaced by a specially designed incoherent diagnosis light system D-LIGHT, the equipment met all the requirements for a daily routine procedure and is used in combination with standard urological endoscopes[25]. Based on a per patient fashion, we found that the patients received a benefit in 150 of 328 (45%) cases of aminolevulinic acid-induced fluorescence endoscopies (AFE). In 82 AFE, additional neoplastic lesions were found which would have been missed under white-light observation alone. In 68 cases of complete fluorescence-negative mucosa, no biopsies would have been necessary due to the high sensitivity of the procedure. Thirty-one percent of the malignant foci, which were found only because of their positive PPIX fluorescence signal in the normal-appearing or non-specific inflamed mucosa, were high-risk lesions, such as carcinoma *in situ* or poorly differentiated papillary tumors. In 30% of the AFE, exclusively false-positive findings were observed. This seems to be acceptable as, in total, the mean number of biopsies was low, at 2.2 per patient. Obviously, this is markedly less than the number of random biopsies, carried out under white light.

AFE-guided biopsies and cytology seem to be complementary methods for the accurate diagnosis of bladder cancer. In 14 of 112 patients who had no exophytic tumors and a negative cytology, a neoplastic lesion was found in fluorescing areas of the bladder wall. In five of 15 patients with complete negative fluorescing mucosa but positive cytology, neoplastic disease was found later due to positive AFE-guided biopsies during follow-up of these patients.

The outcome of the admission study for 5-ALA in urology in Germany is positive[26]. This clinical trial represents a multicenter, parallel-group, phase III design. The study was controlled by reference pathology. Following stratification of the patients according to the participating centers and the EORTC risk score[27], patients were randomized to the AFE group ($n = 83$) or white-light group ($n = 82$). Residual tumor in both groups was evaluated by means of a second transurethral resection 10–14 days later. The analysis was performed according to the intention-to-treat principle, with all patients randomized and followed by a per-protocol analysis.

The intention-to-treat analysis set revealed that, in the white-light group, 40.6% of the patients were resected tumor-free in the primary resection, whereas, with the AFE-controlled transurethral resection, 61.5% of the patients were tumor-free when resected ($p = 0.016$, Fisher's exact test). In the per protocol set, 46.9% of the patients in the white-light arm and 67.3% of the patients in the fluorescence arm were resected tumor-free ($p = 0.031$, Fisher's exact test). There was no difference either in symptoms or in laboratory findings between the AFE group and the white-light group.

Conclusions

5-Aminolevulinic acid-based fluorescence endoscopy facilitates detection of neoplastic lesions within the bladder during transurethral resection. In the case of complete negative fluorescence findings, endoscopy can be performed without biopsies due to the high sensitivity of the procedure. A decrease of the rate of overlooked tumors is expected for transurethral resection supported by 5-aminolevulinic acid-induced fluorescence endoscopy. A resulting relatively decreased number of recurrences has to be documented in prospective randomized trials.

Acknowledgement

Supported by grants from the Deutsche Forschungsgemeinschaft (DFG #Kr1645/1–1).

References

1. Kennedy JC, Pottier RH. Endogenous protoporphyrin IX: a clinically useful photosensitizer for photodynamic therapy. *J Photochem Photobiol B* 1992;14:275–92

2. Kriegmair M, Baumgartner R, Hofstetter AG. Intravesikale Instillation von Delta-Aminolävulinsäure (ALA) – Eine neue Methode zur photodynamischen Diagnostik und Therapie. *Laser Medizin* 1992;8:83

3. Peng O, Warloe T, Berg K, *et al.* 5-Aminolevulinic acid-based photodynamic therapy: clinical research and future challenges. *Cancer* 1997; 79:2282–308

4. Klän R, Loy V, Huland H. Residual tumor discovered in routine second transurethral resection in patients with stage T1 transitional cell carcinoma of the bladder. *J Urol* 1991;146: 316–18

5. Köhrmann KU, Woeste M, Kappes J, Rassweiler J, Alken P. Der Wert der transurethralen Nachresektion beim oberflächlichen Harnblasenkarzinom. *Akt Urol* 1994;25:208

6. Vögeli TA, Grimm MO, Ackermann R. Prospective study for quality control of TUR of bladder tumors by routine 2nd TUR (ReTUR). *J Urol* 1998;159 Suppl:143

7. Mersdorf A, Brauers A, Wolf JM, Schneider V, Jakse G. 2nd TUR for superficial bladder cancer: a must. *J Urol* 1998;159 Suppl:143

8. Fitzpatrick JM, West AB, Butler MR, Lane V, O'Flynn JD. Superficial bladder tumors (stage pTa grades 1 and 2): the importance of recurrence pattern following initial resection. *J Urol* 1986;135:920–2

9. Pryor JP. Factors influencing the survival of patients with transitional cell tumours of the urinary bladder. *Br J Urol* 1973;45:586–92

10. Brausi M, Kurth K-H, Van der Meyden AP, Sylvester RJ. Variability in the three-months recurrence rate after TUR in superficial cell carcinoma (TCC) of the bladder: a combined analysis of 8 EORTC studies. *J Urol* 1998;159 Suppl:143

11. Smith G, Elton RA, Beynon LL, Newsam JE, Chisholm GD, Hargreave TB. Prognostic significance of biopsy results of normal-looking mucosa in cases of superficial bladder cancer. *Br J Urol* 1983;55:665–9

12. Heney NM, Ahmed S, Flanagan MJ, *et al.* Superficial bladder cancer: progression and recurrence. *J Urol* 1983;130:1083–6

13. Flamm J, Dona S. The significance of bladder quadrant biopsies in patients with primary superficial bladder carcinoma. *Eur Urol* 1989;2: 81–5

14. Kiemeney LA, Witjes JA, Heijbroek RP, Verbeek AL, Debruyne FM. Predictability of recurrent and progressive disease in individual patients with primary superficial bladder cancer. *J Urol* 1993;150:60–4

15. Kiemeney LA, Witjes JA, Heijbroek RP, Koper NP, Verbeek AL, Debruyne FM. Should random urothelial biopsies be taken from patients with primary superficial bladder cancer? A decision analysis. Members of the Dutch South-East Co-Operative Urological Group. *Br J Urol* 1994; 73:164–71

16. Sarosdy MF, deVere White RW, Soloway MS, *et al.* Results of a multicenter trial using the BTA test to monitor for and diagnose recurrent bladder cancer. *J Urol* 1995;154:379–83

17. Vicente J, Chechile G, Algaba F. Value of *in vivo* mucosa-staining test with methylene blue in the diagnosis of pretumoral and tumoral lesions of the bladder. *Eur Urol* 1987;13:15–16

18. Kriegmair M, Baumgartner R, Knuechel R, *et al.* Fluorescence photodetection of neoplastic urothelial lesions following intravesical instillation of 5-aminolevulinic acid. *Urology* 1994;44:836–41

19. Kriegmair M, Stepp H, Steinbach P, *et al.* Fluorescence cystoscopy following intravesical instillation of 5-aminolevulinic acid: a new procedure with high sensitivity for detection of hardly visible urothelial neoplasias. *Urol Int* 1995;55:190–6

20. Kriegmair M, Baumgartner R, Knuchel R, Stepp H, Hofstadter F, Hofstetter A. Detection of early bladder cancer by 5-aminolevulinic acid induced porphyrin fluorescence. *J Urol* 1996;155:105–9

21. Rick K, Sroka R, Stepp H, *et al.* Pharmacokinetics of 5-aminolevulinic acid induced protoporphyrin IX in skin and blood. *J Photochem Photobiol B: Biol* 1997;40:313–19

22. Jichlinski P, Forrer M, Mizeret J, *et al.* Clinical evaluation of a method for detecting superficial surgical transitional cell carcinoma of the bladder by light-induced fluorescence of protoporphyrin IX following the topical application of 5-aminolevulinic acid: preliminary results. *Lasers Surg Med* 1997;20:402–8

23. Filbeck T, Rössler W, Straub M, Kiel HJ, Knüchel R, Wieland WF. Clinical results of the transurethral resection and evaluation of superficial bladder carcinomas by means of fluorescence diagnosis after intravesical instillation of 5-aminolevulinic acid. *J Endourol* 1999;13:117–21

24. König F, McGovern FJ, Larne R, Enquist H, Schomacker KT, Deutsch TF. Diagnosis of bladder carcinoma using protoporhyrin IX fluorescence induced by 5-aminolevulinic acid. *BJU Int* 1999;83:129–35

25. Kriegmair M, Zaak D, Stepp H, *et al.* Transurethral resection and surveillance of bladder cancer – supported by 5-aminolevulinic acid induced fluorescence endoscopy. *Eur Urol* 1999;36:386–92

26. Kriegmair M, Mitglieder der AFE-Studiengruppe. Die transurethrale Elektroresektion von Harnblasentumoren mit und ohne 5-Aminolävulinsäure induzierter Fluoreszenz-Endoskopie. *Urologe A* 1998;37:S15

27. Bouffioux Ch, Kurth KH, Bono A, *et al.* Intravesical adjuvant chemotherapy for superficial transitional cell bladder carcinoma: results of 2 European organisations for research and treatment of cancer randomized trials with mitomycin C and doxorubicin comparing early versus delayed instillations and short-term versus long-term treatment. *J Urol* 1995;153:934–41

T$_a$–T$_1$ G$_1$–G$_2$ transitional cell carcinoma

28

D. W. W. Newling

Introduction

The majority of bladder tumors are superficial at their initial presentation. Around 80% of patients presenting with a T$_a$ or T$_1$ tumor will recur at some time and, depending on the grade of the tumor, between 2 and 50% will show evidence of progression[1]. The mainstay of therapy is a thorough transurethral resection. The rate of recurrence can be reduced in all tumors by the use of chemotherapy or immunotherapy. In the case of solitary tumors, a single instillation would seem to be adequate, provided that the tumor is not poorly differentiated and, with multiple tumors, early treatment with weekly instillations for 4 weeks, followed by 5-monthly instillations, appears to be satisfactory. Because of its toxicity, the use of immunotherapy with bacillus Calmette–Guérin (BCG) instillations is mainly restricted to very poorly differentiated tumors, multiple tumors or tumors that recur within the 1st year of transurethral resection. This chapter will be devoted to the treatment of T$_a$–T$_1$, G$_1$ and G$_2$ tumors.

If these tumors present *de novo* as a solitary lesion, they fall into a very good prognostic group, with less than 10% showing progression and only around 40% recurring within the 1st year. If the tumors are grade 2 and multiple, they fall into a different prognostic group and a more intensive therapy is certainly indicated[2].

The transurethral resection of superficial bladder tumors

Transurethral resection of superficial bladder tumors is the mainstay of therapy. The resection must be preceded by a thorough inspection of the bladder, using 30°, 70° and 120° lenses if a rigid cystoscope is employed. With a flexible cystoscope, and an experienced urologist, the use of a rigid instrument will be restricted to the resection itself.

For accuracy and ease of pathological examination, if the tumor is papillary, it is useful to resect the exophytic part of the tumor and send it as a separate specimen from the deeper resection which must include superficial muscle. A bimanual examination must be performed before and after the resection and, after removal of the resectoscope, a further cystoscopic assessment of the bladder should be made. During the resection, any abnormal areas of urothelium should be biopsied and, if the preoperative urine examination revealed malignant cells, then random biopsies may be necessary. In a recent evaluation, the use of random biopsies in superficial bladder tumors, without positive cytology or clear evidence of atypical epithelium, has not been shown to be of benefit. In a recent evaluation of transurethral resection (bladder tumors) carried out during the course of a number of European Organization for Research and Treatment of Cancer (EORTC) studies, there was a worrying incidence of recurrence at 3 months with both solitary and multiple tumors. In solitary tumors, the 3-month recurrence rate varied from 0 to 36% and, with multiple tumors, from 7 to 75%. Many of these tumors were found in difficult areas of the bladder, but, in the case of T$_1$ tumors, a number were found at the site of the original tumor, suggesting an incomplete resection. During the 20 years that the EORTC has been carrying out studies in superficial bladder tumors, the 3-month recurrence rate has diminished from 21 to 44% during

1975–78, to between 3 and 5.3% during 1987 and 1989[3].

Histological examination

From a prognostic standpoint, the histological examination of the resected specimen is of major importance. The difference between T_a and T_1 tumors and between T_{1a} and T_{1b} tumors (depending on the penetration of the muscularis mucosa) will determine the incidence of recurrence and the chance of progression. In the case of recurrent tumors, the pathologist must be in possession of the original tumor histology in order that a direct comparison can be made. Slides of each tumor should be archived and kept for reference. Special staining of superficial bladder tumors for markers of proliferation and specific bladder tumor antigens has not thus far proved particularly useful from a prognostic point of view.

The subsequent treatment of T_a, T_1, G_1 and G_2 tumors will depend upon the prognostic factors identified after the initial resection. There is clear evidence that all patients with T_a or T_1 lesions achieve some benefit in terms of the time to recurrence and the incidence of recurrent tumors from adjuvant chemo- or immunotherapy. The magnitude and type of that treatment will be determined according to the prognostic factor analysis carried out by the EORTC and subsequently mirrored in other analyses.

Superficial bladder tumors may be divided into three groups, the most simple being solitary, primary T_a–T_1 G_1–G_2 tumors and the most sinister being T_1 G_3 tumor, single, multiple or recurrent. Between these two extreme groups fall the majority of superficial bladder tumors, some 60%. Apart from the differentiation between T_a and T_1 lesions, probably the most significant prognostic factor is whether or not the superficial tumor is primary or recurrent, particularly if that recurrence has occurred within the first 3 months following the resection[4].

Subsequent therapy

In patients who have a positive cytology after complete resection of visible lesions, a second-look cystoscopy between 4 and 6 weeks after the initial operation should be carried out. If there is no obvious visible tumor, then random biopsies should be taken to identify the source of the carcinoma in situ. If these biopsies are negative, then more sophisticated investigations of the upper urinary tract, such as retrograde pyelogram with urine sampling from both ureters and ureterorenoscopy, should be considered. In patients where there is suspicion that the tumor has not been completely resected, then a further resection in 4–6 weeks may identify a significant number of patients with a residual malignancy[3].

Since the studies of the EORTC and the Medical Research Council (MRC) have clearly indicated the benefit for a single instillation of a cytotoxic agent after transurethral resection of solitary, well-differentiated tumors, this should be the standard practice in the majority of institutions. There is evidence that the instillation should be carried out within the first 6 h[5]. The instillation has been demonstrated to be effective using adriamycin, epirubicin, mitomycine and thiotepa. The disadvantage with thiotepa is that instillation within 6 h can give rise to absorption through the resected area of the bladder and subsequent myelotoxicity. All cytotoxic agents instilled into the bladder will give rise to symptoms of bladder inflammation. The earlier that instillation is carried out, the more acute the symptoms may be. If patients are warned of this, it rarely constitutes a major problem.

In patients with T_a–T_1 lesions who fall into the second prognostic group, i.e. multiple tumors or recurrent tumors, then a more intensive course of intravesical chemotherapy is indicated. If this is started within 24 h of the transurethral resection, then 4-weekly instillations of a suitable agent, followed by 5-monthly instillations, are probably an adequate treatment. If, for any reason, the instillation cannot be started within 24 h, then the EORTC has demonstrated that longer-term maintenance therapy for up to 1 year is probably of benefit[6].

Until now, no benefit has been accrued for continual maintenance therapy up to 3 years. Patients in the second prognostic group, according to the EORTC, may also benefit from BCG therapy. This should probably be reserved for patients presenting with multiple tumors and patients presenting with T_1 rather than T_a tumors. The disadvantage of BCG therapy is that it cannot be given immediately and there is clear evidence that, for adequate treatment and prophylaxis, the BCG should be administered by weekly instillations, for 6 weeks, followed by three further weekly instillations after the first 3-month cystoscopy, provided there is no evidence of recurrent tumor. From 6 months onwards, 3-weekly instillations should be given at 6-monthly intervals until 3 years have elapsed[7].

The follow-up

Patients who present with a solitary, well-differentiated T_a or T_1 tumor, which has been completely resected, have a much reduced chance of recurrence compared with those with multiple tumors or those in whom the tumor could not be completely resected. If this group of patients does not recur within the 1st year, the chances of recurrence are placed at less than 2%. It has, therefore, been suggested that these patients should, after thorough transurethral resection of the solitary tumor, receive a single instillation of a chemotherapeutic agent. If, at review cystoscopy after 3 months, there is no tumor present, the patient's cystoscopic follow-up can probably be postponed for 1 year. If, at the end of the year, there is no sign of recurrent tumor or positive cytology, then annual cystoscopy by means of a flexible cystoscope under no or topical anesthesia is probably the only follow-up that these patients require. Thus, in spite of the initial cost of an intravesical instillation, the reduced number of cystoscopies and admissions for these patients will result in considerable savings[8].

For patients presenting with multiple or recurrent tumors, the customary rigid follow-up, 3-monthly for the 1st year and 6-monthly subsequent to that, can only be altered when the patient has remained free of tumor for at least 2 years. Depending on the grade of the tumor and its multiplicity, even more intensive therapy may be necessary, particularly if any tumor has been diagnosed stage T_{1b} and is G_2 by grade. Since it is known that around 30% of G_2 tumors are initially given the wrong grade, a significant number of these patients will, in fact, have G_3 tumors and more rigorous therapy, even including cystectomy, may be indicated.

Life-style changes

Clear evidence has been presented by the Southwest Oncology Group (SWOG) that the treatment of patients with superficial bladder cancer with multi-vitamin therapy is of benefit in preventing recurrence. There is no evidence that it has a significant effect on progression[9]. The use of yoghurt preparations has also been shown to be of value and the working mechanism may well be related to changes in the gut flora. Smoking continues to exert a pernicious effect on the bladder, and it is essential that all patients presenting with bladder tumors, at any stage, are persuaded to stop smoking. A high fluid intake, certainly more than 2 liters a day, has also been shown to be of benefit in preventing recurrence, and there is no doubt that the side-effects of intravesical instillations and operative manipulations in the bladder can be considerably reduced if the urine output is maintained above 1500 ml/day.

Summary

The treatment of T_a–T_1 tumors that are well differentiated or even moderately differentiated is a combination of thorough transurethral resection followed by single or multiple chemotherapeutic interventions and, if necessary, a second-look cystoscopy. The reliability of present resection techniques, pathological staging and efficiency of prompt use of intravesical agents mean that, in a substantial number of patients, the traditional follow-up schedule can be modified, with savings of inconvenience to the patient and important financial benefits for the health-care services. In the treatment of superficial bladder cancer, for all the efficiencies of resection and intravesical therapy, there is no more important intervention than stopping these patients smoking.

References

1. Fitzpatrick JM, West AB, Butler MR, *et al.* Superficial bladder tumors (stage pTa, grade 1 and 3): the importance of recurrence pattern following initial resection. *J Urol* 1986;135:920–2

2. Kurth KH, Bouffioux C, Sylvester R, *et al.* and members of the EORTC Genitourinary Group. Treatment of suprficial bladder tumors: achievements and needs. *Eur Urol* 2000;37 (Suppl 3):1–9

3. Brausi M, Kurth KH, van der Meijden APM, *et al.* Variability in the three months recurrence rate after TUR in superficial transitional carcinoma of the bladder: a combined analysis of 8 EORTC studies. *J Urol* 1998;159(Suppl):143

4. Kurth KH, Denis L, Bouffioux C, *et al.* Factors affecting recurrence and progression in superficial bladder tumours. *Eur J Cancer* 1995;31A: 1840–6

5. Oosterlinck W, Kurth KH, Schröder FH, *et al.* and members of the EORTC Genitourinary Group. A prospective EORTC randomized trial comparing transurethral resection followed by a single intravesical instillation of Epirubicin or water in single stage Ta, T1 papillary carcinoma of the bladder. *J Urol* 1993;149:749–52

6. Bouffioux C, Kurth KH, Bono A, *et al.* and members of the EORTC Genitourinary Group. Intravesical adjuvant chemotherapy for superficial transitional cell bladder carcinoma: results of two EORTC randomized trials with mitomycin C and doxorubicin comparing early versus delayed and short-term versus long-term treatment. *J Urol* 1995;153:931–41

7. Lamm DL, Blumenstein BA, Crissman JD, *et al.* Maintenance BCG immunotherapy for recurrent T_a, T_1 and CIS transitional cell carcinoma of the bladder: a randomized SWOG study. *J Urol* 2000;163:1124–9

8. Hall RR, Parmar MKB, Richards AB, *et al.* Proposal for changes in cystoscopic follow-up in patients with bladder cancer and adjuvant intravesical chemotherapy. *Br Med J* 1994;308: 257–60

9. Lamm DL, Rigg D, Shriven J, *et al.* Megadose vitamins in bladder cancer: a double-blind clinical trial. *J Urol* 1994;151:21–6

BCG in transitional cell carcinoma – schedules of application, results and limitations

29

D. L. Lamm

Introduction

Intravesical treatment of superficial bladder cancer began to be popularized in the early 1960s, before the traditional three-phased system for cancer treatment development and evaluation was commonly used. Early treatment doses and schedules for intravesical chemotherapy were largely empiric, based on experience in other tumor systems and convenience rather than systematic testing for toxicity, optimal dose and relative efficacy. Unfortunately, this tradition has continued even today. The initial bacillus Calmette–Guérin (BCG) treatment schedule designed by Alvaro Morales was similarly empiric, based on experience, convenience and intuition.

Remarkably, the initial treatment schedule of six weekly instillations of 120 mg Armand Frappier BCG diluted in 50 cc of physiological saline, retained for 2 h, and associated with percutaneous BCG vaccination, has subsequently proven to be so effective that it has taken decades to demonstrate that any other regimen is superior. Important advances have been made to reduce the toxicity, improve the complete response rate, further reduce the risk of disease progression and to extend the duration of protection afforded by BCG immunotherapy. These advances, as well as the limitations of BCG immunotherapy, are reviewed.

BCG induction

Early investigators began BCG immunotherapy as soon as possible after transurethral resection of bladder tumors[1,2]. This was done in order to increase the direct contact between BCG organisms and any remaining tumor cells. Morales and the current author were concerned that the urothelium could grow over nests of transitional cell carcinoma and prevent juxtaposition of BCG and the tumor. While most patients tolerated early BCG without side-effects, it soon became clear that intravenous absorption of BCG could produce life-threatening sepsis. This observation, plus the historical comparison of early versus delayed (2–4 weeks post-resection) that showed reduced side-effects with no reduction in efficacy, resulted in the universal acceptance of delaying the initiation of intravesical BCG for at least 1 week.

The schedule of six weekly BCG instillations is remarkably effective and immunologically sound. In most patients, immune stimulation as measured by urinary cytokines, for example, peaks at 6 weeks. Continued administration can actually suppress the immune response and result in disappointing antitumor effects, as observed by Ratliff and Catalona in their trial of 12 weekly BCG administrations[3]. In the Southwest Oncology Group (SWOG) study of maintenance BCG, the addition of three weekly BCG administrations at 3 months increased the complete response rate in 217 randomized patients with carcinoma *in situ* from 69% to 84% ($p < 0.01$)[4]. To my knowledge, this is the only controlled study that has demonstrated an improvement over the standard six weekly instillations. The 6-week interval between the sixth and seventh instillations is believed to be essential for avoiding immunosuppression as a result of excess BCG administration.

Percutaneous BCG using the Tine technique of multiple needle puncture was used by Morales and the subsequent two National Cancer Institute-sponsored controlled randomized trials by Lamm[5] and Pinsky and colleagues[6] of intravesical BCG versus surgical resection alone, without BCG. The subsequent highly successful uncontrolled study of weekly followed by monthly intravesical BCG by Brosman clearly showed that percutaneous administration was not necessary[7]. Two subsequent randomized controlled comparisons of intravesical BCG, with or without percutanous administration, failed to show any significant advantage of percutaneous BCG[8,9]. In both studies, however, groups receiving additional percutaneous BCG did slightly better. Since both studies were small, it would be unwise to conclude that systemic administration is of no benefit. Studies confirm that patients who convert from negative protein purified derivative (PPD) skin test to positive have reduced tumor recurrence compared with those who remain skin test negative. Combining the series reported by Lamm[5] and Torrence[10], 17 out of 55 patients (31%) who converted to positive PPD had tumor recurrence, compared with 51 out of 82 patients (62%) who remained PPD skin test negative or were positive before treatment ($p = 0.0225$). In contrast, in very high-risk patients enrolled in the Memorial Sloan Kettering study, patients who were previously skin test positive had the lowest incidence of tumor recurrence[11]. The current author's interpretation of these data is that optimal local immune response may occur in those patients with systemic BCG immunity. In patients at very high risk for tumor recurrence, prior immunization with the attendant accelerated immune response may be beneficial. This is supported by data from the SWOG randomized comparison of induction therapy alone versus 3-week maintenance therapy. In patients with carcinoma *in situ* enrolled in that study, 77% of those who converted to a positive PPD had a complete response, compared to only 49% of those who remained skin test negative. Moreover, the SWOG studies that had the highest disease-free status for the BCG treatment arms (SWOG 8216 and 8507) both used percutaneous BCG administration[4,12]. Therefore, although not confirmed by controlled randomized studies, consideration should be given to the administration of percutaneous BCG at the time of diagnosis in PPD skin test-negative patients who are to receive intravesical BCG.

BCG dose

The dose of BCG has been selected arbitrarily, and may be higher than needed. Dose-reduction studies are difficult to interpret since different BCG preparations with widely varying strengths have been employed. While some dose-reduction studies have failed to show significant differences in response, the general conclusion is that reduced BCG doses do reduce the side-effects of BCG. With highly potent preparations, dose reduction is appropriate. Pagano and co-workers found a 40% reduction in tumor recurrence with half-strength Pasteur BCG when compared with full strength[13]. The CUETO group, however, found no improvement in response with reduced dose Connaught BCG[14].

It is likely that the optimal BCG dose changes not only with BCG preparation, but also with patient immunity, PPD skin-test status, interval since last BCG treatment and a host of factors that are currently unknown. For this reason, the author has adopted O'Donnell's recommendation that the BCG dose be reduced to a one-third, one-tenth, one-thirtieth or one-hundredth dose to reduce the side-effects. By adjusting the dose of BCG according to side-effects, not only is the risk of side-effects reduced, but it is possible that immuno-suppression from excess BCG administration may be avoided.

Principles of BCG immunotherapy

Animal studies, as reviewed by Bast and colleagues[15], have defined a series of principles that generally apply to maximize the response to cancer immunotherapy. These principles are summarized as follows:

(1) Minimize tumor burden (10^3 cells is the maximum number of cells reliably killed by BCG in murine models);

(2) Juxtapose BCG and tumor cells;

(3) Use an optimal number of CFU BCG (1×10^7 in the mouse, 2–20×10^8 intravesically in humans);

(4) An immune competent host is required, so treatment timing and the avoidance of immunosuppressive drugs is important to avoid immunosuppression.

The failure to follow these principles has led to profound failures in immunotherapy, and, indeed, has threatened to eliminate BCG immunotherapy completely. In the 1970s, multiple anecdotal reports of response to BCG in a wide variety of cancers brought widespread enthusiasm for immunotherapy. When controlled trials based on anecdotes and naïve enthusiasm rather than sound principles failed to confirm the benefit of BCG, most considered BCG immunotherapy to be dead. Many of these studies were destined to fail due to what we now know to be faulty design: the use of BCG in combination with immunosuppressive chemotherapy, use in patients with large tumor burden and use in patients with pre-existing immunosuppression. The confirmed success of BCG immunotherapy in carcinoma *in situ*, and T$_a$ and T$_1$ transitional cell carcinoma of the bladder further emphasizes the importance of the principles of BCG immunotherapy, and brings promise that failures based on poorly designed studies may be replaced by the successful application of BCG immunotherapy in other cancers in the future.

Maintenance BCG

It is well known that the immune stimulation induced by BCG is long lasting but wanes with time. In the animal model, additional BCG administration does not improve protection from transitional cell carcinoma 9 months post-treatment, but by 15 months the effect of BCG has waned to the extent that additional BCG improves the response. Studies of the immune response in patients given BCG show that many of the immune effects persist for at least 6 months[16]. In our initial study, examination of bladder biopsies in patients receiving BCG demonstrated that lymphocytic infiltration persisted for up to 6 months after intravesical BCG[17]. Studies of antibody response to BCG and PPD antigens as well as delayed-type cutaneous hypersensitivity responses in these patients revealed that immunity persisted for more than 6 months in most patients[18]. Prescott[19] found that human leukocyte antigen (HLA)-DR expression and increased T-helper/suppressor ratios persisted for 6 months and Zlotta and co-workers[20] found that the immunoproliferative response induced by BCG returns to baseline by 6 months. Since it is known that the risk for tumor recurrence remains increased essentially for life in most patients, it is logical to assume that maintenance BCG immunotherapy would be required to provide long-term protection.

While my initial evaluation of maintenance BCG given as a single instillation every 3 months for 2 years resulted in a four-fold reduction in the rate (though not the incidence) of tumor recurrence when compared with induction therapy alone, subsequent early trials of single instillations given quarterly[21] or monthly[22] provided no evidence of improved response. Similarly, Palou and colleagues in a randomized study found that the '6 + 6' regimen, giving six weekly instillations of BCG as maintenance at 6-month intervals for 2 years, was not significantly better than induction alone[23]. The latter study is particularly important in view of the common recommendation that patients who fail BCG should be given a second 6-week induction course.

In 1985, based on the failure of monthly and single quarterly maintenance schedules and immunological data suggesting that maintenance BCG should in fact be effective, the author designed a maintenance schedule based on repeated series of three weekly instillations[12]. The resultant study, SWOG 8507, enrolled 660 patients and confirmed beyond doubt the superior efficacy of maintenance BCG. With the administration of three weekly BCG treatments

6 weeks after completion of induction, complete response in carcinoma *in situ* increased from 68% to 84% in 130 randomized patients ($p < 0.01$). Three months after the initiation of BCG induction therapy, 384 disease-free patients who had been randomized by central computer to receive BCG maintenance therapy or no BCG maintenance therapy, were evaluable. Patients who received the maintenance BCG ($n = 192$) for 3 weeks given at 3, 6, 12, 18, 24, 30 and 36 months from the initiation of induction therapy had an increased median recurrence-free survival from 35.7 to 76.8 months ($p < 0.0001$) (Figure 1). Overall survival after a 10-year follow-up was 51.5% in the no-maintenance arm compared to 57.8% in the maintenance arm ($p = 0.08$). In addition to a highly significant difference in the recurrence pattern, BCG maintenance significantly increased the time to worsening disease or death to 111.5 months and is not estimable in the maintenance arm ($p < 0.05$). Worsening-free survival increased from 46.3% to 54.7% (Figure 2). This 3-week, 3-year BCG maintenance schedule can now be recommended as the treatment of choice for superficial transitional cell carcinoma, carcinoma *in situ* and high-risk stage T_a and T_1 disease, but, since only 16% of patients received the full eight courses of maintenance therapy, the benefit of maintenance therapy can accrue with less intensive treatment (Figure 3). As illustrated by the failure of every-6-month maintenance therapy to reduce tumor recurrence, excess administration of BCG can be counterproductive. We also suspect that, despite 3 years of maintenance therapy, immune stimulation would still eventually wane. Therefore, although we have no supportive data yet, the maintenance schedule has been extended to include three weekly treatments at 4, 5, 6, 8, 10 and 12 years in patients at high risk of disease

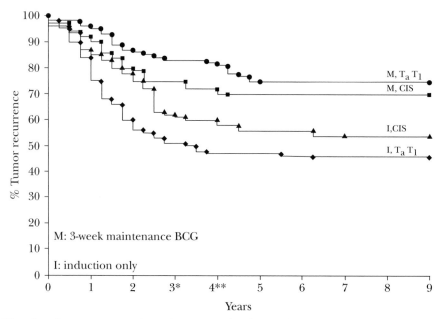

Figure 1 Time free from recurrence for patients treated with 3-week maintenance bacillus Calmette–Guérin (BCG) (top two curves) compared with 6-week induction only (bottom two curves). Note that there is an apparent increase in the rate of recurrence in the maintenance group beginning 1 year following termination of BCG maintenance. Also note that patients with T_a, T_1 and transitional cell carcinoma respond relatively better than carcinoma *in situ* (CIS) patients when maintenance therapy is given. Presumably this is a result of BCG and tumor cell juxtaposition, which occurs commonly in CIS patients, but may require maintenance therapy to occur with T_a, T_1 and transitional cell carcinoma. *Completion of therapy; **apparent increase in rate of recurrence 1 year after completion of maintenance

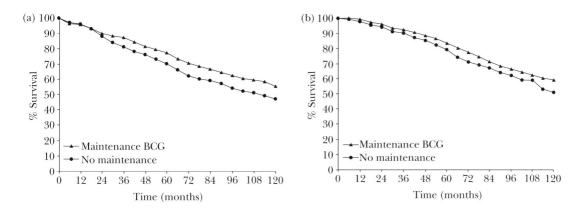

Figure 2 Worsening-free survival (a) and overall survival (b) for patients treated with 3-week maintenance (top curves) or induction only (bottom curves) in Southwest Oncology Group (SWOG) study 8507. Note that a statistically significant ($p < 0.04$) reduction in disease worsening occurred with 3-week maintenance, and this is reflected in an apparent, although not yet statistically significant, improvement in survival. BCG, bacillus Calmette–Guérin

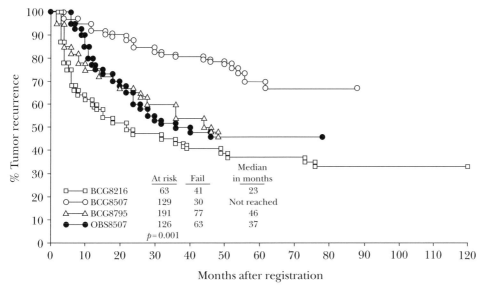

Figure 3 Comparison of bacillus Calmette–Guérin (BCG) treatment arms in Southwest Oncology Group (SWOG) studies with similar entry criteria. Only 3-week maintenance is clearly superior to 6-week induction

progression, i.e. those with carcinoma *in situ* or a grade 3 tumor.

Complications of BCG therapy

The side-effects and complications of BCG immunotherapy can certainly be considered to be one of the limitations of this therapy[24]. While BCG generally produces more side-effects than intravesical therapy, many large studies have failed to show a significant increase in treatment intolerance when compared with chemotherapy. Many of the side-effects of BCG are in fact a consequence of the beneficial immune stimulation, such as frequency, dysuria, and mild malaise and fever. These symptoms can herald a beneficial response to treatment. Cystitis can occur in as many as 90% of patients.

Dysuria, frequency, low-grade fever and malaise usually occur after the third dose. If irritative bladder symptoms, malaise and fever persist or progress, isoniazid 300 mg daily is given until the symptoms resolve. Treatment may then be re-instituted the day prior to BCG instillation and continued for 3 days, but the European Organization for Research and Treatment of Cancer (EORTC) study failed to confirm that prophylactic isoniazid actually reduces the local or systemic side-effects of BCG. Prophylactic isoniazid is clearly not indicated for asymptomatic patients, and has been shown to decrease the immune stimulation of intravesical BCG in animals[25]. Significant reactions to intravesical BCG occur in only 5% of patients. Fever greater than 103°F is the most common reaction, occurring in 3% of all patients. The main concern is the inability to distinguish an uncomplicated febrile episode from the onset of systemic BCG infection or hypersensitivity sepsis. Patients developing a high fever should, therefore, be hospitalized for observation and treated with isoniazid 300 mg and rifampicin 600 mg daily. BCG sepsis has been observed in up to 0.4% of patients treated with intravesical BCG. Current estimates are far lower, but, to date, ten deaths have been attributed to intravesical BCG. Patients initially present with signs and symptoms that are indistinguishable from Gram-negative sepsis and should, therefore, be covered with broad-spectrum antibiotics for Gram-negative sepsis as well as isoniazid 300 mg, rifampicin 600 mg and prednisolone 40 mg daily for BCG sepsis. BCG hypersensitivity is observed in animal models and may occur simultaneously with systemic infection; hence, prednisolone is recommended in addition to isoniazid and rifampicin[26]. Prednisone alone should be avoided since, in our animal study, it resulted in increased mortality. Ethambutol 1200 mg daily may be added to isoniazid and rifampicin; BCG is also sensitive to quinolones and aminoglycosides. In patients with deep BCG infection or sepsis, antibiotic treatment is continued for 3–6 months.

Many of the side-effects of BCG immunotherapy can be avoided by simply reducing the dose of BCG logarithmically when increased symptoms occur. We routinely reduce the dose of BCG to one-third, one-tenth, one-thirtieth or one-hundredth as needed to prevent increased side-effects. A controlled evaluation to confirm the efficacy of this approach has not been carried out, but it appears that side-effects are significantly reduced without altering efficacy.

Combined BCG and interferon immunotherapy

Interferon-α is effective in the treatment of carcinoma *in situ*, and several authors have used BCG in combination with interferon. O'Donnell[27] has recently popularized this approach in the United States, and has reported his results with 52 high-risk patients treated with BCG plus α-2b interferon (Intron A). Overall, after a 2-year follow-up, 53% of patients are free of recurrence, including 45% of 34 patients with carcinoma *in situ* and 58% of 33 patients who had failed previous courses of BCG. O'Donnell added 50 million units of interferon to BCG in his study, but Esuvaranathan[28], who confirmed the superiority of combination therapy over BCG alone in a controlled trial, added just 10 million units. Studies of urinary cytokines suggest that immunosuppression induced by excess BCG administration can be reversed by the addition of interferon.

Combined BCG and vitamins

Oncovite (Mission Pharmacal, San Antonio, Texas, USA), a preparation of high doses of vitamins A (40 000 IU), B_6 (100 mg), C (1000 mg) and E (400 IU) plus zinc (90 mg) taken by mouth daily in patients treated with BCG reduced long-term tumor recurrence by 40% in a double-blind comparison with vitamins in the recommended daily allowance[29] (Figure 4). Immunological studies demonstrated a statistically significant increase in NK-cell activity in patients on Oncovite compared with those taking standard dose vitamins. Surprisingly, the benefit in terms of reduction in tumor recurrence is greater than that in the combined BCG plus interferon study reported above.

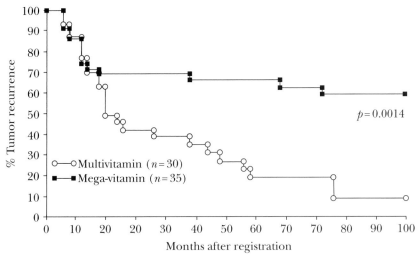

Figure 4 Kaplan–Meier estimate of 5-year tumor-free period in patients receiving vitamin supplements and bacillus Calmette–Guérin (BCG) therapy for bladder carcinoma. In patients given suboptimal BCG treatment, prevention of tumor recurrence is markedly improved with the addition of high doses of vitamins A, B_6, C and E (Oncovite, Mission Pharmacal, San Antonio, Texas)

Conclusions

Suboptimal BCG treatment schedules have been found to be superior to standard intravesical chemotherapy and, unlike chemotherapy, appear to reduce disease progression. A single 6-week course of BCG is highly effective and quite long lasting, but the effect does diminish with time. The addition of three weekly BCG instillations at 3 months significantly increases the complete response rate in patients with carcinoma *in situ*, and maintenance therapy in patients who are disease-free following induction significantly reduces subsequent tumor recurrence and progression. To achieve these results, the schedule of up to three weekly instillations at 3, 6, 12, 18, 24, 30 and 36 months must be used, since studies of single quarterly or monthly instillations did not show significantly better results than induction alone. The treatment schedule should be individualized according to the patient's side-effects and as few as 16% of patients may require the full compliment of scheduled treatments. Side-effects can be reduced by cutting the dose of BCG logarithmically. The benefit of BCG may be enhanced by the addition of vitamins A, B_6, C and E, and many patients who fail BCG can be rescued by adding interferon-α to the instillation.

References

1. Morales A, Eidinger D, Bruce AW. Intracavitary bacillus Calmette-Guérin in the treatment of superficial bladder tumors. *J Urol* 1976; 116:180–3

2. Lamm DL, Thor DE, Harris SC, *et al.* Bacillus Calmette-Guérin immunotherapy of superficial bladder cancer. *J Urol* 1980;124:38–40

3. Ratliff TL, Catalona WJ. Depressed proliferative responses in patients treated with 12 weeks of intravesical BCG. *J Urol* 1989;141:230A

4. Lamm DL, Blumenstein BA, Crissman JD, *et al.* Maintenance bacillus Calmette-Guerin immunotherapy for recurrent TA, T1 and carcinoma *in situ* transitional cell carcinoma of the bladder: a randomized Southwest Oncology Group Study. *J Urol* 2000;163:1124–9

5. Lamm DL. Bacillus Calmette-Guérin immunotherapy for bladder cancer. *J Urol* 1985;134:40

6. Pinsky CM, Camacho FJ, Kerr D, *et al.* Intravesical administration of bacillus Calmette-Guerin in patients with recurrent superficial carcinoma of the urinary bladder: report of a prospective, randomized trial. *Cancer Treatm Rep* 1985;69: 47–53

7. Brosman SA. Experience with bacillus Calmette-Guerin in patients with superficial bladder cancer. *J Urol* 1982;128:27–30

8. Lamm DL, DeHaven JI, Shriver JS, *et al.* A randomized prospective comparison of oral versus intravesical and percutaneous Bacillus Calmette-Guerin for superficial bladder cancer. *J Urol* 1990;144:65–7

9. Luftenegger W, Ackermann DK, Futterlieb A, *et al.* Intravesical versus intravesical plus intradermal bacillus Calmette-Guerin: a prospective randomized study in patients with recurrent superficial bladder tumors. *J Urol* 1996;155: 483–7

10. Torrence RJ, Kavoussi LR, Catalona WJ, *et al.* Prognostic factors in patients with intravesical bacillus Calmette-Guerin for superficial bladder cancer. *J Urol* 1988;139:941–4

11. Herr HW, Laudone VP, Badalament RA, *et al.* Bacillus Calmette-Guérin therapy alters the progression of superficial bladder cancer. *J Clin Oncol* 1988;6:1450

12. Lamm DL, Blumenstein BA, Crawford ED, *et al.* A randomized trial of intravesical doxorubicin and immunotherapy with Bacille Calmette-Guérin for transitional cell carcinoma of the bladder. *N Engl J Med* 1991;325:1205–9

13. Pagano F, Bassi P, Milani C, *et al.* A low dose bacillus Calmette-Guérin regimen in superficial bladder cancer therapy: is it effective? *J Urol* 1991;146:32–5

14. Martinez-Pineiro JA, Solsona E, Flores N, *et al.* Improving the safety of BCG immunotherapy by dose reduction. Cooperative Group CUETO. *Eur Urol* 1995;27 (Suppl 1):13–18

15. Bast RC Jr, Zbar B, Borsos T, *et al.* BCG and Cancer 1. *N Engl J Med* 1974;290:1413

16. Reichert DF, Lamm DL. Long-term protection in bladder cancer following intralesional therapy. *J Urol* 1984;132:570–3

17. Lamm DL, Thor DE, Harris SC, *et al.* BCG immunotherapy of superficial bladder cancer. *J Urol* 1980;124:38–40

18. Winters WD, Lamm DL. Antibody responses to Bacillus Calmette-Guérin during immunotherapy in bladder cancer patients. *Cancer Res* 1981;41:2672–6

19. Prescott S, James K, Busuttil A, *et al.* HLA-DR expression by high grade superficial bladder cancer treated with BCG. *Br J Urol* 1989;63:264–9

20. Zlotta AR, van Vooren JP, Huygen K, *et al.* What is the optimal regimen for BCG intravesical therapy? Are six weekly instillations necessary? *Eur Urol* 2000;37:470–7

21. Hudson MA, Ratliff TL, Gillen DP, *et al.* Single course versus maintenance Bacillus Calmette-Guérin therapy for superficial bladder tumors: a prospective, randomized trial. *J Urol* 1987; 138:295

22. Badalament RA, Herr HW, Wong GY, *et al.* A prospective randomized trial of maintenance versus nonmaintenance intravesical Bacillus Calmette-Guérin therapy of superficial bladder cancer. *J Clin Oncol* 1987;5:441

23. Palou J, Laguna P, Algaba F, *et al.* High grade superficial transitional cell carcinoma of the bladder and/or CIS treated with BCG: control vs maintenance treatment. *Br J Urol* 1997; 80(Suppl):32

24. Lamm DL. Complications of Bacillus Calmette-Guerin immunotherapy. *Urol Clin N Am* 1992;19:565–72

25. De Boer EC, Steerenberg PA, van der Meijden AP, *et al.* Impaired immune response by isoniazid treatment during intravesical BCG administration in the guinea pig. *J Urol* 1992;148:1577–82

26. DeHaven JI, Traynelis C, Riggs DR, *et al.* Antibiotic and steroid therapy of massive systemic Bacillus Calmette-Guérin toxicity. *J Urol* 1992;147:738–42

27. O'Donnell MA, Downs TM, De Wolf WC. Preliminary phase 2 results of combination BCG plus interferon-alfa-2B (IFN-α) in high risk patients with superficial bladder cancer. *J Urol* 1999;161(Suppl: pt 2):286

28. Esuvaranathan K, Cheng C, Chia SJ, *et al.* A phase IIB trial of BCG combined with interferon alpha for bladder cancer. *Br J Urol* 2000;86 (Suppl 3):4

29. Lamm DL, Riggs DR, Shriver JS, *et al.* Megadose vitamins in bladder cancer: a double-blind clinical trial. *J Urol* 1994;151:21–6

30

The approach to high-grade transitional cell carcinoma in T_a, CIS and T_1 stages

M. S. Soloway and M. Sofer

Transitional cell carcinoma (TCC) is the second most common malignancy of the genitourinary tract and the second most common cause of death among the genitourinary tumors[1]. Although 75–85% of TCC is confined to the mucosa at presentation, 70% of patients with multiple or high-grade tumors develop a true recurrence or a new occurrence following the initial transurethral resection (TUR) and 10–15% will progress to muscle-invasive disease[2]. The purpose of this chapter is to review the present knowledge regarding high-grade superficial TCC outlining ways that may contribute to a reduction in the rate of progression together with subsequent improvement in survival.

Staging and grading

Bladder cancer staging (Union Internationale Contre le Cancer TNM 1997) is based on a combined assessment of the depth of bladder penetration, lymph node invasion and meta-stasis. Although, histologically, lamina propria represents a submucosal component and, there-fore, bladder cancer at this level is considered 'superficial', its biological behavior differs from that of tumors confined to the urothelium. Discrepancy in biological behavior also characterizes different forms of TCC confined to the mucosa. The term 'superficial' TCC, commonly used for tumors involving the bladder mucosa and submucosa, should be avoided and replaced by a pathological classifi-cation, i.e. T_a, T_1, carcinoma *in situ* (CIS). T_a tumors involve only the urothelium, forming papillary fronds around a central vascular stalk that protrudes into the bladder lumen. T_1 stage is characterized by tumors that are usually more sessile and that penetrate the lamina propria. A subdivision of stage T_1 into T_{1a}, invasion superficial to the muscularis mucosae, and T_{1b}, extension through the muscularis mucosae but still confined to the lamina propria, was proposed based on reports showing a different prognosis between these groups[3]. This sub-division is not formally included in the current TNM staging system. CIS is a high-grade cancer confined to the urothelium and is flat.

Histological grading provides prognostic information regarding biological behavior. The most widely used grading was proposed by Mostofi and colleagues[4] and adopted by the World Health Organization (WHO) in 1973. This classification defines three histological grades and is presented in Table 1.

Pathogenesis

Many etiological factors have been associated with bladder cancer. These include cigarette smoking, occupational factors (aniline dyes and aromatic amines), local irritating factors (bacterial and parasitic infections, cysto-lithiasis), carcinogens (cyclophosphamide) and pelvic irradiation. The carcinogenetic process involves DNA damage and alteration of cellular replication control.

It has been hypothesized that bladder cancer development follows two distinct pathways, both

Table 1 Histological grading of transitional cell carcinoma (WHO)

Grade	Papillary form	Nuclear pleomorphism	Chromatin	Nucleoli	Mitoses
Papilloma	absent	absent	fine	absent or inconspicuous	absent
1	present	absent to minimal	fine	inconspicuous	absent or rare
2	usually present	mild to moderate	granular to coarse	distinct	occasional
3	possibly present	marked	coarse and irregularly distributed	prominent	numerous

beginning with a proliferative diathesis expressed as atypical hyperplasia and dysplasia within the normal urothelium. The low-grade pathway is characterized by atypical hyperplasia and generates papillary low-grade carcinoma. It is believed to be associated with a defect in either the long or short arm of chromosome 9 and increased vascular endothelial growth factor (VEGF) expression. As a result of this dysplastic process, the grade of these tumors may progress from low to high with further implications in the invasive potential[5]. The high-grade pathway generates CIS and implies urothelial dysplasia associated with defects in chromosome 17p53. This lesion has higher invasive potential and is able to progress both to papillary high-grade cancer or to a solid muscle-invasive tumor. It appears that a chromosome 17p53 defect also plays an essential role in promoting the invasive ability of high-grade papillary carcinomas[5].

Evaluation and transurethral resection

Early diagnosis is critical especially for high-grade TCC. A prompt urological work-up is recommended when suspected signs and symptoms such as hematuria and/or irritative urinary symptoms occur. The endoscopic evaluation is essential for the diagnosis. With the advent of the modern flexible endoscopes, the initial endoscopy is often performed in the office with minimal patient discomfort. This allows a complete and systematic endoscopic survey including the entire urethra and the bladder. The ureteral orifices should be inspected and the efflux of urine should be observed. Bladder filling should allow differentiation between true pathological findings and trabeculations but, on the other hand, overfilling may lead to subsequent loss of the ability to identify CIS. Papillary and solid tumors are easily recognized while erythematous areas should be suspected for the presence of CIS. All the pathological findings should be described, preferably by a schematic drawing, or, when possible, by picture acquisition. This simple practice permits easy orientation and complete identification of the lesions when a subsequent endoscopic procedure is necessary. It is also advantageous when the patient is evaluated by other clinicians.

Bladder washing should be sent for cytological assessment if a high-grade tumor is suspected. Cytology has a sensitivity of 70–90% and a specificity of 98% for high-grade cells[6]. Synchronous upper urinary tract tumors that occur in 2–5% of cases should be excluded by intravenous urography. The value of initial intravenous pyelograms (IVP) has been questioned by Goessl and co-workers[7] who considered ultrasonography to be equivalent to IVP but less expensive and without side-effects. Recently, Herranz-Amo and colleagues[8] considered IVP unnecessary in patients with newly diagnosed bladder carcinoma because the incidence of upper tract tumors was only 1.1% and an IVP diagnosed only 66% of these cases. However, IVP is still widely used in practice for the screening of the upper urinary tract while retrograde pyelography with washing cytology is reserved for assessment of suspicious or poorly imaged regions.

Abnormal endoscopic findings indicate the need for biopsy under anesthesia. In our practice, the procedure is initiated using an optical dilator with a 0° or 12° telescope which allows urethral dilatation under vision, avoiding complications related to blind dilatation. Following urethral dilatation, a 27 or 28 Fr continuous flow resectoscope sheath is placed in the urethra and the entire bladder is assessed using the 70° telescope. During endoscopic resection, one should maintain the bladder at a capacity of 50–75% to diminish the risk of bladder perforation or excitation of the obturator nerve. Overdistension also limits the ability to detect CIS. All evident tumor should be removed, if possible, by TUR. When necessary, suprapubic pressure or digital rectal or vaginal motion allow the surgeon to improve the accessibility for difficult locations. In order to permit accurate pathological staging, the retrieved specimen should include not only the obvious tumor, but also the underlining muscle if invasion of the bladder wall is a possibility. Better control of the excision depth can be achieved using a bladder wall loop for tumors located on the posterior and lateral walls and a video system which magnifies and improves the image. The coagulation current should be reduced in order to minimize the electrical carbonization that leads to inadequate pathological assessment. Cold cup biopsies should be taken from areas suspicious for CIS.

A bladder wash should be sent for cytology if the patient has a history of, or is suspected of, having a high-grade tumor. A bimanual examination should be carried out pre- and postoperatively to compare findings such as mobility, palpable mass and consistency. Co-operation with the pathologist is essential in assuring a precise pathological diagnosis. The specimen should be accompanied by a note to the pathologist describing a brief clinical history including previous tumors and related treatments, e.g. radiation or chemotherapy, which might influence the diagnosis. In a multicenter study of 1400 patients, Van Der Meijden and colleagues[9] showed that pathological reassessment of T_1 G_3 TCC resulted in an overall 50% change of diagnosis, of which 10% were re-classified as muscle invasions.

Intravesical therapy

Once diagnosed and pathologically defined, the superficial bladder cancer should be evaluated for its potential to recur and progress. While low-grade tumors recur frequently but rarely progress, high-grade tumors are aggressive and tend to progress and lead to almost the entire disease-related mortality of bladder cancer. In addition to high grade, factors associated with increased risk for recurrence and progression are tumor size, multifocality, positive postoperative cytology, prostatic urethral involvement, presence of CIS and lamina propria invasion[10]. When one of these factors, or a combination of these factors, is present, measures to reduce recurrence and delay progression are recommended.

Intravesical therapy, using either chemotherapeutic or immunological agents in an adjuvant fashion following endoscopic resection, has been shown to reduce the recurrence of superficial TCC. Bacillus Calmette–Guérin (BCG) has gained acceptability as the most effective agent in preventing or delaying recurrence of CIS and T_1G_3 tumors. The mechanism of action is a local immunological host response resulting in immunocompetent cytotoxic cell activation as well as release of cytokines, such as interleukins, that have antineoplastic activity[11,12]. In practice, it appears that T_1G_3 tumors behave either as BCG-sensitive, responding to treatment after initial therapy, or BCG-refractory, continuing to recur or progress. None of the intravesical treatments have been found to be helpful in terms of preventing progression despite a probable more durable effect of BCG. Other intravesical chemotherapeutic agents which show benefit in the prophylaxis of recurrence are thiotepa, adriamycin (doxorubicin), mitomycin C and epirubicin[13]. Some authors have suggested using the combination of BCG with a chemotherapeutic agent. This was found to result in a slightly better outcome especially in patients with CIS. However, trials using combination chemotherapy resulted in modest outcome improvement with increased local side-effects which made its use unjustified[14,15].

Intravesical therapy works optimally when used as prophylaxis. We believe that the completeness of the resection has an important impact on the evolution of the disease. Our routine protocol for patients with high-grade TCC, with or without CIS, consists of immediate instillation of mitomycin C after a complete TUR, followed by BCG instillations weekly for 6 weeks, beginning 10–14 days after surgery. The rationale behind the immediate administration of mitomycin C is to avoid tumor implantation and provide immediate treatment for microscopic residual disease after TUR. It has been shown that a single immediate instillation of mitomycin C decreases the recurrence rates and increases the recurrence-free interval[16,17].

Many studies have evaluated which of the adjuvant treatments and regimens, single or combined with maintenance protocols, result in less recurrence and progression. The Southwest Oncology Group reported promising results with a maintenance protocol of a 6-week induction course followed by three weekly instillations at 3 and 6 months and every 6 months for 3 years. However, only 16% of the patients could tolerate the complete regimen[18].

Prognostic factors, early detection and follow-up

Efforts have been made to define predictors for responders to adjuvant BCG treatment and/or patients at high risk for progression. Proposed prognostic factors such as depth of lamina propria invasion, vascular invasion, increasing grade of anaplasia and flow cytometry have been studied, but as yet do not have enough specificity for clinical use[19–22].

Llopis and co-workers[23] showed in a case–control study that $p53$ expression analyzed at a cut-off point of 20% positivity is a significant predictor of progression. In contrast, Steiner and colleagues[24] denied the helpfulness of $p53$ in selection of candidates for radical cystectomy. Promising results were reported using the presence of chromosomes 7 and 17 aneusomy for prediction of pT_a/pT_1 recurrence and expression of thymidine phosphorylase for prediction of progression[25,26]. However, these parameters are still in a preliminary stage of analysis.

To date, the most accepted predictors of progression are clinical and pathological. These include early recurrence of high-grade TCC following BCG, the association of CIS, invasion and depth of lamina propria invasion and grade 3 classification. In a series of 166 patients who underwent radical cystectomy for invasive TCC in our institution, 43% had a prior non-invasive tumor while 57% had muscle invasion at presentation. Among the prior non-invasive TCC group, half were stage T_a, 90% of them were high grade (G_3), 20% had CIS and 30% were stage T_1 of which 90% had associated CIS. In this prior non-invasive group, 25% were operated on for high-grade refractory superficial bladder cancer but, in all cases, the final pathology indicated muscle invasion. When comparing patients who had either $> T_2$ or $< T_2$ stage bladder cancer at their initial diagnosis, we found a 2-year disease-free survival of 49% and 79%, respectively. This emphasizes the aggressive behavior of high-grade TCC and the need for close follow-up and the crucial timing for radical cystectomy. In addition, we found a decrease in the rate of *de novo* T_2 stage TCC in comparison to the series from the 1980s, which suggests some improvement in early detection[27]. This change may be attributed to a better recognition of the need of primary physicians to refer patients with hematuria and voiding symptoms. Diagnosis of TCC at an earlier stage might lead to either eradication of the tumor before muscle invasion or consideration of cystectomy before muscle invasion in the presence of adverse risk factors.

Despite a lower overall incidence of TCC, women are more likely to be diagnosed at a more advanced stage. A possible reason is that a healthy female may not seek medical attention for hematuria or irritative symptoms or the primary physician may attribute these signs to a urinary tract infection, deferring referral for endoscopy.

In addition to improving the health education of the entire population, screening of high-risk populations, e.g. cigarette smokers, with early detection might contribute to a decrease in bladder cancer mortality.

During the past decade an impressive number of molecular markers of TCC have been identified. These include the BTA Stat, NMP22 and, recently described, telomerase and HA-Haase[28,29]. However, there is still a need for better tumor markers because none of the current markers when used alone has enough sensitivity and specificity to be used for screening purposes[30].

Early recognition of high-risk factors implies a rigorous surveillance protocol combining periodic cystoscopy and bladder-wash cytology. Our surveillance program differs according to the initial stage and grade. Low-grade tumors such as T_a G_1 are followed with cystoscopy and cytology at 3 months. If the first cystoscopy is negative, the interval is progressively lengthened. Cytology may be used in lieu of endoscopy. Although cytology will not detect a low-grade tumor 'recurrence', a delay of 6 months in the diagnosis of a low-grade tumor will not adversely affect the patient. Cytology serves to minimize the likelihood of missing a high-grade tumor. If the initial tumor is high grade, the patient is treated and is placed in the high-risk group, which is monitored more rigorously.

The high-risk group includes patients with grade 2 or 3 disease, CIS and/or stage T_1. These patients undergo cystoscopy and cytology at 3, 6, 9 and 12 months. If they remain tumor-free, they are followed every 3–6 months thereafter, with an option for cytology at 3-month intervals if endoscopy is not performed. A restaging TUR under anesthesia may be performed for an initial T_1, G_{2-3} TCC, in order to exclude understaging and ensure complete resection. All patients in this group

should be followed for life since their risk of progression does not diminish over time and may materialize even after a 10–15-year disease-free interval[31].

Rationale and timing of radical cystectomy

The high progression potential of T_1 G_3 and its related morbidity and mortality emphasize the need for aggressive treatment. Some have suggested early radical cystectomy without a trial of TUR plus adjuvant therapy. Supporters of this approach argue that the 5-year survival rate of 90% falls to 50–60% if the radical cystectomy is delayed until recurrence or progression[32]. On the other hand, since the reported progression rates are approximately 25% with TUR plus BCG and 50% with TUR alone, it seems that, with this aggressive regimen, 50–75% of patients will be over-treated. Furthermore, the morbidity and mortality associated with radical cystectomy are 30% and 1–4%, respectively, and, despite advanced techniques of orthotopic replacement, the quality of life is altered[33].

Therefore, the most important issue is how to restrict the radical cystectomy to selective high-risk patients, choosing an initial conservative approach without affecting survival. We think that this goal can be achieved by combining a complete TUR with BCG adjuvant therapy but remaining prepared to recognize the appropriate time for radical cystectomy.

The dilemma of continuation of bladder sparing arises with the failure of adjuvant treatment and recurrence of T_1 G_3 TCC with or without CIS. We usually suggest radical cystectomy. If the recurrence is T_a or CIS alone, a second 6-week course of BCG may be used. It has been shown that 38–50% of patients whose tumors recur after the initial induction BCG course may benefit from a second course of BCG[34,35].

In the last decade, the role of radical cystectomy as an efficient prophylactic and curative treatment of high-grade superficial TCC was widely analyzed. The amplitude of this operation in regards to its possible benefit was taken into consideration and criteria for decision and timing were elaborated. Controversial opinions regarding the timing for radical cystectomy were published in the early 1990s. However, survival rates in the range 77–84% were reported with either early radical cystectomy or radical cystectomy carried out after failed conservative treatment[32,36]. A similar outcome with superficial high-grade TCC has been outlined by Serretta and co-workers[37] who concluded that an initial bladder-sparing approach is legitimate and radical cystectomy should be postponed until the appearance of CIS, recurrence of same grade and stage tumors, or progression to muscle invasion. This approach has been supported recently by Brake and colleagues[38]. In a series of 44 patients with initial T_1 TCC treated with TUR and BCG, they were able to limit the radical cystectomy rate to 9% and to achieve a disease-free survival rate of 89% at a median follow-up of 28 months. As mentioned previously, early recurrence following BCG is an adverse factor. In this context, Herr[31] concluded that T_1G_3 TCC that is refractory to conservative treatment, especially within the first year, is best treated with radical cystectomy. We are in agreement with this, and consider the results of the first cystoscopy at 3 months after TUR and BCG as crucial for

deciding further treatment. If this is negative, the patient enters a maintenance intravesical program. However, recognition of recurrence of the same grade/stage TCC and appearance of CIS in association lead to a recommendation for radical cystectomy.

Our experience with T_1G_3 TCC treated initially in a conservative manner concurs with most of the contemporary series. In 61 cases, we found recurrence and progression rates of 23% and 15%, respectively, while the overall survival rate was 93% at a median follow-up of 37 months.

Based on this experience and other contemporary results, we have adopted the initial bladder-sparing approach (Figure 1), contemplating radical cystectomy in the presence of the criteria listed in Table 2.

Table 2 Indications for radical cystectomy in the treatment of superficial bladder tumors

Number	Indication
1	progression to G_3 after BCG
2	recurrence of $T_1 G_3$ with CIS
3	appearance of CIS after BCG
4	muscle invasion

CIS, carcinoma *in situ*

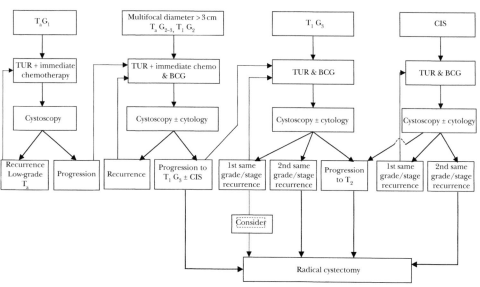

Figure 1 Follow-up and therapeutic flow-chart of transitional cell carcinoma (TCC) in stage T_a, T_1 and carcinoma *in situ* (CIS). BCG, bacillus Calmette–Guérin; TUR, transurethral resection

We believe that rigorous surveillance with long-term follow-up is crucial in managing these patients. The goal is to spare bladders when possible but *not* at the risk of mortality from metastatic TCC.

References

1. Bandis SH, Muray T, Borden S. Cancer statistics. *CA Cancer J Clin* 1999;49:8–31
2. Catalona WJ, Dresner SM, Haaff EO. Management of superficial bladder cancer. In Skinner DG, Lieskovsky G, eds. *Diagnosis and Management of Genitourinary Cancer*. Philadelphia: WB Saunders Co., 1988:281–94
3. Angulo JC, Lopez JI, Grignon DJ, *et al.* Muscularis mucosa differentiates two populations with different prognosis in stage T1 bladder cancer. *Urology* 1995;45:47–53
4. Mostofi FK, Sobin LH, Torloni H. Histological typing of urinary bladder tumors. *International Classification of Tumors*. No. 10. Geneva: World Health Organization, 1973
5. Lee R, Droller MJ. The natural history of bladder cancer. Implications for therapy. *Urol Clin N Am* 2000;27:1–14
6. Brown FM. Urine cytology. Is it still the gold standard for screening? *Urol Clin N Am* 2000;27:25–38
7. Goessl C, Knispel HH, Miller K, *et al.* Is routine excretory urography necessary at first diagnosis of bladder cancer? *J Urol* 1997;157:480–1
8. Herranz-Amo F, Diez-Cordero JM, Verd-Tartajo F, *et al.* Need for intravenous urography in patients with primary transitional carcinoma of the bladder? *Eur Urol* 1999;36:221–4
9. Van Der Meijden A, Sylvester R, Collette L, *et al.* The role and impact of pathology review on stage and grade assessment of stages Ta and T1 bladder tumors: a combined analysis of 5 European organizations for research and treatment of cancer trials. *J Urol* 2000;164:1533–7
10. Badalament RA, Farah RN. Treatment of superficial bladder cancer with intravesical chemotherapy. *Semin Surg Oncol* 1997;13:335–41
11. Bohle A, Thanhauser A, Ulmer AJ. Dissecting the immunobiological effects of bacillus Calmette-Guerin (BCG) *in vitro*: evidence of a distinct BCG-activated killer (BAK) cell phenomenon. *J Urol* 1993;150:1932–7
12. Ratliff TL, Haaff EO, Catalona WJ. Interleukin-2 production during intravesical bacille Calmette-Guerin therapy for bladder cancer. *Clin Immunol Immunopathol* 1986;40:375–9
13. Duque JLF, Loughlin KR. An overview of the treatment of superficial bladder cancer: intravesical therapy. *Urol Clin North Am* 2000;27:125–35
14. Isaka S, Okano T, Abe K, *et al.* Sequential instillation therapy with mitomycin C and adryamicin for superficial bladder cancer. *Cancer Chemother Pharmacol* 1992;30(Suppl):41–4
15. Sekine H, Fukui I, Yamada T, *et al.* Intravesical mitomycin C and doxorubicin sequential therapy for carcinoma *in situ* of the bladder: a longer follow-up result. *J Urol* 1994;151:27–30
16. Solsona E, Iborra I, Ricos M, *et al.* Effectiveness of a single immediate mitomycin C instillation in patients with low risk superficial bladder cancer: short and long-term follow-up. *J Urol* 1999;161:1120–3
17. Tolley DA, Parmar MK, Grigor KM, *et al.* The effect of intravesical mitomycin C on recurrence of newly diagnosed superficial bladder cancer: a further report with 7 years of follow-up. *J Urol* 1996;155:1233
18. Lamm DL, Blumenstein BA, Crissman JD, *et al.* Maintenance bacillus Calmette-Guerin immunotherapy for recurrent Ta, T1 and carcinoma *in situ* TCC of the bladder: a randomized SWOG study. *J Urol* 2000;163:1124–9
19. Hermann GG, Horn T, Steven K. The influence of the level of lamina propria invasion and the prevalence of p53 nuclear accumulation on survival in stage T1 transitional cell bladder cancer. *J Urol* 1998;159:91–4
20. Lopez JL, Angulo JC. The prognostic significance of vascular invasion in stage T1 bladder cancer. *Histopathology* 1995;27:27–33
21. Sanchez de la Muela P, Rossel D, Aguera L, *et al.* Multivariate analysis of progression in superficial bladder cancer. *Br J Urol* 1993;71:284–9
22. Thomas DJ, Robinson MC, Charlton R, *et al.* p53 expression, ploidy and progression in pT1 transitional cell carcinoma of the bladder. *Br J Urol* 1993;73:533–7

23. Llopis J, Alcaraz A, Ribal MJ, *et al.* p53 expression predicts progression and poor survival in T1 bladder tumors. *Eur Urol* 2000;37:644–53

24. Steiner G, Bierhoff E, Schmidt D, *et al.* p53 immunoreactivity in biopsy specimens of T1G3 transitional cell carcinoma of the bladder – a helpful parameter in guiding the decision for or against cystectomy? *Eur J Cancer* 2000;36:610–14

25. Watters AD, Ballantyne SA, Going JJ, *et al.* Aneusomy of chromosomes 7 and 17 predicts the recurrence of transitional cell carcinoma of the urinary bladder. *BJU Int* 2000; 85:42–7

26. Arima J, Imazono Y, Takebayashi Y, *et al.* Expression of thymidine phosphorylase as an indicator of poor prognosis for patients with transitional cell carcinoma of the bladder. *Cancer* 2000;88:1131–8

27. Vaidya A, Soloway MS, Hawke C, *et al.* De novo muscle invasive bladder cancer: is there a change in trend? *J Urol* 2001;165:47–50

28. Landman J, Kavaler E, Droller M, *et al.* Application of telomerase in urologic oncology. *World J Urol* 1997;15:120–4

29. Lokeshar V, Pham H, Obek C. Ha-Haase urine test for detecting bladder cancer and evaluating its grade. *J Urol* 1997;157:341

30. Lamm LD. Bladder cancer: twenty years of progress and the challenges that remain. *CA Cancer J Clin* 1998;48:263–8

31. Herr HW. Tumor progression and survival in patients with T1G3 bladder tumours: 15-year outcome. *Br J Urol* 1997;80:762–5

32. Malkowicz BS, Nicholas P, Lieskovsky G, *et al.* The role of radical cystectomy in the management of high grade superficial bladder cancer. *J Urol* 1990;144:641–5

33. Hautman RE, dePetricini R, Gottfried HW, *et al.* The ileal neobladder: complications and functional results in 363 patients after 11 years of follow-up. *J Urol* 1999;161:422–7

34. Catalona WJ, Hudson MA, Gillen DP, *et al.* Risks and benefits of repeated courses of intravesical bacillus Calmette-Guérin therapy for superficial bladder cancer. *J Urol* 1987;137:220–4

35. Baniel J, Grauss D, Engelstein D, *et al.* Intravesical bacillus Calmette-Guérin treatment for stage T1 grade 3 transitional cell carcinoma of the bladder. *Urology* 1998;52:785–9

36. Amling CL, Thraser JB, Frazier HA, *et al.* Radical cystectomy for stages Ta, Tis and T1 transitional cell carcinoma of the bladder. *J Urol* 1994;151:31–6

37. Serretta V, Piazza S, Pavone C, *et al.* Results of conservative treatment (transurethral resection plus adjuvant intravesical chemotherapy) in patients with primary T1, G3 transitional cell carcinoma of the bladder. *Urology* 1996;47:647–51

38. Brake M, Loertzer H, Horsch R, *et al.* Recurrence and progression of stage T1, grade 3 transitional cell carcinoma of the bladder following intravesical immunotherapy with bacillus Calmette-Guerin. *J Urol* 2000;163:1697–701

Brachytherapy for transitional cell carcinoma of the bladder (category $\geq T_1 G_3$): an alternative to cystectomy?

31

K. H. Kurth, H. J. van der Veen and L. E. C. M. Blank

Introduction

In selected patients with bladder cancer, durable local control can be achieved with radiotherapy[1]. However, in small, randomized trials comparing radical radiotherapy with pre-operative radiotherapy followed by cystectomy, better outcome was achieved by the combined treatment, although, due to the sample size, differences were not significant[2,3]. In selected patients with small T_2 and T_{3a} tumors (< 5–7 cm) and without co-existent diffuse carcinoma *in situ*, treatment has been shown to result in a 60% complete response rate[4] and patients can have normal bladder function and a good quality of life[5]. While higher radiotherapy doses produce higher response rates, the rate of late toxicity will likewise increase, thus limiting the dose of definitive radiotherapy. In an unselected patient population, definitive radiotherapy is associated with a local failure rate of 70%[1]. The majority of patients with poor local control are at a high risk of distant failure. In advanced disease ($\geq T_{3b}$), radiotherapy can be considered only as a palliative therapy.

Intravesical isotope application

Intravesical application of isotopes such as bromine-60, sodium-24, cobalt-60, arsenic-76, yttrium-90, cesium-137 and gold-198 through a balloon (filled with fluid radioisotope) or directly into the bladder, was initiated in the early 1950s and applied up to the 1980s. However, this technique had to be abandoned,

mainly due to severe complications such as extensive necrosis or contracted bladder[6–11]. The method of intracavitary irradiation for bladder cancer was considered useful for localizing the radiation dose to the tumor. It could be used for multiple scattered superficial tumors (T_a/T_1) resistant to other local measures. When radiocolloids are used – allowing a homogeneous distribution of the dose to the urothelium – it can prove difficult to handle with regard to radiation safety for the patient and medical staff. With intracavitary isotopes, complete response rates of 50–70% have been achieved; however, rates free of recurrence were found to be lower. It is surprising that patients with recurrent non-invasive disease following the intracavitary isotope treatment were able to have further transurethral tumor resections without complications[10].

Intraoperative radiotherapy by electron beams

Intraoperative radiotherapy (IORT) by electron beams has been performed most extensively in Japan[12–17]. IORT is given by open cystotomy without resection or fulguration of the tumor. A single dose of 25–30 Gy by 3.5–7.5 MeV electron beam is delivered to the tumor area through cylinders with an internal diameter of 4, 5 or 6 cm. Generally, additional external irradiation is given postoperatively to the whole urinary bladder up to a total dose of 30–40 Gy. For tumor categories T_a, T_1 and T_2, freedom from local recurrence was achieved in up to 94%, 88% and 82% of cases, respectively. Combined IORT and external irradiation to the whole pelvis appeared to be well tolerated. Experience is limited; the good results with IORT may be due to the direct inspection of the bladder tumor by open cystotomy, allowing minimal irradiation of the surrounding tissue[13].

Interstitial radiotherapy

Interstitial radiotherapy makes possible the delivery of a high dose of radiation to a limited area of the body within a short period of time. For brachytherapy in the bladder, the permanent implantation of radon seeds and gold grains has been used, temporary implantation being achieved by applying radium- or cesium-containing needles or iridium wires[18,19]. In 1910, Pasteau and colleagues reported the first radium implant in bladder cancer[20]. Both American[21-23] and French investigators[24] have described their experiences with implanted radium or radon through the suprapubic cystotomy route.

The technique was supposed to have become old fashioned with the introduction of megavoltage therapy. However, to eradicate bladder cancer high doses are required with the risk of damage to surrounding healthy tissue. Radioactive material inserted interstitially, on the other hand, can deliver high doses to the bladder and still spare vulnerable adjacent tissues and organs. The implantation technique has been popularized by van der Werf-Messing and co-workers in the Netherlands who have treated more than 1000 patients since 1951[25]. The use of interstitial radiation (IRT) in patients with bladder cancer is more common in Europe than in North America and, at present, is routinely applied in France and the Netherlands. Close co-operation between urologists and radiation oncologists is required to ensure optimal patient selection and high quality of treatment. The bladder cancer should be solitary and the tumor should belong to categories T_1, T_2 and T_{3a} with a limited diameter (≤ 5 cm). Depending on tumor stage, IRT is preceded by a short course or longer course of

external beam radiotherapy (EBRT) (to prevent tumor implantation due to perioperative tumor spill). In French centers, the majority of patients undergo (when feasible) a partial cystectomy prior to the IRT. The theoretical advantage of a brachytherapy-based treatment is the possibility of delivering a very high radiation dose (70 Gy) to a limited area of the bladder, thereby increasing the chance of obtaining tumor control without increasing the incidence of severe toxicity. As only parts of the bladder are treated with high-dose radiation, the development of tumors in the untreated part cannot be excluded. Lesions extending outside the bladder (T_{3b}) are considered unsuitable for implantation because the tumor coverage using a single-plane implant would be insufficient[26]. Treatment of large areas of the bladder (> 5 cm) would result in badly healing wounds and even necrosis of the bladder wall.

Pretreatment investigations

Cystoscopy and bimanual palpation under general anesthesia prior to and immediately after transurethral resection of the exophytic part of the malignancy are performed together by a urologist and a radiation therapist. In our institution, routinely random biopsies are taken in order to exclude associated carcinoma *in situ* (CIS). Arguments against performing bladder biopsies have been raised by van der Werf-Messing and colleagues[25]:

(1) Interstitial therapy also kills CIS adjacent to the apparent malignancy;

(2) The radium implant will kill or suppress the growth of potential cancer cells elsewhere in the bladder since the bladder will collapse on the implanted area;

(3) Transurethral resection, which is an additional mechanical trauma, might act as a promoting agent to the bladder mucosa;

(4) Malignant cells might be implanted in mucosal lesions[25].

Whereas one can agree with the first argument and, undoubtedly, the mechanisms referred to in arguments three and four are important for tumor recurrence, it has not yet been demonstrated in controlled studies whether or not isotope implants will suppress or even kill short- and long-term CIS distant from the exophytic tumor. Therefore, for the time being patients with proven CIS are excluded from brachytherapy in our institution. Routine laboratory tests and imaging examination are done for staging.

Iridium-192

Permanent implantion of radon seeds or gold grains, or temporary insertion of radium or cobalt needles, tantalum or iridium wires were found to have the serious disadvantage of being a radiation hazard[27]. This problem was solved by the development of an afterloading system which decreased the radiation exposure of paramedical and medical staff. In 1953, Henschke and colleagues introduced the concept of afterloading through surgically inserted plastic tubes[28]; Pierquin and co-workers developed this method further[29]. Use of iridium wires for applying the afterloading method was first described in 1969 for the treatment of bladder tumors[30]. Today, the iridium remote-controlled afterloading technique is considered standard in IRT for bladder cancer[27,31–34]. Besides the reduction in radiation exposure, this technique, to some extent, allows for dose optimization by the selection of wires of different activity or by using different application times within the implanted volume. A new type of IRT is pulsed-dose rate brachytherapy using a single iridium source and 'stepping' through a range of dwell positions, simulating a continuous low-dose rate treatment by a series of pulses of short duration with time intervals between fractions of 1 h to a few hours[35]. Iridium-192, a low-energy gamma emitter, is supplied in the form of flexible wires. Platinum sheets absorb the beta rays. Isotopic iridium-192 wires have a half-life period of 74 days, a low-energy gamma irradiation of 0.3 MeV and a half-attenuation constant (value layer) of only 0.3 mm of lead (Table 1). Because of these physical properties and also because of the relatively low costs of this radioisotope,

Table 1 Physical properties of isotopes used for interstitial radiotherapy

Isotope	Half-life time	MeV	HVL*
Radium-226	1620 years	1.4	1.2
Cesium-137	30 years	0.66	0.65
Tantalum-182	115 days	1.1	1.0
Iridium-192	74 days	0.3	0.3
Gold-198	2.7 days	0.4	0.33

* HVL, half-value layer (cmPb)

iridium-192 was chosen as the best interstitial irradiation agent for treatment of bladder tumors which do not exceed 5 cm in diameter.

Interstitial radiation with iridium-192

Method and materials

The procedure described below is that performed in the Academic Medical Center, University of Amsterdam. Four centers in the Netherlands participated in this study. From 1984 to 1998, 251 patients were treated by IRT. Conditions for use of IRT were that there was a possibility of covering the tumor area by a single-plane implant, and that the patient's condition permitted surgery. CIS distant from the tumor, a history of bladder tumors at different sites, earlier radiation of the pelvic area and small bladder capacity were excluded. Complete resection of the exophytic tumor parts was generally performed; however, residual palpable tumor was not an exclusion criterion. Partial cystectomy was performed in the few cases of urachus carcinoma located in the bladder dome or for tumors in mobile parts of the bladder (and/or tumors located in a diverticulum). Tumors of the upper urinary tract were excluded by IVP and computerized tomography (CT). The latter allowed additional imaging of grossly enlarged lymph nodes in the retroperitoneal space or possible metastases to the liver.

T_1 G_3 and small T_2 tumors were treated with EBRT 3×3.5 Gy followed by IRT at 60 Gy. Larger (but always < 5 cm) T_2 tumors and T_3 tumors were subjected to EBRT 20×2.0 Gy in conjunction with IRT 30 Gy. The EBRT target area is the true pelvis, radiation being given through opposed anterior and posterior fields (dose calculation in the midplane) or four-field box technique. Surgery and insertion of catheters were performed under general anesthesia. A lymph node dissection of the internal iliac region and the fossa obturatoria was performed prior to cystotomy (more recently only selecting some lymph nodes or resectioning enlarged lymph nodes). The bladder was opened in the midline of the anterior wall, unless the tumor site required a paramedian incision. Using a curved needle, appropriate to the anatomical conditions and dimensions of the target volume, the location of the radioactive source was established by passing the needle through the bladder wall corresponding with the palpable, visible or documented area of bladder malignancy. After partial cystectomy, the needle was passed through the wall next to the suture line. The point of the needle was passed through the bladder mucosa at the opposite side of the target volume. A plastic tube was then introduced over the point of the needle, and the needle carrying the plastic tube was extracted. Each plastic tube was left long enough to enable it to be brought out through a separate incision in the abdominal wall. The spacing between the tubes was determined by the thickness of the target volume. To maintain the parallel position between the tubes, plastic spacers were used. By puncturing the bladder wall, abdominal muscles and skin, the tubes, fed with the nylon fibers, were brought out at both sides of the incision and carefully secured to the skin. Bladder and skin were closed leaving a drain paravesically. The spacers were tied to the top of an indwelling catheter and later removed through the urethra. On the first postoperative day, patients were transferred to the department of radiotherapy. IRT was started within 24 h after insertion of the catheters. Computerized dose calculation was performed after three-dimensional reconstruction of the implant.

The catheters were loaded remotely with iridium. After completion of the calculated application time, the iridium was retracted, the catheters removed and, subsequently, the patient returned to the urological ward. Patients were seen for follow-up and cystoscopy, thereafter, every 3 months in the first year, every 4 months in the second year and then every 6 months provided there was freedom from recurrence. Recurrent tumors of categories T_a and $T_1 < G_3$ were treated by transurethral resection followed in some cases by adjuvant chemo- or immunotherapy. Salvage cystectomy was performed – when feasible – in cases of muscle-invasive recurrence.

Results of IRT with iridium-192

Of the 251 patients treated, 27 were staged $T_1 G_3$ and 223 $\geq T_2$; in one patient with a tumor staged $T_1 G_3 N_1$, lymph node metastases were diagnosed only in the paraffin-embedded material. Histologically, all patients, except six with adenocarcinoma, had transitional cell carcinoma. Mean size of the tumors was 2.5 cm. Partial cystectomy was performed in 53 patients. The mean follow-up period was 48 months (ranging from 1 month to 157 months). Local failure was observed in 29 patients and distant metastases without bladder relapse in 34 patients. Globally, the 5-year survival rate (according to the Kaplan–Meier method) was 62%, and disease-specific survival was 76%. Our own results, as earlier reported by van der Veen[36,42], and results reported by other authors, are listed in Tables 2–6.

Complications

EBRT caused no serious bowel/rectum or skin toxicity. Almost all patients complained of transient urgency and bladder spasm after IRT. A late complication of small bladder capacity occurred in two patients. Radiation cystitis with repeated gross hematuria was seen in four patients and successfully treated in three patients in a hyperbaric oxygen chamber. Two more patients suffered from high micturition frequency (≥ 10/day) due to reduced bladder capacity (< 200 ml).

Table 2 Five-year disease-specific survival after surgery, external beam and interstitial radiation for bladder cancer $\geq T_1 G_3$

Author	Implant	Number of patients	5-year survival (%)	Follow-up
van der Werf-Messing et al.[25]	Ra-226	391	75	≥ 2 years (2–17 years)
Batterman et al.[37]	Ra-226	123	72	36 months median
de Neve et al.[38]	Ce-137	32	76	81 months median
Botto et al.[39]	Ir-192	19	89	36 months
Mazeron et al.[41]	Ir-192	55	67	5 years
Mazeron et al.[40]	Ir-192	66	74	5 years
Rozan et al.[34]	Ir-192	205	83	51 months mean
Moonen et al.[32]	Ir-192	40	86	40 months mean
Moonen et al.[31]	Ir-192	63	66	4.2 years median
Pernot et al.[33]	Ir-192	85	71	84 months median
Wijnmaalen et al.[27]	Ir-192	66	69	26 months mean
Schlosser et al.[42]	Ir-192	24	75	5 years
van der Veen et al.[36]	Ir-192	251	76	48 months mean
Van Poppel et al.[43]	Ir-192	28	57	6.9 years mean

Ra, radium; Ce, cesium; Ir, iridium

Table 3 Five-year disease-specific survival related to stage after surgery, external beam and interstitial radiation

Author	T_1		T_2		T_3		Follow-up
	%	n	%	n	%	n	
van der Werf-Messing et al.[25]	—	—	75	328	62	63	≥ 2 years
Battermann et al.[37]	74	34	56	89	—	—	36 months median
Mazeron et al.[40]	79	36	69	20	25	4	≥ 5 years
Rozan et al.[34]	77	98	63	66	47	35	51 months mean
de Neve et al.[38]	62	13	89.5	19	—	—	81 months median
Pernot et al.[33]	85	27	76	31	72	27	84 months median
Wijnmaalen et al.[27]	—	—	69	66	—	—	26 months median

Table 4 Bladder recurrence after surgery, external beam and interstitial radiation

Author	Implant	Number of patients	Recurrence
van der Werf-Messing et al.[25]	Ra-226	391	18%
Mazeron et al.[40]	Ir-192	85	15%
Straus et al.[46]	Ir-192	14	3/14
Grossman et al.[45]	Ir-192	7 (T_{3a})	2/7
Moonen et al.[32]	Ir-192	40	22.5%
Moonen et al.[31]	Ir-192	66	24%
Pernot et al.[33]	Ir-192	85	27%
Schlosser et al.[42]	Ir-192	24	16.6%
Wijnmaalen et al.[27]	Ir-192	66	10.6%
van der Veen et al.[36]	Ir-192	251	11.5%
Van Poppel et al.[43]	Ir-192	28	17.8%

Ra, radium; Ir, iridium

Conclusion

The treatment of bladder carcinoma by IRT using iridium-192 is a well-defined technique routinely used in many Dutch centers. The method is limited to patients with small (≤ 5 cm), solitary (by preference primary) bladder tumors of categories T_1, T_2 and T_{3a}. Close co-operation between the urologist and radiotherapist is required. In this selected group of patients, IRT gives comparable survival rates to radical cystectomy without the mutilating sequelae. Technical improvements may further improve local control and increase tolerance. In the absence of controlled, randomized trials comparing EBRT with IRT, it is imposible to conclude whether brachytherapy offers a significant advantage to that provided by EBRT in a group of patients with favorable characteristics, as presented here.

Table 5 Bladder recurrence related to stage, duration of follow-up and implant

Author	Follow-up	Implant	T_1	T_2	T_3
van der Werf-Messing et al.[25]	≥ 2 years	Ra-226	—	16%	28%
Mazeron et al.[40]	> 5 years	Ir-192	24%	6%	8%
Grossman et al.[45]	≥ 5 years	Ir-192	—	—	2/7
Moonen et al.[32]	40 months mean	Ir-192	0/12 (T_1G_3)	21% (6/28) (T_2,T_{3a})	
Pernot et al.[33]	84 months median	Ir-192	15%	30%	30%*
Wijnmaalen et al.[27]	26 months mean	Ir-192	—	7/62	0/4
Van Poppel et al.[43]	6.9 years mean	Ir-192	1/4	0/12	4/12

*$2pT_4$, $3pT_x$; Ra, radium; Ir, iridium

Table 6 Systemic failure after interstitial radiotherapy

Author	Number of patients	Follow-up	Implant	Failure rate		
				T_1	T_2	T_3
Battermann et al.[37]	119	36 months mean	Ra-226	2/34	11/85	
Mazeron et al.[40]	66	> 5 years	Ir-192	4/36	4/20	2/10
Grossman et al.[45]	7	≥ 5 years	Ir-192		2/7	
Moonen et al.[32]	40	40 months mean	Ir-192	0/12	7/28 (T_2,T_{3a})	
Pernot et al.[33]	85	84 months median	Ir-192		all stages 14%	
Rozan et al.[34]	205	51 months mean	Ir-192		all stages 10.2%	
Wijnmaalen et al.[29]	66	26 months median	Ir-192		31% (T_2/T_3)	
van der Veen et al.[36]	251	48 months mean	Ir-192		all stages 13.5%	
Van Poppel et al.[43]	28	6.9 years mean	Ir-192	0/4	0/12	2/12

Ra, radium; Ir, iridium

References

1. Duncan W, Quilty PM. The results of a series of 963 patients with transitional cell carcinoma of the urinary bladder primarily treated by radical megavoltage x-ray therapy. *Radiother Oncol* 1986;7:299–310
2. Sell A, Jakobsen A, Nerstrom B, *et al.* Treatment of advanced bladder cancer category T2, T3 and T4a. *Scand J Urol Nephrol* 1991;138(Suppl): 193–201
3. Horwich A. Commentary 1. In Hall RR, ed. *Clinical Mangement of Bladder Cancer.* New York: Arnold/Oxford Press, 1999:236–8
4. Fung CY, Shipley WU, Young RH, *et al.* Prognostic factors in invasive bladder carcinoma in a prospective trial of preoperative adjuvant chemotherapy and radiotherapy. *J Clin Oncol* 1991;9:1533–42
5. Lynch WJ, Jenkins BJ, Fowler CG, *et al.* The quality of life after radiotherapy for bladder cancer. *Br J Urol* 1992;70:519–21
6. Becker J. Die Strahlenbehandlung des Blasenkarzinoms. *Strahlentherapie* 1956;101:208–16
7. Durrant KR, Laing AH. Treatment of multiple superficial papillary tumors of the bladder by intracavitary yttrium 90. *J Urol* 1975;113:480–2
8. Russel KJ, Koh WJ, Russel AH, *et al.* Combined intracavitary and external beam irradiation for superficial transitional cell carcinoma of the bladder: an alternative to cystectomy for patients with recurrence after intravesical chemotherapy. *J Urol* 1989;141:30–2
9. Van der Werf-Messing B. Carcinoma of the bladder treated with intracavitary application of cobalt-60 beads. *Clin Radiol* 1971;22:101–10
10. Hewitt CB, Babiszewski JF, Antunez AR. Update on intracavitary radiation in the treatment of bladder tumours. *J Urol* 1981;126:323–5
11. Bex A, Rübben H, Feldmann HJ, *et al.* A system for focal intracavitary irradiation of bladder cancer with remote iridium-p192 afterloading. *Eur Urol* 1992;21:245–9
12. Gerard JP, Hulewicz G, Marechal JM, *et al.* Pilot study of IORT for bladder carcinoma. *Front Radiat Ther Oncol* 1997;31:250–2

13. Calvo FA, Henriquez I, Santos M, *et al.* Intraoperative and external beam radiotherapy in invasive bladder cancer: pathological findings following cystectomy. *Am J Clin Oncol* 1990;13:101–6

14. Shipley W. Intraoperative electron-beam therapy and other bladder-sparing approaches to bladder carcinoma. *Urology* 1988;31(Suppl 2):18–21

15. Martinez A, Gunderson LL. Intraoperative radiation therapy for bladder cancer. *Urol Clin North Am* 1984;11:693–8

16. Abe M, Takahashi M. Intraoperative radiotherapy: the Japanese experience. *Int J Radiat Oncol Biol Phys* 1981;7:863–8

17. Fuchs G, Überall R. Intraoperative radiotherapy of bladder carcinoma. *Strahlentherapie* 1968;135:280–4

18. van der Werf-Messing B, Menon RS, Hop WC. Carcinoma of the urinary bladder category T3N×Mo treated by the combination of radium implant and external irradiation: second report. *Int J Radiat Oncol Biol Phys* 1983;9:177–80

19. van der Werf-Messing BHP. Interstitial radiation therapy of carcinoma of the urinary bladder. *Endocurie Hypertherm Oncol* 1988;4:1–6

20. Pasteau O, Wickham L, Degrais A. Presented at *2ᵉ Conférence Internal pour l'Étude du Cancer.* Paris, 1910:707–12

21. Barringer BS. Radium treatment of cancer of the bladder. *J Am Med Assoc* 1930;95:1734–6

22. Braasch WF, Scholl AJ. Preoperative treatment by radium of malignant tumors of the bladder. *Arch Surg* 1922;5:334–47

23. Smith GG. The treatment of cancer of the bladder by radium implantation. *J Urol* 1922;9:217–26

24. Darget R, Lange J. Résultats du traitement des cancers de la vessie par l'implantation d'aiguilles de radium a vessie ouverte en un temps. *J Urol* 1939;47:273–86

25. van der Werf-Messing B, Menon RS, Hop WC. Cancer of the urinary bladder category T2, T3, (N×Mo) treated by interstitial radium implant: second report. *Int J Radiat Oncol Biol Phys* 1983;9:481–5

26. Moonen LMF. Commentary 2. In Hall RR, ed. *Clinical Management of Bladder Cancer.* New York: Arnold/Oxford Press, 1999:239–40

27. Wijnmaalen A, Helle PA, Koper PC, *et al.* Muscle invasive bladder cancer treated by transurethral resection, followed by external beam radiation and interstitial iridium-192. *Int J Radiat Oncol Biol Phys* 1997;39:1043–5

28. Henschke UK, Hilaris BS, Mahan GD. After loading in interstitial and intracavitary radiation therapy. *Am J Roentgenol* 1961;90:386–95

29. Pirquin B, Chassagne DJ, Chahbazian CM, *et al. Brachytherapy.* St. Louis, MO: Warren H. Green, Inc., 1978

30. Gros CH, Bollack C, Keiling R. Curietherapie par Iridium 192. Préparation inactive des petits cancers de la vessie. *J Radiol Electrol* 1969;50:437–9

31. Moonen LM, Horenblas S, Pos F, *et al.* Good results of bladder-preserving treatment in poorly differentiated and invasive bladder carcinoma using interstitial Iridium-192 radiotherapy. *Ned Tijdschr Geneeskd* 1996;140:1406–10

32. Moonen LM, Horenblas S, van der Voet JC, *et al.* Bladder conservation in selected T1G3 and muscle-invasive T2–T3a bladder carcinoma using combination therapy of surgery and iridium-192 implantation. *Br J Urol* 1994;74:322–7

33. Pernot M, Hubert J, Guillemin F, *et al.* Combined surgery and brachytherapy in the treatment of some cancers of the bladder (partial cystectomy and interstitial iridium-192). *Radiother Oncol* 1996;38:115–20

34. Rozan R, Albuisson E, Donnarieix D, *et al.* Interstitial iridium-192 for bladder cancer (a multicentric survey: 205 patients). *Int J Radiat Oncol Biol Phys* 1992;24:469–77

35. Brenner DJ, Hall EJ. Conditions for the equivalence of continuous to pulsed low dose rate brachytherapy. *Int J Radiat Oncol Biol Phys* 1991;20:181–90

36. Van der Veen HJ, Blank LECM, Kurth KH, *et al.* Bladder preservation by brachytherapy in a selected group of patients with TCC ≥ T1G3 bladder cancer. *Radiother Oncol* 1990;51(Suppl 2):11(abstr)

37. Battermann JJ, Tierie AH. Results of implantation for T1 and T2 bladder tumors. *Radiother Oncol* 1986;5:85–90

38. De Neve W, Lybeert MLM, Goor C, *et al.* T1 and T2 carcinoma of the urinary bladder: long term results with external preoperative, or interstitial radiotherapy. *Int J Radiat Biol Phys* 1992;23:299–304

39. Botto H, Perrin JL, Auvert J, *et al.* Treatment of malignant bladder tumors by iridium-192 wiring. *Urology* 1980;16:467–9

40. Mazeron JJ, Crook J, Chopin D, *et al.* Conservative treatment of bladder carcinoma by partial cystectomy and interstitial iridium 192. *Int J Radiat Oncol Biol Phys* 1988;15:1323–30

41. Mazeron JJ, Marinello G, Leung S, *et al.* Treatment of bladder tumors by iridium 192 implantation. The Creteil technique. *Radiother Oncol* 1985;4:111–19

42. Schlosser J, Hubert J, Hofstetter S, *et al.* Chirurgie conservatrice et iridium 192 pour tumeurs vésicale de stade pT2. Résultats à 5 ans. *Prog Urol* 1997;7:953–9

43. Van Poppel H, Lievens Y, Van Limbergen E, *et al.* Brachytherapy with iridium-192 for bladder cancer. *Eur Urol* 2000;37:605–8

44. Gonzalez D, Van der Veen HJ, Ypma AF, *et al.* Brachytherapy for urinary bladder cancer. *Arch Esp Urol* 1999;52:655–61

45. Grossman HB, Sandler HM, Perez-Tamayo C. Treatment of T3a bladder cancer with iridium implantation. *Urology* 1993;41:217–20

46. Straus KL, Littman P, Wein AJ, *et al.* Treatment of bladder cancer with interstitial iridium-192 implantation and external beam irradiation. *Int J Radiat Oncol Biol Phys* 1988;14:265–71

Current status of systemic treatment in locally advanced and metastatic bladder cancer

32

P. H. M. De Mulder

Introduction

Bladder cancer is the fifth most common malignancy in Europe and the fourth most common malignancy in the United States. About 75% of patients with bladder cancer are men. The most established risk factors for bladder cancer are cigarette smoking and occupational exposure to certain carcinogens. About 80% of bladder tumors are confined to the bladder mucosa, the so-called superficial tumors, and 20% invade the muscle layer. The management and prognosis of the two types of cancer are completely different: superficial tumors are fairly benign and invasive tumors are highly malignant. Worldwide, the vast proportion of bladder cancer is of the transitional cell type[1]. The topic of this chapter will be mainly restricted to the transitional cell type and will focus on the invasive and metastatic variants.

Of the patients who present with clinically localized, muscle-invasive transitional cell carcinoma, 20–80% can be cured with adequate local treatment, consisting of either cystectomy with pelvic lymphadenectomy or various radiotherapeutic approaches. The others will develop either local relapse or metastatic disease, with only a minute chance of cure. Most patients will relapse at distant sites, reflecting occult metastatic disease at the time of local treatment. Only about one-third of the patients relapse in the pelvis alone. The most important prognostic factor for survival is the pathological stage of the disease. The relatively high rate of response observed with combination chemotherapy in metastatic disease has led to the use of

chemotherapy earlier in the disease. Three approaches have been used:

(1) Concurrent radiation and chemotherapy;

(2) Neoadjuvant chemotherapy given before local treatment;

(3) Adjuvant chemotherapy given after local therapy.

Next to the place of chemotherapy in metastatic disease, these approaches will be discussed in this contribution.

Concurrent radiotherapy and chemotherapy

The rationale for combining radiotherapy and chemotherapy is two-fold: first, the spatial co-operation of the two treatments (radiotherapy treats the primary and chemotherapy the micrometastases, with differing dose-limiting toxicities) and, second, the potential effect of the combination to improve local tumor control. Several agents have been studied in small, single-arm trials and cisplatin as a single agent appears to be the drug of choice. It has been shown to improve survival when used concurrently with radiation for other indications such as cervical or esophageal cancer. Cisplatin is also one of the best single agents for treatment of metastatic transitional cell carcinoma. The optimal timing and dosage of cisplatin in relation to irradiation have not been evaluated and the dose and schedule of administration of cisplatin in most protocols

281

have been selected arbitrarily. The only randomized trial comparing radical radiotherapy to concomitant radio-chemotherapy, carried out by the Canadian National Cancer Institute, could not include the pre-planned number of patients[2]. A total of 99 patients were randomized to receive radiation alone or radiation with three courses of cisplatin, 100 mg/m^2 given concurrently at 2–3-week intervals; the radiotherapy was planned either to be definitive local treatment or preoperative. The trial did not demonstrate an advantage in survival, but the arm treated with concurrent cisplatin had a significantly lower rate of pelvic failure than the control arm (33 vs. 55%; $p = 0.034$). While these data are encouraging, and appear to have been achieved with minimal increase in toxicity, further randomized trials indicating improvement in tumor control and survival are needed before concurrent radiation and chemotherapy can be considered as a standard approach to bladder cancer. In addition, the quality of the preserved bladder, acute and delayed toxicity, and cost-effectiveness can only be assessed through appropriate clinical trials.

Neoadjuvant chemotherapy

This form of treatment is defined as chemotherapy given prior to definitive local treatment. The advantages of this approach are the availability of an *in vivo* marker to evaluate the response to chemotherapy, enabling both continuation of treatment to maximal response, or discontinuation of ineffective therapy. Furthermore, locoregional drug delivery is probably better without prior radiotherapy and/or surgery; compliance with planned chemotherapy is more likely, and the treatment of occult metastases starts as early as possible. The disadvantages of this approach include delay of potentially curative local treatment, the lack of full pathological staging prior to the start of any treatment, possible effects of chemotherapy in stimulating the seeding of metastases from circulating tumor cells, and possible effects of stimulating repopulation if radiotherapy is given subsequently. Neoadjuvant

chemotherapy may have the goal of improving survival and/or to render patients operable, or to perform an organ-preserving procedure. Many data are available from single-arm, pilot studies. The following conclusions can be drawn from these studies: an overall response rate of 60–70% with a complete remission rate of about 30% can be achieved[3–5]. A clinically complete remission does not imply a pathologically complete response. About 30% of bladder tumors staged as T_0 after neoadjuvant chemotherapy will have muscle-invasive disease on pathological examination after cystectomy. It is clear that lower-staged tumors respond better than more advanced stages. A pathological complete response was reported in 30% of cases with a T_2 or T_{3a} tumor versus 9% when a T_{3b} or T_4 tumor was diagnosed[6]. A response to chemotherapy predicts a more favorable outcome. In collected series, 91% of responders, defined as pT_1 or lower stage at cystectomy, were disease-free at a median follow-up of 25 months versus 37% of non-responders ($> pT_1$)[5–7]. Response was also shown to be an independent prognostic factor for survival. Finally, nontransitional cell histology is generally insensitive to chemotherapy. Therefore, adenocarcinomas and squamous cell carcinoma should not be considered for this approach. The true value of this approach can only be established in randomized trials.

Various randomized studies have been performed (Table 1)[8–12] and the main endpoint of these studies has been survival. Two major flaws limit the interpretation of the majority of these studies. First, the number of patients entered was too small to detect a difference in survival of at least 10% that might reasonably be expected as a result of such treatment. Second, both the type of chemotherapy and the number of courses given were often suboptimal. The only reported study with enough power to detect a 10% difference in 3-year survival is that reported by Hall[12] which evaluated three cycles of cisplatin, methotrexate and vinblastine (CMV), followed by definitive local treatment, as compared to local treatment alone. Local treatment was either cystectomy, or radiotherapy, or preoperative radiation and

Table 1 Randomized trials of neoadjuvant chemotherapy

Authors	Number of patients	Chemotherapy	Local treatment	Result
Shearer, et al.[8]	376	methotrexate (pre and post local rx)	RT ± cystectomy	no difference
Wallace, et al.[9]	255	cisplatin (2 or 3 courses)	RT	no difference
Martinez-Pineiro, et al.[10]	122	cisplatin	cystectomy	no difference
Malmstrom, et al.[11]	325	doxorubicin/cisplatin (2 courses)	RT + cystectomy	5-year survival, 59% vs. 51% favoring chemotherapy ($p = 0.1$)
International Collaboration of Trialists[12]	976	cisplatin/methotrexate/vinblastine (3 courses)	RT, cystectomy, or both	3-year survival, 55.5% vs. 50.0% favoring chemotherapy ($p = 0.075$)

RT, radiotherapy

cystectomy, and was predetermined by the center. A total of 976 patients with $T_2 G_3$, T_3, T_{4a}, $N_0–N_x$ or M_0 transitional cell carcinoma of the bladder were randomized to receive chemotherapy or no chemotherapy. The median follow-up of patients still alive was 4 years. A total of 485 patients have died, and 78.6% of the deaths were due to cancer. Mortality due to chemotherapy was 1% and due to surgery, 3.7%. The calculated absolute difference in 3-year survival rate was 5.5% (95% confidence interval (CI) –0.5–11.0, $p = 0.075$), 55.5% for CMV versus 50.0% for no chemotherapy. About one-third (32.5%) of cystectomy specimens contained no evidence of tumor following neoadjuvant CMV, which is consistent with the earlier mentioned phase II data. The study shows that neoadjuvant CMV chemotherapy has, at most, a small influence on survival; it was not designed to detect a 5% survival difference and a further 2500 patients would be required for a trial designed to show or rule out such a difference. In the reported study, 34% of patients were staged T_2 (with grade 3 disease) and N+ patients were excluded, resulting in recruitment of patients with a relatively good prognosis. In a subgroup analysis, however, a similar reduction in the relative risk of death was observed for patients with T_2, T_3 and T_{4a} tumors. The concern that neoadjuvant chemotherapy might compromise local treatment was not

supported by the experience within this study. There was no difference in locoregional control ($p = 0.74$). A total of 518 patients developed metastases or died, with an absolute difference in metastasis-free survival of 8% (53% for CMV and 45% for the control group; $p = 0.007$).

The Nordic study[11] randomized 325 patients to receive two cycles of doxorubicin and cisplatin or no chemotherapy prior to preoperative radiotherapy and cystectomy. Overall, no significant difference in survival was found, with 59% (chemotherapy) versus 51% of patients surviving at 5 years. The power of this study to detect a difference in survival was limited by the low number of patients randomized. A subset analysis suggested a 15% overall survival benefit for patients ($n = 137$) with T_{3a} and T_4 tumors, but cannot be accepted as proof of a real advantage, because the study was not designed for this subgroup analysis. A multivariate analysis showed that tumor stage and chemotherapy were independent prognostic factors for survival. This result is surprising in view of the suboptimal chemotherapy given and the limited number of courses. The recently closed Southwest Oncology Group trial, comparing three cycles of methotrexate, vinblastine, adriamycin and cisplatin (M-VAC) prior to cystectomy versus cystectomy alone, might shed additional light on the impact of neoadjuvant chemotherapy on survival. M-VAC is considered to be optimal chemotherapy but the study randomized just over 300 patients and can, therefore, only detect or rule out a survival advantage of the order of 15%.

Neoadjuvant chemotherapy cannot presently be recommended as standard treatment for locally advanced bladder cancer when the goal is improvement of survival.

Another possible reason to use neoadjuvant chemotherapy is to allow organ preservation. There is interest in the approach of treating patients with radio-chemotherapy first and selecting, on the basis of the response, those patients whose tumor is fit for bladder preservation and those who might rather benefit from an immediate cystectomy. Adequate patient selection is mandatory: recognized criteria for selection are a small tumor size, the possibility of complete transurethral resection of all visible disease, the absence of hydronephrosis, and the achievement of complete remission after induction chemotherapy and radiation. In a small, randomized trial undertaken by the RTOG, neoadjuvant methotrexate, cisplatin and vinblastine (MCV) was given prior to radiotherapy plus concurrent cisplatin, versus radiotherapy and cisplatin alone[13]. Only 74% of the patients completed the protocol, 81% in the arm without and 67% in the arm with MCV, mainly because of systemic toxicity. The trial failed to demonstrate any benefit for neoadjuvant treatment: the rates of metastasis, of bladder conservation, and of 5-year survival were nearly identical[13]. It is important to recognize that there is no level 1 or 2 evidence that such an approach does not compromise survival in some patients, or that it is a better alternative than primary radiotherapy for bladder preservation. If used, frequent cystoscopy is indicated to detect residual or recurrent disease.

Adjuvant chemotherapy

Adjuvant chemotherapy is defined as any planned chemotherapy given after definitive local treatment with the aim of improving survival. The advantage of adjuvant chemotherapy used after cystectomy is the known pathological staging that can be used to predict risk of recurrence prior to the start of chemotherapy. Known adverse prognostic features are the presence of nodal metastases, extravesical extension of tumor, lymphatic and or vascular permeation of the primary tumor, and pelvic visceral invasion[14]. Furthermore, adequate local and potentially curative treatment is not delayed. A disadvantage is the lack of an indicator lesion to judge response and reduced patient compliance for delivering sufficient courses of chemotherapy. The concept is of proven benefit in breast and colon cancer, but, in bladder cancer, the published studies lack statistical power to detect or rule out a difference in survival that might reasonably be expected. Six randomized studies have been completed and reported[15–21] (Table 2), although they were small and several used suboptimal chemotherapy. In the study of Skinner and colleagues[16], pT_{3-4} or N+ patients were randomized to either cystectomy ($n = 47$) or cystectomy followed by four cycles of cyclophosphamide, doxorubicin and cisplatin ($n = 44$). In this small study, there was a non-significant trend to improved survival with chemotherapy but no evidence of long-term benefit. Major flaws in this study were the number of patients included ($n = 91$), non-standardized chemotherapy, the statistical methodology, and the premature closure of the study. A second study initially recruited 49 patients in a prospective, two-center randomized study[17,18]. Only patients with pT_{3b}, T_{4a}, and/or positive pelvic nodes were treated, with either three courses of methotrexate, vinblastine, cisplatin, doxorubicin, or epirubicin, or no treatment. In the observation arm, 18 of 23 patients relapsed (82%) versus three of 18 who received chemotherapy (17%; $p = 0.0007$); seven randomized patients refused chemotherapy. An analysis performed on an intention-to-treat basis revealed a tumor progression rate of 42% (11/26) versus 87% (20/23), but there has been no report of a difference in overall survival despite several publications. In another very small, randomized

Table 2 Randomized trials of adjuvant chemotherapy

Authors	Number of patients	Chemotherapy	Local treatment	Result
Richards, et al.[15]	129	doxorubicin/5-fluorouracil	radiotherapy	no difference
Skinner, et al.[16]	91	cyclophosphamide/doxorubicin/ cisplatin	cystectomy	non-significant trend to better survival
Stöckle, et al.[17,18]	49	methotrexate/vinblastine/cisplatin/ doxorubicin or epirubicin	cystectomy	better progression-free survival. No survival data
Studer, et al.[19]	77	cisplatin	cystectomy	no difference
Freiha, et al.[20]	50	cisplatin/vinblastine/methotrexate	cystectomy	better progression-free survival. No difference in survival
Bono, et al.[21]	83	cisplatin/methotrexate	cystectomy	no difference

study, 25 patients received four cycles of CMV as adjuvant treatment and 25 patients were followed closely and chemotherapy was offered at the time of relapse[20]. All patients had T_{3a-4} transitional cell carcinoma, with or without nodal involvement. The progression-free survival was better for the immediately treated group, but the overall survival was similar.

The published data on adjuvant chemotherapy, although heavily criticized[22], are in the public domain and have influenced daily practice. Given the very poor prognosis of patients with N+ disease or lymphovascular invasion after local treatment alone, some oncologists have elected to use adjuvant chemotherapy, even though high-level evidence of benefit is lacking. For patients with pT_{2-3a}, N_0 tumors, adjuvant chemotherapy should not be given outside the framework of a clinical study. For patients with pT_{3b}, pT_4, and pN+ tumors, the risk of relapse is very high and the pros and cons of early versus delayed treatment should be discussed with the patient. Priority should be given to an adequately powered, randomized, controlled trial of adjuvant chemotherapy following cystectomy[22]. The toxicity of protocols that include both chemotherapy and local treatment leads to a substantial proportion of dropouts and, in some series, of toxic death. These protocols are therefore reserved for patients with a good performance status and usually exclude elderly patients. Although some encouraging results have been reported in non-randomized and small, randomized trials, the selection of patients to participate in these trials prevents definitive conclusions about benefit, and limits their generalizability to a less selected population.

Chemotherapy for metastatic disease

Metastatic transitional cell carcinoma is moderately sensitive to chemotherapy. Many cytotoxic agents, alone and in combination, have been evaluated. Among older drugs, the most efficacious single agents for advanced bladder cancer are cisplatin and methotrexate. Other compounds with activity include doxorubicin, vinblastine, mitomycin-C, and the newer agents paclitaxel and gemcitabine.

The M-VAC combination developed at Memorial Sloan Kettering Cancer Center in New York produced high response rates in the initial study, with objective remissions in more than 70% of the patients treated[23]. Thirty-six per cent of patients attained a complete response. Long-term survival was achieved in those patients who attained complete response. Patients who achieved a complete response to chemotherapy plus surgery had twice the survival of patients who had partial response alone. Two prospective, randomized trials have established the value of M-VAC[24–26]. In a multicenter, international trial of 239 evaluable patients, response was observed in 11% treated with single-agent cisplatin compared to 36% treated with M-VAC chemotherapy. The median survival with M-VAC was 13.5 months, compared to 8.2 months in patients treated with cisplatin ($p = 0.04$)[24,25]. At the MD Anderson Hospital, M-VAC was also found to be superior to cisplatin, adriamycin and cyclophosphamide (CISCA)[26]. The median survival was 11.2 months after M-VAC, compared to 8.4 months with CISCA. The complete plus partial response rate was 65% with M-VAC and 46% with CISCA (cisplatin, cyclophosphamide, adriamycin) ($p < 0.05$). Predictive factors for poor outcome were non-transitional cell histology, the presence of bone and liver metastases, and a low performance status. After 6 years, only 3.7% of the M-VAC-treated patients were alive and continuously disease-free. This trial confirms the experience in several centers that aggressive chemotherapy can lead to long-term control or cure of metastatic disease in a small proportion ($< 5\%$) of patients.

While M-VAC is currently regarded as the gold standard, it is associated with substantial toxicity. Delays or omission on days 15 and 22 of the schedule are often necessary because of insufficient bone marrow recovery, and chemotherapy-induced mortality is in the range of 2–5% in most series. Other aggressive regimens, such as CMV (doxorubicin is omitted, but with a higher dose intensity of the other drugs), are associated with comparable rates of response and toxicity in non-randomized studies.

Several studies have tried to improve on the results of M-VAC by dose escalation. In a recent analysis of single-agent studies, a steep dose–response relationship was suggested for cisplatin and, to a lesser extent, for doxorubicin, but evaluation of 132 M-VAC-treated patients at Memorial Sloan Kettering Cancer Center showed no effect of received dose intensity on survival[27]. Several authors have evaluated the use of hematological growth factors with M-VAC in attempts to deliver more of the prescribed treatment or to escalate the dose or frequency of drugs in the regimen in order to improve the complete response rate[28–31,33–36]. In an early study, M-VAC was given with granulocyte macrophage colony-stimulating factors (GM-CSF), and both mucositis and myelosuppression were ameliorated[32]. After initial favorable reports of responses in heavily pretreated patients with escalated M-VAC and growth factors[33], several groups began phase II trials of escalated chemotherapy[34–36]. In the United States, this approach has been largely abandoned because of excessive toxicity. In Europe, a novel every 2-week schedule of escalated dosage M-VAC and GM-CSF was evaluated in previously untreated patients. A 70% response rate was encouraging[30]. Based upon this preliminary trial, the Genitourinary Group of the European Organization for Research and Treatment of Cancer (EORTC) began a randomized trial in which the dose intensities of cisplatin and doxorubicin were increased[36]. This study was initiated in order to study whether or not increasing the dose intensity of M-VAC (HD-M-VAC) by adding GM-CSF could lead to an improvement in overall survival. This co-operative trial is the only study that addresses the issue of dose intensity in a randomized trial compared to standard M-VAC.

A total of 121 patients on the M-VAC arm and 127 on the HD-M-VAC arm had bidimensionally measurable TCC and were eligible for response assessment. The complete and partial response rate for HD-M-VAC was 72% (95% confidence interval (CI) 65–81%), as compared to 58% (95% CI 48–67%) for M-VAC. The complete response rate was 25% (95% CI 17–33%) with HD-M-VAC as compared to 11% with M-VAC (95% CI 5–16%). The p value for the difference in complete response rate was $p = 0.006$ and for the difference in overall response rate (complete + partial) was 0.016.

A statistically significant difference in terms of complete response rate and progression-free survival in favor of HD-M-VAC was observed in this patient population in which the Bajorin risk factors were well-balanced. No statistically significant difference in overall survival was seen. All of the survival curves seem to diverge in favor of the HD-M-VAC arm; however, the small number of patients in the tail of the curves do not enable a precise estimation. However, there is the potential for a cohort of long-term survivors in this study. When comparing the dose intensity delivered per week of HD-M-VAC compared to M-VAC, twice the dose intensities of cisplatin (205%) and doxorubicin (201%) were delivered on the high-dose regimen. Less dose intensity of methotrexate (86%) and vinblastine (81%) were achieved in the HD-M-VAC arm.

On the HD-M-VAC arm, the total doses of doxorubicin and cisplatin were higher. The total dose of methotrexate and vinblastine were higher, however, on the M-VAC arm. The total duration of treatment was also much longer on the M-VAC arm. The HD-M-VAC regimen is, therefore, a more dose-dense regimen in terms of doxorubicin and cisplatin.

It was possible to give more cycles in a shorter period of time in the HD-M-VAC arm than on the M-VAC arm. This is probably due to the fact that there was less white blood cell toxicity and mucositis due to the GM-CSF and the fact that less methotrexate was given in this arm. HD-M-VAC is an interesting regimen to be used in both the neoadjuvant and adjuvant setting, as the chemotherapy is finished in half the time of classic M-VAC.

Although the gold standard of chemotherapy for patients with metastatic transitional cell carcinoma and better performance status is M-VAC, it results in a median survival of approximately 1 year and the toxicity is substantial. Therefore, new approaches are needed. Newer agents such as gemcitabine[37–40] and the taxanes[41–43] show promising results in single-agent phase I and II studies. Other recently evaluated compounds, such as ifosfamide[44] and gallium nitrate[45], also have promising activity. Gemcitabine is a deoxycytidine analog with structural and metabolic similarities to cytarabine, an antimetabolite interfering with DNA synthesis. Gemcitabine is usually given weekly for three consecutive weeks, every 4 weeks, and in most patients is well-tolerated. Substantial activity has been found in phase II studies when gemcitabine was given to chemotherapy-naive patients, with response rates in the range of 24–30%[37,38]. The toxicity was mild and primarily hematological. Several phase II trials have also evaluated the combination of gemcitabine and cisplatin, with response rates in the range of 40–60% (similar to those achieved with M-VAC), and some sustained complete response (e.g. Moore and colleagues[39]). Responses were seen in extra-nodal sites such as lung and liver. Based on these results, a randomized trial comparing gemcitabine and cisplatin with M-VAC has been completed[40]. This is the largest study ever completed in metastatic bladder cancer with 405 patients randomized. Overall survival was similar on both arms (HR, 1.04; 95% CI, 0.82–1.32; $p = 0.75$). The median survivals were 13.8 versus 14.8 months, respectively. Times to progressive disease and treatment failure were also similar in both groups. More patients on the gemcitabine/cisplatin arm completed six cycles. The incidence of anemia requiring blood transfusions and asymptomatic thrombocytopenia was higher in the gemcitabine arm. However, the incidence of neutropenic fever and sepsis was higher on the M-VAC arm (14% vs. 2% and 12% vs. 1%). Furthermore, grade 3/4 mucositis and alopecia was lower (22% vs. 1% and 55% vs. 11%, respectively) on the gemcitabine/cisplatin arm. The study was not designed to prove equivalence between the two arms and cannot be proclaimed equal on scientific data. Based on the toxicity profile, it is an alternative for M-VAC. Paclitaxel is also active as a single agent in bladder cancer. At a high dose of $250 mg/m^2$ over 24 h, 11 of 26 patients demonstrated an objective response (42%), with seven complete responses in a phase II trial[41], and similarly encouraging results have been reported from some but not other trials. Paclitaxel is cleared primarily via hepatic metabolism which might be of relevance for patients with compromised renal function. It is probable that combinations including gemcitabine and/or taxanes will lead to improvement in the treatment of transitional cancer of the urothelial tract.

Other regimens that have become increasingly popular for metastatic transitional cell tumors include the use of paclitaxel and carboplatin. Most studies report response rates around 50%, with median survivals of 8–9 months[42–44]. In a recently published multi-center study, the response rate in 29 patients was only 20.7% (95% CI 8–40%)[45]. An ongoing ECOG phase III trial compares paclitaxel/ carboplatin and M-VAC.

For patients who tolerate cisplatin-based therapy, other new and interesting regimens include paclitaxel, ifosfomide and gemcitabine[46]. None of these new regimens has been evaluated in the phase III setting compared to M-VAC. In a recently published phase I–II study of paclitaxel, cisplatin and gemcitabine, a 27.6% complete response rate and 50% partial response rate were found in 58 assessable patients[47]. A prospective, randomized study will be initiated shortly to evaluate its true relevance for this disease.

Conclusion

Chemotherapy has a definite role in the treatment of metastatic disease. Induction chemotherapy has not yet been shown to convey benefit, and is best administered in the context of a clinical trial; adjuvant chemotherapy may be an option in patients with node-positive disease and others at very high risk of relapse. It should be realized that there is no proven impact on overall survival in this setting. A worldwide, randomized study addressing this question will be activated later in 2001. Patients with metastatic or recurrent disease and reasonable performance status should receive a trial of chemotherapy, and a very small proportion may be cured ($< 5\%$). M-VAC is still the standard regimen. Escalated M-VAC and gemcitabine/cisplatin can be considered as an alternative in view of the significantly better toxicity profile.

References

1. Parkin DM, Muir CS, Whelan S, Ferlay J, Raymond L, Young J. *Cancer Incidence in Five Continents*, Vol VII. Lyon: International Agency for Research on Cancer, 1997
2. Coppin C, *et al.* The NCI-Canada trial of concurrent cisplatin and radiotherapy for muscle invasive bladder cancer. *J Clin Oncol* 1996;14:2901–7
3. Marini L, Sternberg C. Neoadjuvant and adjuvant chemotherapy in locally advanced bladder cancer. *Urol Oncol* 1997;3:133–40
4. Herr H, Scher H. Neoadjuvant chemotherapy and partial cystectomy for invasive bladder cancer. *J Clin Oncol* 1994;12:975–80
5. Splinter TAW, *et al.* A European organisation for research and treatment of cancer. Genitourinary Group Phase II study of chemotherapy in Stage T3-4NO-XMO transitional cell cancer of the bladder: evaluation of clinical response. *J Urol* 1992;148:1793–6
6. Splinter T, *et al.* The prognostic value of the pathological response to combination chemo-

therapy before cystectomy in patients with invasive bladder cancer. *J Urol* 1992;147:606–8
7. Schultz T, *et al.* Neoadjuvant chemotherapy for invasive bladder cancer: prognostic factors for survival of patients treated with M-VAC with 5 year follow-up. *J Clin Oncol* 1994;12:1394–401
8. Shearer RJ, Chilvers CED, Bloom HJG, *et al.* Adjuvant chemotherapy in T3 carcinoma of the bladder. *Br J Urol* 1988;62:558–64
9. Wallace DM, Raghavan D, Kelly KA, *et al.* Neo-adjuvant (pre-emptive) cisplatin therapy in invasive transitional cell carcinoma of the bladder. *Br J Urol* 1991;67:608–15
10. Martinez-Pineiro JA, Gonzalez Martin M, Arocena F, *et al.* Neoadjuvant cisplatin chemotherapy before radical cystectomy in invasive transitional cell carcinoma of the bladder: prospective randomized phase III study. *J Urol* 1995;153:964–73
11. Malmstrom PU, Rintala ER, Wahlqvist R, Hellstrom P, Hellsten S, Hannisdal E. Five year follow-up of a prospective trial of radical

cystectomy and neoadjuvant chemotherapy. *J Urol* 1996;155:1903–6

12. International Collaboration of Trialists. Neoadjuvant cisplatin, methotrexate and vinblastine chemotherapy for muscle invasive bladder cancer: a randomised controlled trial. *Lancet* 1999;354:533–40

13. Shipley WU, Winter KA, Kaufman DS, *et al*. Phase III trial of neo adjuvant chemotherapy in patients with invasive bladder cancer treated with selective bladder preservation by combined radiation and chemotherapy: initial results of Radiation Therapy Oncology Group 89–03. *J Clin Oncol* 1998;16:3576–83

14. Logothetis CJ, Johnson DE, Chong C, *et al*. Adjuvant cyclophosphamide, doxorubicin, and cisplatin chemotherapy for bladder cancer: an update. *J Clin Oncol* 1988;6:1590–6

15. Richards B, Bastable JRG, Freedman L, *et al*. Adjuvant chemotherapy with doxorubicin (Adriamycin) and 5-fluorouracil in T3, NX, MO bladder cancer treated with radiotherapy. *Br J Urol* 1983;55:386–91

16. Skinner DG, Daniels JR, Russell CA, *et al*. The role of adjuvant chemotherapy following cystectomy for invasive bladder cancer: a prospective comparative trial. *J Urol* 1991;145:459–67

17. Stöckle M, Meyenburg W, Wellek S, *et al*. Advanced bladder cancer (stages pT3b, pT4a, pN1 and pN2): improved survival after radical cystectomy and 3 adjuvant cycles of chemotherapy, results of a controlled prospective study. *J Urol* 1992;148:302–7

18. Stöckle M, Meyenburg W, Wellek S, *et al*. Adjuvant poly chemotherapy of non organ confined bladder cancer after radical cystectomy revisited: long term results of a controlled prospective study and further clinical experience. *J Urol* 1995;153:47–52

19. Studer UE, Bacchi M, Biedermann C, *et al*. Adjuvant cisplatin chemotherapy following cystectomy for bladder cancer: results of a prospective randomized trial. *J Urol* 1994;152:81–4

20. Freiha F, Reese J, Torti FM, Scher HI. A randomized trial of radical cystectomy versus radical cystectomy plus cisplatin, vinblastine and methotrexate chemotherapy for muscle invasive bladder. *J Urol* 1996;155:495–500

21. Bono AV, Benvenutti C, Gibbaa A, *et al*. Adjuvant chemotherapy in locally advanced bladder cancer. Final analysis of a controlled multicentre study. *Acta Urol Ital* 1997;11:5–8

22. Sylvester R, Sternberg C. The role of adjuvant combination chemotherapy after cystectomy in locally advanced bladder cancer: what we do not know and why. *Ann Oncol* 2000;11:851–6

23. Sternberg CN, Yagoda A, Scher HI, *et al*. Methotrexate, vinblastine, doxorubicin and cisplatin for advanced transitional cell carcinoma of the urothelium: efficacy patterns of response and relapse. *Cancer* 1989;64:2448–58

24. Loehrer PJ, Einhorn LH, Elson PJ, *et al*. A randomized comparison of cisplatin alone or in combination with methotrexate, vinblastine, and doxorubicin in patients with metastatic urothelial carcinoma: a cooperative group study. *J Clin Oncol* 1992;10:1066–73

25. Saxman SB, Propert KJ, Einhorn LH, *et al*. Long-term follow-up of phase III intergroup study of cisplatin alone or in combination with methotrexate, vinblastine and doxorubicin in patients with metastatic urothelial carcinoma. A cooperative group study. *J Clin Oncol* 1997;15:2564–9

26. Logothetis CJ, Dexeus FH, Finn L, *et al*. A prospective randomized trial comparing M-VAC and CISCA chemotherapy for patients with metastatic urothelial tumors. *J Clin Oncol* 1990;8:1050–5

27. Scher HI, Geller NL, Curley T, *et al*. Effect of relative cumulative dose-intensity on survival of patients with urothelial cancer treated with M-VAC. *J Clin Oncol* 1993;11:400–7

28. Moore MJ, Iscoe N, Tannock IF. A phase II study of methotrexate, vinblastine, doxorubicin and cisplatin plus recombinant human granulocyte-macrophage colony stimulating factors in patients with advanced transitional cell carcinoma. *J Urol* 1993;150:1131–4

29. Seidman AD, Scher HI, Gabrilove JL, *et al*. Dose intensification of M-VAC with recombinant granulocyte colony stimulating factor as initial therapy in advanced urothelial cancer. *J Clin Oncol* 1993;11:408–14

30. Sternberg CN, De Mulder PHM, van Oosterom AT, *et al*. Escalated M-VAC chemotherapy and recombinant human granulocyte-macrophage colony stimulating factor (GM-CSF) in patients with advanced urothelial tract tumors. *Ann Oncol* 1993;4:403–8

31. Logothetis CJ, Finn LD, Smith T, *et al*. Escalated M-VAC with or without recombinant human granulocyte-macrophage colony-stimulating factor for the initial treatment of advanced malignant urothelial tumors: results of a randomized trial. *J Clin Oncol* 1995;13:2272–7

32. Gabrilove JL, Jakubowski A, Scher H, *et al*. Effect of granulocyte colony-stimulating factor on neutropenia and associated morbidity due to chemotherapy for transitional-cell carcinoma of the urothelium. *N Engl J Med* 1988;318:1414–22

33. Logothetis CJ, Dexeus FH, Sella A, *et al*. Escalated therapy for refractory urothelial tumors: methotrexate-vinblastine-doxorubicin-cisplatin

plus unglycosylated recombinant human granulocyte-macrophage colony-stimulating factor. *J Natl Cancer Inst* 1990;82:667–72

34. Loehrer PJS, Elson P, Dreicer R, *et al.* Escalated dosages of methotrexate, vinblastine, doxorubicin, and cisplatin plus recombinant human granulocyte colony-stimulating factor in advanced urothelial carcinoma: an Eastern Cooperative Oncology Group trial. *J Clin Oncol* 1994;12:483–8

35. Seidman AD, Scher HI, Gabrilove JL, *et al.* Dose-intensification of methotrexate, vinblastine, doxorubicin, and cisplatin with recombinant granulocyte-colony stimulating factor as initial therapy in advanced urothelial cancer. *J Clin Oncol* 1992;11:414–20

36. Sternberg CN, de Mulder P, Schornagel J, *et al.* and the Genitourinary Group EORTC BB. Randomized phase III trial in advanced urothelial tract tumors of high dose intensity: M-VAC chemotherapy and G-CSF versus classic M-VAC. *Proc Am Soc Clin Oncol* 2000;19:320a (abstr 1292)

37. Moore MJ, Tannock I, Ernst S, Auan S, Murray N. Gemcitabine: a promising new agent in treatment of advanced urothelial cell cancer. *J Clin Oncol* 1997;15:3441–5

38. Stadler WWM, Kuzel T, Roth B, Raghavan D, Dorr FA. A phase II study of single-agent gemcitabine in previously untreated patients with metastatic urothelial cancer. *J Clin Oncol* 1997;15:3394–8

39. Moore MJ, Winquist EW, Murray N, *et al.* Gemcitabine plus cisplatin, an active regimen in advanced urothelial cancer: a phase II trial of the National Cancer Institute of Canada Clinical Trials Group. *J Clin Oncol* 1999;11:2876–81

40. von der Maase H, Hansen SW, Roberts JJ, *et al.* Gemcitabine and cisplatin versus methotrexate, vinblastine, doxorubicin, and cisplatin in advanced or metastatic bladder cancer: results of a large, randomized, multinational, multicenter, phase III study. *J Clin Oncol* 2000;18:3068–77

41. Roth BJ, Dreicer R, Einhorn LA, *et al.* Significant activity of paclitaxel in advanced transitional cell carcinoma of the urothelium: a phase II trial of the Eastern Cooperative Oncology Group. *J Clin Oncol* 1994;12:2264–70

42. Vaughn DJ, Malkowicz SB, Zoltick B, *et al.* Paclitaxel plus carboplatin in advanced carcinoma of the urothelium: an active and tolerable outpatient regiment. *J Clin Oncol* 1998;16:255–60

43. Small EJ, Lew D, Petrylak DP, Crawford ED. Carboplatin and paclitaxel (Carbo/Tax) for advanced transitional cell carcinoma (TCC) of the urothelium. *Proc Am Soc Clin Oncol* 1999; 18:333a (abstr 1280)

44. Redman BG, Smith DC, Flaherty L, Du W, Hussain M. Phase II trial of paclitaxel and carboplatin in the treatment of advanced urothelial carcinoma. *J Clin Oncol* 1998;16: 1844–8

45. McCaffrey JA, Hilton S, Mazumdar M, *et al.* Phase II randomized trial of gallium nitrate plus fluorouracil versus methotrexate, vinblastine, doxorubicin, and cisplatin in patients with advanced transitional cell carcinoma. *J Clin Oncol* 1997;15:2449–55

46. Bajorin DF, McCaffrey JA, Dodd PM, *et al.* Ifosfamide, paclitaxel, and cisplatin for patients with advanced transitional cell carcinoma of the urothelial tract: final report of a phase II trial evaluating two dosing schedules. *Cancer* 2000; 88:1671–8

47. Bellmunt J, Guillem V, Paz-Ares L, *et al.* Phase I–II study of paclitaxel, cisplatin, and gemcitabine in advanced transitional-cell carcinoma of the urothelium. *J Clin Oncol* 2000;18:3247–55

Index